Current Topics in Microbiology and Immunology

Volume 344

Current Topics in Microbiology and Immunology

Previously published volumes
Further volumes can be found at springer.com

Vol. 318: **Rodriguez, Moses (Ed.):**
Advances in Multiple Sclerosis and Experimental Demyelinating Diseases. 2008. XIV, 376 pp. ISBN 978-3-540-73679-9

Vol. 319: **Manser, Tim (Ed.):**
Specialization and Complementation of Humoral Immune Responses to Infection. 2008. XII, 174 pp. ISBN 978-3-540-73899-2

Vol. 320: **Paddison, Patrick J.; Vogt, Peter K.(Eds.):** RNA Interference. 2008. VIII, 273 pp. ISBN 978-3-540-75156-4

Vol. 321: **Beutler, Bruce (Ed.):**
Immunology, Phenotype First: How Mutations Have Established New Principles and Pathways in Immunology. 2008. XIV, 221 pp. ISBN 978-3-540-75202-8

Vol. 322: **Romeo, Tony (Ed.):**
Bacterial Biofilms. 2008. XII, 299. ISBN 978-3-540-75417-6

Vol. 323: **Tracy, Steven; Oberste, M. Steven; Drescher, Kristen M. (Eds.):**
Group B Coxsackieviruses. 2008. ISBN 978-3-540-75545-6

Vol. 324: **Nomura, Tatsuji; Watanabe, Takeshi; Habu, Sonoko (Eds.):**
Humanized Mice. 2008. ISBN 978-3-540-75646-0

Vol. 325: **Shenk, Thomas E.; Stinski, Mark F. (Eds.):**
Human Cytomegalovirus. 2008. ISBN 978-3-540-77348-1

Vol. 326: **Reddy, Anireddy S.N; Golovkin, Maxim (Eds.):**
Nuclear pre-mRNA processing in plants. 2008. ISBN 978-3-540-76775-6

Vol. 327: **Manchester, Marianne; Steinmetz, Nicole F. (Eds.):**
Viruses and Nanotechnology. 2008. ISBN 978-3-540-69376-5

Vol. 328: **van Etten, (Ed.):**
Lesser Known Large dsDNA Viruses. 2008. ISBN 978-3-540-68617-0

Vol. 329: **Griffin, Diane E.; Oldstone, Michael B.A. (Eds.):** Measles. 2009. ISBN 978-3-540-70522-2

Vol. 330: **Griffin, Diane E.; Oldstone, Michael B.A. (Eds.):** Measles. 2009. ISBN 978-3-540-70616-8

Vol. 331: **Villiers, E. M. de (Ed.):**
TT Viruses. 2009. ISBN 978-3-540-70917-8

Vol. 332: **Karasev A. (Ed.):**
Plant produced Microbial Vaccines. 2009. ISBN 978-3-540-70857-5

Vol. 333: **Compans, Richard W.; Orenstein, Walter A. (Eds.):**
Vaccines for Pandemic Influenza. 2009. ISBN 978-3-540-92164-6

Vol. 334: **McGavern, Dorian; Dustin, Micheal (Eds.):**
Visualizing Immunity. 2009. ISBN 978-3-540-93862-0

Vol. 335: **Levine, Beth; Yoshimori, Tamotsu; Deretic, Vojo (Eds.):**
Autophagy in Infection and Immunity. 2009. ISBN 978-3-642-00301-1

Vol. 336: **Kielian, Tammy (Ed.):**
Toll-like Receptors: Roles in Infection and Neuropathology. 2009. ISBN 978-3-642-00548-0

Vol. 337: **Sasakawa, Chihiro (Ed.):**
Molecular Mechanisms of Bacterial Infection via the Gut. 2009. ISBN 978-3-642-01845-9

Vol. 338: **Rothman, Alan L. (Ed.):**
Dengue Virus. 2009. ISBN 978-3-642-02214-2

Vol. 339: **Spearman, Paul; Freed, Eric O. (Eds.):**
HIV Interactions with Host Cell Proteins. 2009. ISBN 978-3-642-02174-9

Vol. 340: **Saito, Takashi; Batista, Facundo D. (Eds.):**
Immunological Synapse. 2010. ISBN 978-3-642-03857-0

Vol. 341: **Bruserud, Øystein (Ed.):**
The Chemokine System in Clinical and Experimental Hematology. 2010. ISBN 978-3-642-12638-3

Vol. 342: **Arvin, Ann M. (Ed.):**
Varicella-zoster Virus. 2010. ISBN 978-3-642-12727-4

Vol. 343: **Johnson, John E. (Ed.):**
Cell Entry by Non-Enveloped Viruses. 2010. ISBN 978-3-642-13331-2

Glenn Dranoff
Editor

Cancer Immunology and Immunotherapy

Springer

Editor
Glenn Dranoff, MD
Dana-Farber Cancer Institute
Dana Building, Room 520 C
44 Binney Street
Boston, MA 02115
USA

ISSN 0070-217X
ISBN: 978-3-642-14135-5 e-ISBN: 978-3-642-14136-2
DOI 10.1007/978-3-642-14136-2
Springer Heidelberg Dordrecht London New York

Library of Congress Control Number: 2011926592

Cover design: WMXDesign, Heidelberg

Printed on acid-free paper

Springer is part of Springer Science+Business Media (www.springer.com)

Preface

The recent FDA approval of Provenge® as the first therapeutic cancer vaccine together with the recent demonstration that Ipilimumab®, a monoclonal antibody that blocks a negative immune checkpoint called cytotoxic T lymphocyte-associated antigen-4 (CTLA-4), prolongs patient survival are major achievements that usher in a new era of cancer immunotherapy (Hodi et al. 2010; Kantoff et al. 2010). These "first-into-class" treatments reflect the substantive progress that basic and translational scientists have made toward understanding the mechanisms underlying protective tumor immunity in cancer patients.

Immunotherapies were first explored at the turn of the twentieth century, but the crafting of potent treatments required more detailed knowledge of how the immune system responds to cancer. Advances in genetic, cellular, and biochemical technologies have begun to yield this critical information, which has stimulated the development and widespread application of monoclonal antibodies and bone marrow transplantation as highly beneficial therapies for many solid and hematologic malignancies. Moreover, recognition of the pathogenic involvement of microbial agents in cancer resulted in the generation of effective preventive vaccines against hepatitis B virus and human papilloma virus, which have and will significantly reduce the incidence of liver and cervical cancer, respectively.

The success of Provenge®, Ipilimumab®, and likely other cancer immunotherapies in the near future derives from a richer characterization of the processes of immune recognition and immune regulation. Dendritic cells are specialized to present cancer antigens to effector lymphocytes through a pathway that involves both positive and negative signals. In turn, the activities of effector lymphocytes are modified in the tumor microenvironment through mechanisms that normally contribute to the maintenance of self-tolerance. Moreover, in the context of an ineffectual host response, tumors evolve to exploit factors present in the microenvironment that facilitate disease progression. Thus, therapeutic manipulation of immune recognition, immune regulation, and tumor-promoting inflammation should prove decisive in triggering immune-mediated tumor destruction.

This volume brings together 13 groups that have made major contributions to the study of endogenous and therapeutic tumor immunity in model systems and patients. Collectively, these investigations have generated remarkable insights into the complex cross-talk between the tumor and host. This knowledge should render possible the identification of specific molecular mechanisms that restrain protective immunity in individual patients; this information will thereby guide the administration of appropriate immunotherapeutics to overcome these limitations and markedly impact patient outcome. It is likely that a combination of immune approaches that address complementary defects will prove most potent, and that immune treatments will be effectively integrated with other strategies for cancer therapy.

Glenn Dranoff
Dana-Farber Cancer Institute
and Harvard Medical School

References

Hodi FS, O'Day SJ, McDermott DF, Weber RW, Sosman JA, Haanen JB, Gonzalez R, Robert C, Schadendorf D, Hassel JC, Akerley W, van den Eertwegh AJ, Lutzky J, Lorigan P, Vaubel JM, Linette GP, Hogg D, Ottensmeier CH, Lebbe C, Peschel C, Quirt I, Clark JI, Wolchok JD, Weber JS, Tian J, Yellin MJ, Nichol GM, Hoos A, Urba WJ (2010) N Engl J Med 363:711–723

Kantoff PW, Higano CS, Shore ND, Berger ER, Small EJ, Penson DF, Redfern CH, Ferrari AC, Dreicer R, Sims RB, Xu Y, Frohlich MW, Schellhammer PF (2010) N Engl J Med 363:411–422

Contents

Immune Infiltration in Human Cancer: Prognostic Significance and Disease Control 1
Wolf H. Fridman, Jérome Galon, Marie-Caroline Dieu-Nosjean, Isabelle Cremer, Sylvain Fisson, Diane Damotte, Franck Pagès, Eric Tartour, and Catherine Sautès-Fridman

Subversion and Coercion: The Art of Redirecting Tumor Immune Surveillance 25
John B. Mumm and Martin Oft

STAT3: A Target to Enhance Antitumor Immune Response 41
Heehyoung Lee, Sumanta Kumar Pal, Karen Reckamp, Robert A. Figlin, and Hua Yu

Biology and Clinical Observations of Regulatory T Cells in Cancer Immunology 61
Michele W.L. Teng, David S. Ritchie, Paul Neeson, and Mark J. Smyth

Concepts and Ways to Amplify the Antitumor Immune Response 97
Bent Rubin and Jean Edouard Gairin

Angiogenesis and the Tumor Vasculature as Antitumor Immune Modulators: The Role of Vascular Endothelial Growth Factor and Endothelin 129
Lana E. Kandalaft, Gregory T. Motz, Johanna Busch, and George Coukos

Adoptive Cellular Therapy 149
Stephan A. Grupp and Carl H. June

Dendritic Cell Subsets as Vectors and Targets for Improved Cancer Therapy 173
Karolina Palucka, Hideki Ueno, Lee Roberts, Joseph Fay, and Jacques Banchereau

Identification of Human Idiotype-Specific T Cells in Lymphoma and Myeloma 193
Jinsheng Weng, Sattva S. Neelapu, Alison F. Woo, and Larry W. Kwak

Modulation of CTLA-4 and GITR for Cancer Immunotherapy 211
Francesca Avogadri, Jianda Yuan, Arvin Yang, David Schaer, and Jedd D. Wolchok

Immunobiology of Cancer Therapies Targeting CD137 and B7-H1/PD-1 Cosignal Pathways 245
Shengdian Wang and Lieping Chen

LAG-3 in Cancer Immunotherapy 269
Monica V. Goldberg and Charles G. Drake

Immunologically Active Biomaterials for Cancer Therapy 279
Omar A. Ali and David J. Mooney

Erratum: Identification of Human Idiotype-Specific T Cells in Lymphoma and Myeloma 299
Jinsheng Weng, Sattva S. Neelapu, Alison F. Woo, and Larry W. Kwak

Index 301

Contributors

Omar A. Ali Harvard School of Engineering and Applied Sciences, Harvard University, 58 Oxford St., 415, Cambridge, MA 02138, USA and Wyss Institute for Biologically Inspired Engineering, Cambridge, MA, USA and InCytu Inc, 701 George Washington Hwy, Lincoln, RI 02865, USA, alio@seas.harvard.edu

Francesca Avogadri Immunology Program, Sloan-Kettering Institute, New York, NY 10065, USA

Jacques Banchereau Baylor Institute for Immunology Research, 3434 Live Oak, Dallas, TX 75204, USA and Department of Gene and Cell Medicine, Mount Sinai School of Medicine, New York, NY, USA

Johanna Busch Ovarian Cancer Research Center, University of Pennsylvania, Philadelphia, PA 19104, USA

Lieping Chen Sidney Kimmel Comprehensive Cancer Center and Department of Oncology, Johns Hopkins University School of Medicine, Baltimore, MD, USA, lchen42@jhmi.edu

George Coukos Ovarian Cancer Research Center, University of Pennsylvania, Philadelphia, PA 19104, USA, gcks@mail.med.upenn.edu

Isabelle Cremer INSERM U872, Centre de Recherche des Cordeliers, Paris 75006, France and Université Pierre et Marie Curie–Paris 6, UMRS 872, Paris 75006, France and Université Paris Descartes, UMRS 872, Paris 75006, France

Diane Damotte INSERM U872, Centre de Recherche des Cordeliers, Paris 75006, France and Université Pierre et Marie Curie–Paris 6, UMRS 872, Paris 75006, France and Université Paris Descartes, UMRS 872, Paris 75006, France

Marie-Caroline Dieu-Nosjean INSERM U872, Centre de Recherche des Cordeliers, Paris 75006, France and Université Pierre et Marie Curie–Paris 6, UMRS 872, Paris 75006, France and Université Paris Descartes, UMRS 872, Paris 75006, France

Charles G. Drake Johns Hopkins Kimmel Cancer Center, 1650 Orleans Street – CRB 423, Baltimore, MD 21231, USA

Joseph Fay Sammons Cancer Center, Baylor University Medical Center, Dallas, TX, USA

Robert A. Figlin Department of Medical Oncology and Experimental Therapeutics, City of Hope Comprehensive Cancer Center, 1500 East Duarte Road, Duarte, CA 91010, USA

Sylvain Fisson INSERM U872, Centre de Recherche des Cordeliers, Paris 75006, France and Université Pierre et Marie Curie–Paris 6, UMRS 872, Paris 75006, France and Université Paris Descartes, UMRS 872, Paris 75006, France

Wolf H. Fridman INSERM U872, Centre de Recherche des Cordeliers, Paris 75006, France and Université Pierre et Marie Curie–Paris 6, UMRS 872, Paris 75006, France and Université Paris Descartes, UMRS 872, Paris 75006, France and Service d'Immunologie Biologique Hôpital Européen Georges Pompidou, AP-HP, Paris 75015, France and INSERM U872, Centre de Recherche des Cordeliers, 15 rue de l'Ecole de Médecine, Paris 75006, France, herve.fridman@crc.jussieu.fr

Jean Edouard Gairin Institut de Sciences et Technologies du Médicament de Toulouse, UMR 2587 CNRS-Pierre Fabre, 3, rue des Satellites, 31400 Toulouse, France and Faculté de Pharmacie, Université Paul Sabatier, 31400 Toulouse, France, jean-edouard.gairin@istmt.cnrs.fr

Jérome Galon Université Pierre et Marie Curie–Paris 6, UMRS 872, Paris 75006, France and Université Paris Descartes, UMRS 872, Paris 75006, France and INSERM U872, Centre de Recherche des Cordeliers, 15 rue de l'Ecole de Médecine, Paris 75006, France

Monica V. Goldberg Johns Hopkins Kimmel Cancer Center, 1650 Orleans Street – CRB 423, Baltimore, MD 21231, USA

Stephan A. Grupp Division of Oncology and Department of Pathology and Laboratory Medicine, University of Pennsylvania School of Medicine, Philadelphia, PA, USA and Department of Pediatrics, The Children's

Hospital of Philadelphia, University of Pennsylvania School of Medicine, Philadelphia, PA, USA

Carl H. June Abramson Family Cancer Research Institute and the Department of Pathology and Laboratory Medicine, University of Pennsylvania, 554 Biomedical Research Building II/III, 421 Curie Blvd., Philadelphia, PA, USA, cjune@exchange.upenn.edu

Lana E. Kandalaft Ovarian Cancer Research Center, University of Pennsylvania, Philadelphia, PA 19104, USA

Larry W. Kwak Department of Lymphoma and Myeloma, The University of Texas M.D. Anderson Cancer Center, Houston, TX 77030, USA

Heehyoung Lee Beckman Research Institute, City of Hope Comprehensive Cancer Center, 1500 East Duarte Road, Duarte, CA 91010, USA

David J. Mooney Harvard School of Engineering and Applied Sciences, Harvard University, 58 Oxford St., 415, Cambridge, MA 02138, USA and Wyss Institute for Biologically Inspired Engineering, Cambridge, MA, USA

Gregory T. Motz Ovarian Cancer Research Center, University of Pennsylvania, Philadelphia, PA 19104, USA

John B. Mumm Merck Research Labs (formerly DNAX), 901 California Avenue, Palo Alto, CA 94303, USA

Sattva S. Neelapu Department of Lymphoma and Myeloma, The University of Texas M.D. Anderson Cancer Center, Houston, TX 77030, USA

Paul Neeson Cancer Immunology Program, Peter MacCallum Cancer Centre, East Melbourne 3002, VIC, Australia

Martin Oft Merck Research Labs (formerly DNAX), 901 California Avenue, Palo Alto, CA 94303, USA, martin.oft@spcorp.com

Franck Pagès Université Pierre et Marie Curie–Paris 6, UMRS 872, Paris 75006, France and Université Paris Descartes, UMRS 872, Paris 75006, France and Service d'Immunologie Biologique Hôpital Européen Georges Pompidou, AP-HP, Paris 75015, France and INSERM U872, Centre de Recherche des Cordeliers, 15 rue de l'Ecole de Médecine, Paris 75006, France

Sumanta Kumar Pal Division of Genitourinary Malignancies, Department of Medical Oncology and Experimental Therapeutics, City of Hope

Comprehensive Cancer Center, 1500 East Duarte Road, Duarte, CA 91010, USA

Karolina Palucka Baylor Institute for Immunology Research, 3434 Live Oak, Dallas, TX 75204, USA and Department of Gene and Cell Medicine, Mount Sinai School of Medicine, New York, NY, USA, karolinp@baylor health.edu

Karen Reckamp Division of Thoracic Malignancies, Department of Medical Oncology and Experimental Therapeutics, City of Hope Comprehensive Cancer Center, 1500 East Duarte Road, Duarte, CA 91010, USA

David S. Ritchie Division of Haematology and Medical Oncology, Peter MacCallum Cancer Centre, Locked Bag 1, A'Beckett St., East Melbourne 3002, VIC, Australia and Department of Health Sciences, University of Melbourne, Parkville 3010, VIC, Australia

Lee Roberts Baylor Institute for Immunology Research, 3434 Live Oak, Dallas, TX 75204, USA

Bent Rubin Institut de Sciences et Technologies du Médicament de Toulouse, UMR 2587 CNRS-Pierre Fabre, 3, rue des Satellites, 31400 Toulouse, France

Catherine Sautès-Fridman INSERM U872, Centre de Recherche des Cordeliers, Paris 75006, France and Université Pierre et Marie Curie–Paris 6, UMRS 872, Paris 75006, France and Université Paris Descartes, UMRS 872, Paris 75006, France

David Schaer Immunology Program, Sloan-Kettering Institute, New York, NY 10065, USA

Mark J. Smyth Cancer Immunology Program, Peter MacCallum Cancer Centre, East Melbourne 3002, VIC, Australia and Department of Pathology, University of Melbourne, Parkville 3010, VIC, Australia

Eric Tartour Service d'Immunologie Biologique Hôpital Européen Georges Pompidou, AP-HP, Paris 75015, France and INSERM U872, Centre de Recherche des Cordeliers, 15 rue de l'Ecole de Médecine, Paris 75006, France

Michele W.L. Teng Cancer Immunology Program, Peter MacCallum Cancer Centre, East Melbourne 3002, VIC, Australia and Department of Pathology, University of Melbourne, Parkville 3010, VIC, Australia

Hideki Ueno Baylor Institute for Immunology Research, 3434 Live Oak, Dallas, TX 75204, USA

Shengdian Wang Center for Infection and Immunity, Institute for Biophysics, Chinese Academy of Sciences, Beijing, China

Jinsheng Weng Department of Lymphoma and Myeloma, The University of Texas M.D. Anderson Cancer Center, Houston, TX 77030, USA, jweng@mdanderson.org

Jedd D. Wolchok Immunology Program, Sloan-Kettering Institute, New York, NY 10065, USA and Melanoma/Sarcoma Service, Department of Medicine, Memorial Sloan-Kettering Cancer Center, New York, NY 10065, USA and Ludwig Center for Cancer Immunotherapy, Immunology Program, Sloan-Kettering Institute, New York, NY 10065, USA, wolchokj@mskcc.org

Alison F. Woo Department of Lymphoma and Myeloma, The University of Texas M.D. Anderson Cancer Center, Houston, TX 77030, USA

Arvin Yang Immunology Program, Sloan-Kettering Institute, New York, NY 10065, USA and Melanoma/Sarcoma Service, Department of Medicine, Memorial Sloan-Kettering Cancer Center, New York, NY 10065, USA and Ludwig Center for Cancer Immunotherapy, Immunology Program, Sloan-Kettering Institute, New York, NY 10065, USA

Hua Yu Cancer Immunotherapeutics and Tumor Immunology, City of Hope Comprehensive Cancer Center, 1500 East Duarte Road, Duarte, CA 91010, USA, hyu@coh.org

Jianda Yuan Immunology Program, Sloan-Kettering Institute, New York, NY 10065, USA and Ludwig Center for Cancer Immunotherapy, Immunology Program, Sloan-Kettering Institute, New York, NY 10065, USA

Immune Infiltration in Human Cancer: Prognostic Significance and Disease Control

Wolf H. Fridman, Jérome Galon, Marie-Caroline Dieu-Nosjean, Isabelle Cremer, Sylvain Fisson, Diane Damotte, Franck Pagès, Eric Tartour, and Catherine Sautès-Fridman

Contents

1 Introduction 2
2 "In Situ" Immune Contexture, the Strongest Prognostic Factor for Recurrence and Overall Survival: The Case of Colorectal Cancer 4
3 Induction of Functionally Active Tertiary Lymphoid Structures in the Vicinity of Tumoral Beds as Potential Sites of "In Situ" Immune Reactions: The Example of Lung Carcinoma 8
4 Subversion of Innate Immunity Receptors: Stimulation of Toll Like Receptors on Lung Carcinoma Cells Modulates Cell Survival and Response to Chemotherapy 11
5 "Paradoxical" Control of Inflammation Influences Clinical Outcome in Head and Neck Cancer 13
6 The Immune Reaction in a Tumor Developing in an Immuno-Priviledged Site: The Case of Primary Intraocular Lymphoma 16
7 Conclusions 18
References 19

Abstract The interplay between tumors and their immunologic microenvironment is complex and difficult to decipher, but its understanding is of seminal importance for the development of novel prognostic markers and therapeutic strategies.

W.H. Fridman (✉), J. Galon, M.-C.-D.-Nosjean, I. Cremer, S. Fisson, D. Damotte, F. Pagès, and C. Sautès-Fridman
INSERM U872, Centre de Recherche des Cordeliers, Paris 75006, France
Université Pierre et Marie Curie–Paris 6, UMRS 872, Paris 75006, France
Université Paris Descartes, UMRS 872, Paris 75006, France
e-mail: herve.fridman@crc.jussieu.fr

W.H. Fridman, F. Pagès, and E. Tartour
Service d'Immunologie Biologique Hôpital Européen Georges Pompidou, AP-HP, Paris 75015, France

INSERM U872, Centre de Recherche des Cordeliers, 15 rue de l'Ecole de Médecine, Paris 75006, France

G. Dranoff (ed.), *Cancer Immunology and Immunotherapy*,
Current Topics in Microbiology and Immunology 344, DOI 10.1007/82_2010_46

This chapter discusses tumor–immune interactions in several human cancers that illustrate various aspects of this complexity and proposes an integrated scheme of the impact of local immune reactions on clinical outcome. Thus, the fact that a strong infiltration of memory T cells with a Th1 and cytotoxic pattern is the strongest predictor for recurrence and metastasis is exemplified in colorectal cancer in which intratumoral chemokines shape an efficient immune reaction. Based on these data, we propose an immune score that predicts recurrence in early stage (UICC-TNM stage I-II) cancers. Studies on non-small lung cancers have confirmed findings of colorectal cancers and have addressed the question of the sites where antitumor immune reactions may take place. Tertiary lymphoid structures (TLS) adjacent to the tumor nest are sites of intense activity with mature dendritic cells in contact with T cells and germinal-like centers with proliferating B cells. The large number of these TLS being correlated with disease specific and overall survival tempts to postulate that they are privileged sites to mount an efficient antitumor reaction. Inflammation is a major component of human tumors and chronic inflammation is generally of bad prognosis. Head and neck cancers are highly inflammatory and two ways to modulate inflammation in these diseases are presented here: soluble IL-15 receptor α (IL-15 Rα) increases the pro-inflammatory effect of IL-15 and aggravates inflammation resulting in poor prognosis when found at high levels in the plasma of patients. By contrast, infiltration of regulatory T cells is paradoxically beneficial for local control of head and neck tumors, probably by "cooling down" the inflammatory process. The modulation of other aspects of innate immunity may also result in paradoxical effects such as the signaling through Toll like receptors 7 and 8 expressed on lung tumor cells which induce an aggressive tumoral phenotype. Finally, the analysis of primary intraocular lymphoma, which develops in the eye, exemplifies the induction of an antitumor immune reaction in an "immune sanctuary," presenting all the complexities of the tumor–immune interplay in "open" tissues such as the colon or the lung.

1 Introduction

The fact that the immune system may prevent the occurrence of tumors has been largely documented in immunodeficient mice (Shankaran et al. 2001) and individuals in whom cancer incidence is much higher than in immunocompetent hosts (Van der Meer et al. 1993; Birkeland et al. 1995). Although demonstrative of the concept that nascent cancer cells can be viewed as "foreign" or "danger" by a competent immune system, these observations are of little clinical interest for treating clinically established cancer. They indeed support the concept of immunosurveillance (Burnet 1970) and prompt to treat immunodeficiency to restore the best immunocompetence to prevent infections and potential cancers rather than providing clues for immunotherapy of cancers that have already reached a clinical stage.

However, in the recent years, it appeared that the immune system may also influence the clinical outcome of patients with established tumors. The demonstration in mice that the dormancy stage of a cancer, i.e., a period of months or years during which cancer cells are present in the body usually after reductive surgical and/or radio-chemo therapy, is controlled in great part by interferon-responsive immune cells, creating an equilibrium between immunity and cancer (Koebel et al. 2007), provided the scientific bases for adjuvant immunotherapies. In humans, it is well known that tumors with a similar histopathologic stage, referred as TNM (Greene and Sobin 2009) (T (extension of the primary tumor), N (lymph node invasion), M (distant metastasis)) may behave differently in terms of recurrence and survival. Thus, although the TNM classification utilized worldwide is a good prognostic staging system since cancers with no lymph node invasion or distant metastasis (T1-4, N0, M0) have a better clinical outcome than advanced cancers (T1-4, N+, M+), there are frequent discrepancies. Indeed, some patients with small tumor burden experience rapid recurrence even after curative treatment, while others with advanced cancers show surprisingly good prognosis. Thus, in colorectal cancer, patients with lymph node invasion (UICC-TNM stage III) have a likelihood of recurrence of 50–60% within 5 years, but a significant proportion of patients (about 30%) with no detectable lymph node or distant metastasis (UICC-TNM stages I/II) present with recurrent disease within few years (O'Connell et al. 2004; Pagès et al. 2005).

Whether an immune control is responsible for keeping potentially metastatic or invading cancer cells in hold ("equilibrium") in humans is also an intensive field of investigation as it would provide novel prognostic markers as well as new therapeutic avenues. When quantitative and functional analyses of intratumoral immune reactions became available, data accumulated to show that a high lymphocytic infiltration in the primary tumor usually correlates with a better clinical outcome in patients with cancer (reviewed in Pagès et al. 2010). Moreover, the functional orientation of the infiltrating lymphocytes seems to be instrumental for the control of recurrence. For instance, quantification of cytokine gene expression in uterine cervical tumors, resected from early-stage patients, revealed that low levels of interferon (IFNγ) transcripts at the tumor site were associated with recurrence within 2 years after surgery (Tartour et al. 1998). Similar data were reported in colorectal (Pagès et al. 1999) and prostatic cancers (Lebel-Binay et al. 2000). These observations are reminiscent of the findings of Schreiber and Smyth (Koebel et al. 2007; Dunn et al. 2006; Smyth et al. 2006) demonstrating in mice that the equilibrium phase was largely dependent on IFNγ. Altogether these data suggest that the presence of a strong Th1 compartment in a primary tumor is associated with, and putatively controls, metastatic cells release, circulation and / or nidation. However, the immune reaction in tumors is complex with the recruitment of many cells playing opposite effects, Th1 versus Th2, T reg *versus* cytotoxic T cells, NK, and NK-T cells, etc... Moreover, tumors are sites of intense inflammation, which is often detrimental for the host when macrophages support tumor growth and neovascularization (Balkwill and Mantovani 2001; Coussens and Werb 2002), but is sometimes beneficial when acute inflammation, such as in bladder cancer following acute infections or therapy by BCG (Lamm 1992), results in cancer cell destruction. In the recent years, comprehensive analyses of the intratumoral immune cells and molecules gave new insights into the understanding of the role of the immune system in controlling tumor growth and spreading to other organs (Galon et al. 2007; Pagès et al. 2008; Bindea et al. 2009). They permitted the identification of immunological prognostic markers (Pagès et al. 2009, 2010) and should eventually provide new ways to refine cancer therapy. In this chapter, we mainly discuss our own data on the analysis of the intratumoral immune infiltrates in human cancers, their functional orientation, the respective importance of Th1, T reg, cytotoxic, and memory T cells, as well as the formation of tertiary lymphoid structures (TLS), composed of mature dendritic cells (DC) and T and B lymphocytes, adjacent to the tumor, in view of their prognostic value and their dynamic interactions. To illustrate the general character of the host–immune interactions, four examples of human tumors will be addressed: colorectal cancer, a visceral disease open to diet and bacterial antigens ; lung carcinoma, a tumor open to airways ; head and neck inflammatory cancer; and primary intra-ocular lymphoma, an hematological cancer developing in an immunopriviledged site. Finally, we will propose some new insights on how some cancer cells may divert innate immune reactions to protect themselves from acute inflammation and chemotherapy.

2 "In Situ" Immune Contexture, the Strongest Prognostic Factor for Recurrence and Overall Survival: The Case of Colorectal Cancer

Histopathological analysis of colorectal cancers shows that these tumors are infiltrated by inflammatory and lymphocytic cells, in variable quantities (Dalerba et al. 2003). A closer look reveals that the latter is not distributed randomly, but seem to be organized in more or less dense infiltrations in the tumoral zone, referred to as center of the tumor (CT), in boarding edges at the invasive margin (IM) of tumoral nests (Fig. 1a), and in lymphoid islets adjacent to the tumor. This organization is seen in many other solid tumors and the potential role of the lymphoid islets will be discussed later when presenting the example of lung carcinoma.

We have extensively analyzed the impact of the quantity, the functional orientation, and the location of the immune cells of the tumor microenvironment – that we propose to call the "immune contexture" – on cancer recurrence, metastasis, and patient survival. In a retrospective study of 959 colorectal tumors, followed for over 15 years in the digestive surgery ward of European Hospital Georges Pompidou, we first searched for early signs of metastasis in the primary tumor. We observed venous emboli (VE), lymphatic invasion (LI), and perineural infiltration (PI) in 27% of the tumors. Applying univariate and multivariate Cox analysis, we found that the presence of one early sign of metastasis (VE or LI or PI) was associated with bad prognosis both in terms of disease free survival (DFS) and overall survival (OS). The presence of the three signs was of even worse prognosis. We, then, asked the question of whether the "in situ" immune infiltrates were different in VELIPI

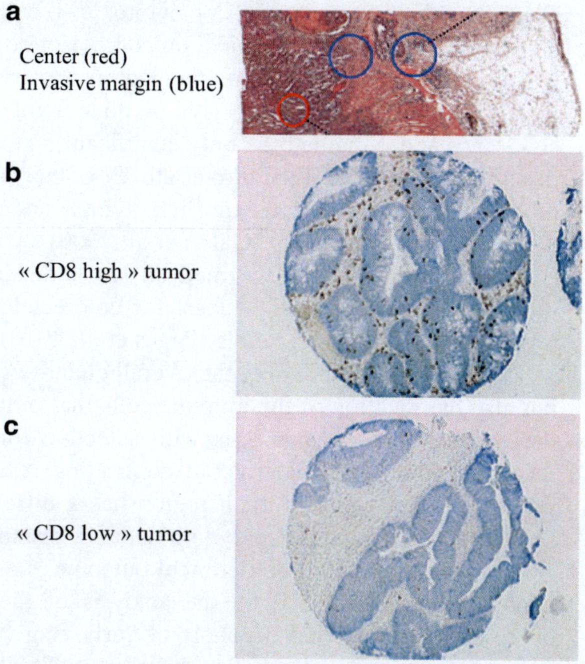

Fig. 1 Characterization of immune infiltrates in colon cancer: The center (*red circle*) and the invasive margin (*blue circle*) of colon tumor (Hematoxylin and eosin staining, original magnification 40×) (**a**), Tumors with high (**b**) or low (**c**) densities of CD8+T cells (original magnification 100×)

(−) and VELIPI (+) tumors. For this purpose, we undertook a comprehensive quantification of immune gene expression by Q-PCR, immune cell identification by flow cytometry of extracted living cells, and tissue micro-array of tumors using antibodies recognizing immune cell subsets. The conclusion of this analysis was that high numbers of memory T cells, particularly effector/memory T cells correlated with lack of early signs of metastasis (VELIPI (−)) and that tumors with low numbers of memory T cells had local (VELIPI(+)) or distant (N+ or M+) metastasis (Pagès et al. 2005). Not only is there a particular immune pattern associated with metastasis at the time of surgery but, more importantly, the "in situ" immune reaction is associated with DFS and OS. Thus, we found that expression of genes associated with adaptive immunity (T-bet, IRF1, IFNγ, CD8α, granzyme B, granulysin) and not genes associated with inflammation (IL-8, VEGF, CEACAM-1, MMP-7) or immuno-suppression (TGFβ, IL-10, B7-H3, CD32b) were associated with lack of metastasis and recurrence (Pagès et al. 2005). Enumeration of cells of adaptive immunity within the tumors revealed an interesting aspect: even if all the T cells or CD8 cells or granulysin-expressing cells or memory (CD45RO) cells were associated with good prognosis, taking into account their location and combining two markers greatly improved their prognostic impact. By combining the analysis of several zones in the CT and in the IM, we found that high infiltrates of memory T cells (CD3/CD45RO) or potential cytotoxic T cells (CD8/CD45RO/granulysin +) (Fig. 1b) both in the center and the IM were highly significantly ($p < 10^{-11}$) associated with very good prognosis, both in terms of DFS and OS.

Tumors with low memory T or cytotoxic T cells in both zones (Fig. 1c) were associated with very bad clinical outcome. Heterogenous (Hi-Lo or Lo-Hi) tumors were intermediate but rather on the bad prognosis side. These differences hold true for all T (tumor extension), N (lymph node involvement), and M (distant metastasis) stages and remained the only significant factor – with bowel perforation – for disease free and OS in multivariate Cox analysis when classically used histoprognostic factors (tumor extension, lymph node metastasis and differentiation) were no longer significant (Galon et al. 2006).

These observations, confirmed on two independent cohorts, change the paradigm of cancer prognosis at least for colorectal cancer (Galon et al. 2007), and propose novel prognostic tools (Pagès et al. 2010) that may guide cancer therapy.

The fact that it is not only the overall quantity or even the functional orientation but also the location of the immune cells that influence tumor recurrence supports the concept that distinct cells with selective functions may, at different tumor locations, play a crucial role in controlling metastasis escape. Analysis are in progress to determine if each region has a different influence on cancer-related progression i.e., tumor size, lymph node, or distant metastasis.

A second indication that clinical outcome is associated with selective immune contexture was provided by the analysis of the coordination of immune gene expression. We studied a cohort of early stage colorectal cancers in which we confirmed the association of high memory T cell infiltration in CT and IM and good prognosis. We, then, performed a gene expression screening (108 genes) looking for immune, inflammation, and angiogenesis-associated genes whose expression correlated, or not, with high CD3/CD45RO infiltration in CT and IM. The results were straightforward: not surprisingly, genes associated with T cell memory were found overexpressed in CD3/CD45RO high tumors and under-expressed in the others ; strikingly, two other clusters of genes were coordinatively coexpressed in tumors with high CD3/CD45RO infiltration: genes involved in Th1 and cytotoxic T cell functions. Genes associated with Th2 functions, suppression, inflammation, and vascularization were not associated with memory T cell infiltration (Pagès et al. 2009).

These data show that a coordinated immune reaction is associated with the immune pattern which predicts clinical outcome. It is therefore likely that Th1 and cytotoxic T cells contribute to keep in hold potential metastatic cells at early stages of the metastatic process. This hypothesis is supported by the fact that, although of no statistic influence by itself, high expression of VEGF gene counteracts the beneficial effect of IRF1 (Th1-associated) or granulysin (cytotoxic granules) high gene expression (Camus et al. 2009). We therefore postulate that the presence of high numbers of memory Th1 and cytotoxic T cells in the center and the IM of primary tumors controls the attempts of metastatic cells to leave through vascular or lymphatic vessels. When the tumor grows, with zones of hypoxia, VEGF is produced that increases the tumor neovascularization offering more emigration possibilities to metastatic cells overcoming even a strong coordinated immune reaction. VEGF also inhibits DC maturation that may result in an increase of Treg in the tumor microenvironment (reviewed in Johnson et al. 2009).

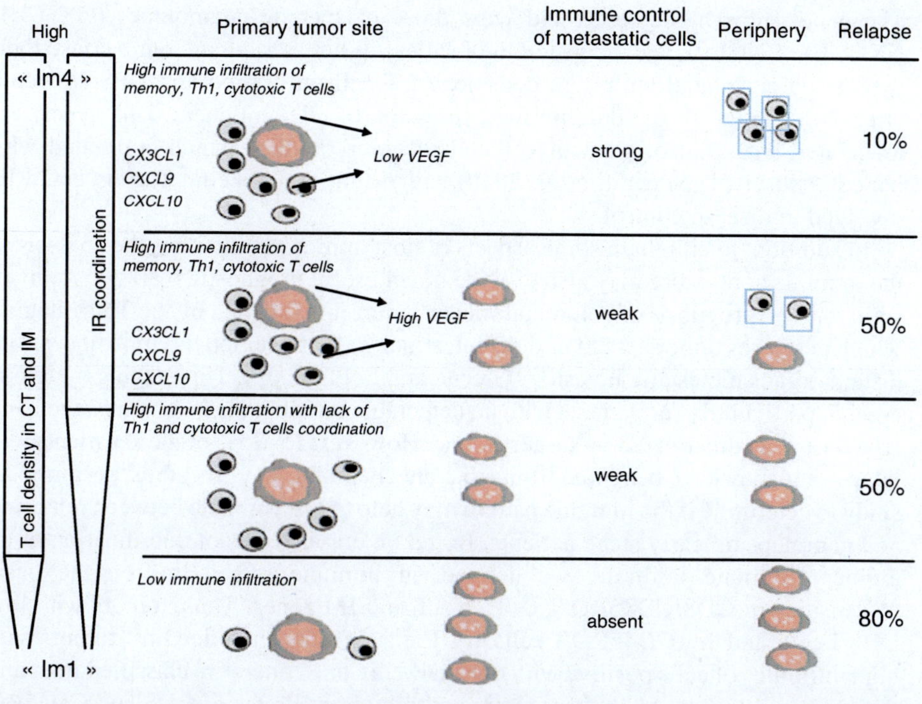

Fig. 2 Immune control of metastasis: Coordinated high T cell density in the CT and at its invasive margin controls metastatic cell dissemination. Four major immune profiles within primary tumors of colorectal cancers are found: (1) strong and coordinated immune response with memory Th1 and cytotoxic T cells control cancer metastasis ("Im4," 10% relapse) (2) same conditions with additional angiogenesis which favors tumor cell dissemination ("Im3," 50% relapse) (3) low coordination of the immune response ("Im2," 50% relapse) (4) weak or low immune response and coordination ("Im0, Im1," 80% relapse). Potential antitumor circulating memory T cells generated in the primary tumor may control metastatic cells and prevent recurrence after surgery

Finally, when the immune contexture is disrupted, no effective control of metastasis and therefore recurrence and survival can anymore be carried out by the immune infiltrate, even it is still present in the tumor (Fig. 2) (Camus et al. 2009). This hypothesis is supported by the analysis of patients who were metastatic at the time of diagnosis and surgery, despite high tumor infiltration by memory T cells. Strikingly, even if the total numbers of memory T cells in these tumors were similar to those of tumors of patients with no metastasis, they lacked the effector/memory T cell subset (Camus et al. 2009). This observation provides a third indication of the need of a finely tuned immune pattern to control tumor spread and invasion.

The identification of factors involved in shaping an efficient immune pattern was approached by using informatic tools and biomolecular networks (Bindea et al. 2009). Databases were explored looking for genes with the following characteristics: conserved genomic neighborhood, phylogenetic profiling, coexpression analysis, literature co-occurrence, and encoded proteins interactions with the subset of genes that had been experimentally shown to be associated with recurrence and DFS.

The genes most highly predicted were those of specific chemokines (CX3CL1, CXCL10, CXCL9) and adhesion molecules. When tested on our series, their expression correlated with high densities of T cell infiltration and DFS (Mlecnik et al. 2010) (Fig. 2). In addition, the expression of relevant chemokine genes was associated with that of particular T cell receptor families which correlated with patient's survival (Mlecnik et al. 2010) suggesting that specific T cells could be involved in disease control.

In addition, to enlighten some aspects of host–tumor interactions, the analysis of the immune contexture may also provide novel useful prognostic markers. As in all solid tumors, prognosis of colorectal cancer is currently defined by the TNM staging which describes tumor spread into the intestinal wall, the regional lymph nodes, and distant organs metastatic invasion (Greene and Sobin 2009). This staging system is crucial, particularly for patients with no detectable lymph node invasion (stage I and II) who are usually treated by surgery alone. However, 15–25% of these patients will relapse and may have benefited from adjuvant chemotherapy. We, thus, performed a study to determine if the immune pattern may help to discriminate between relapsing and nonrelapsing early stage patients. Based on our analyses of coordination of an efficient immune infiltrate, we defined an immune score (Im) on the basis of densities of CD8/CD45RO T cells in CT and IM zones. Thus, tumors with low CD8 T cells and low CD45RO T cells in CT and IM were classified Im0, tumors with high infiltrates of cells positive with one marker in one zone were classified Im1, and then Im2 and Im3 up to Im4 for tumors with high infiltrates of CD8 and CD45RO cells in both CT and IM. The analysis of 353 early-stage (stages I and II) colorectal cancers using the immune score revealed a highly significant correlation between DFS and OS and the immune scoring. Thus, patients with a low immune score (Im0) were of very bad prognosis (75% recurrence at 5-year), whereas patients with a high immune score (Im4) experienced a very low level of recurrence (5% at 5-year) and 86% remained alive. The immune scoring, that was significant over TNM staging, therefore provides a precise prognostic staging to predict recurrence and may therefore encourage to treat patients with low immune score with adjuvant therapies (Fig. 2) (Pagès et al. 2009).

3 Induction of Functionally Active Tertiary Lymphoid Structures in the Vicinity of Tumoral Beds as Potential Sites of "In Situ" Immune Reactions: The Example of Lung Carcinoma

Lung carcinoma is the first cause of death by cancer worldwide with an incidence of over 1.2 million cases/year and a death rate of c.a. 1.1 million cases/year. Curative treatment is surgical for early-stage cancers, followed or not by adjuvant radiotherapy and/or chemotherapy. Lung carcinoma develops in a context of chronic inflammation, in most cases induced by tobacco smoking, but also by asbestos, chronic pulmonary infections, or bronchial obstructive diseases. Lung is at the interface of airways, filtering polluants, bacteria, or viruses that create acute inflammation which may influence clinical outcome of established lung cancers. Lung carcinoma therefore represents a very suitable model to study immune-cancer cell interactions taking place in an adaptive and innate inflammatory microenvironment. A first cohort of 74 early-stage (T1 or T2, N0 or N1, M0) lung cancer patients, without any neo-adjuvant therapy, was analyzed for their immune contexture and the prognostic impact of various immune compartments. Lymphocytic infiltration was found to be a heterogeneously distributed variable between tumors and distributed, as in colorectal cancers, in the center, the IM, and in lymphoid islets adjacent to the tumor nests (Fig. 3a). In addition to T and B cells, we particularly analyzed the quantity and the distribution of DC subsets. The different populations of DC were found diversely located within the tumor. The CD1a+ Langerhans cells were scattered inside the tumor beds showing tight functions with cancer cells, whereas the $CD14^{+/-}$ $CD68^{low}$ Factor XIIIa+ interstitial DC slipped into the interstices of tumor cells and CD123+ plasmacytoid DC concentrated at the IM of tumor nodules. Intratumoral DC were in an immature stage since they lacked the expression of the maturation markers DC-Lamp and CD83. Mature DC-$Lamp^{+}$ cells were found only in the lymphoid islets adjacent to the tumor nests. The extremely low number of DC in nontumoral lung suggests that factors produced by the tumor microenvironment allow the recruitment of DC precursors into the tumor bed without inhibiting their differentiation or maturation. A careful analysis of these lymphoid islets revealed that they resemble canonical secondary lymphoid structures with a T cell zone containing the mature DC in close contact with T cells (Fig. 3b), and a B-cell follicle characterized by the presence of proliferating Ki67+ B cells and the presence of CD21+ follicular DC network (Dieu-Nosjean et al. 2008; Kawamata et al. 2009). These lymphoid islets have therefore the characteristics of functionally active TLS where an ongoing immune reaction takes place. Similar structures have been described in the lungs of human fetuses and infants (Gould and Isaacson 1993) and disappear in normal adult lungs (Tschernig and Pabst 2000). They have been called Bronchus-Associated Lymphoid Tissues (BALT) and, in adults, they reappear in inflammatory lung diseases, such as fibrosis, pneumonia, pneumonitis, or smoking. In patients with tumors, we searched for the presence of TLS at a distance from the tumor and rarely found any. We therefore propose that they are induced by the tumor or the tumor-associated inflammation and call them tumor-induced BALT (Ti-BALT). It is tempting to postulate that Ti-BALT are a location where an efficient immune reaction is shaped before, or in addition to, a response in the draining lymph nodes, where it could be subverted by metastatic cell establishment. Indeed, immune subversion or suppression must be postulated to explain why lymph nodes are the first metastatic sites and why invasion of the sentinel lymph node is a strong deleterious prognostic factor despite the fact that it should be the site of an intense immune reaction. There are indeed examples of immune responses that are not dependent on secondary lymphoid organs. For example, splenectomized alymphoblastic mice can reject xenografts (Tesar et al. 2004), clear viral infections (Moyron-Quiroz et al. 2004), or develop an allergic response

Fig. 3 Characterization of Ti-BALT in NSCLC: Presence of Ti-BALT (*arrow*) in lung tumor section counterstained with hematoxylin and eosin (**a**). DC-Lamp+ mature DC (*red*) home exclusively into CD3+ T –cell (*blue*) rich area of Ti-BALT (**b**). Kaplan-Meier curves of disease-specific survival (Log-rank test) for 74 patients with early-stage NSCLC according to the density of tumor-infiltrating mature DC-Lamp + DC (**c**). Original magnification: A, ×100; B, ×200. T, tumor nest

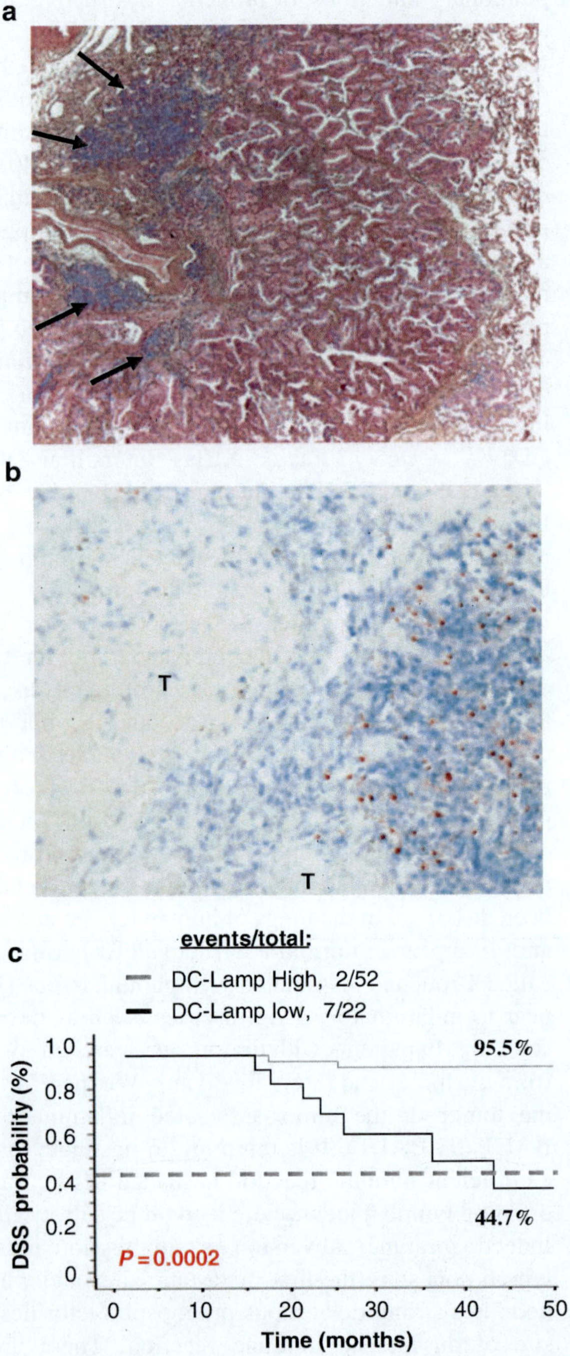

(Gajewska et al. 2001; Halle et al. 2009). If Ti-BALT are sites where an efficient tumor-associated immune response is generated, they should be associated with relevant immune cell infiltration and impact cancer prognosis. Indeed the density of Ti-BALT is heterogeneous between tumors, some presenting with high densities, others with low. We took advantage of the fact that Ti-BALT were the only sites where mature DC-Lamp $^{+}$ DC were present to precisely assess the density of DC-Lamp^{+} cells as a surrogate marker for Ti-BALT. We established that there was a strong correlation between the number of Ti-BALT and that of DC-Lamp^{+} DC in the same fields. We, then, correlated the density of mature DC to other immunological and clinical parameters. The density of mature DC, T, and B lymphocytes correlated with each other. A precise analysis of correlations between high and low DC-Lamp densities and intra-tumoral lymphocyte populations revealed a significant positive correlation with T cell infiltration in CT and IM of the tumors, as well as with T cells with Th1 orientation (T-bet positive). Interestingly, a strong correlation was also found with B cell infiltration in CT and IM and the potential significance of this observation is currently under investigation. In contrast, there was no correlation between high and low DC-Lamp density and clinical parameters such as gender, age, smoking history, histological type (adenocarcinoma or squamous cell carcinoma), histopathological staging (T1, T2, N0, N1), or tumor differentiation. When the patients' cohort was followed for DFS and OS over a period of 4 years, the DC-Lamp^{+} DC density strongly correlated with a favorable clinical outcome. Thus, DFS was 88% in patients with high DC-Lamp^{+} DC infiltration versus 51% in patients with low DC-Lamp^{+} DC density (Dieu-Nosjean et al. 2008). It was even more striking when DSS with 95% of patients not dying from their cancer in DC-Lamp high tumors compared to 45% in DC-Lamp low tumors (Fig. 3c).

These data confirm the observations in colorectal cancer and extend them by showing that TLS adjacent to, and potentially induced by, the tumor could be the first sites of shaping an efficient antitumor reaction. The interaction of mature DC with T cells may result in the generation of memory T cells some with cytotoxic efficiency, that prevent potentially metastatic cells to leave the primary tumor. There may also be sites where circulating memory T cells are generated that are long lived and may control cancer cells disseminating in the periphery (blood, bone narrow) or when they search nidation in distant organs. Finally, the density of mature DC may identify patients with early-stage lung cancer with high risk of relapse.

4 Subversion of Innate Immunity Receptors: Stimulation of Toll Like Receptors on Lung Carcinoma Cells Modulates Cell Survival and Response to Chemotherapy

Lung being a site of frequent inflammation and lung cancers often developing in a context of chronic inflammation, we investigated the presence and the role of Toll Like Receptors (TLR) on lung cancer specimens from Non Small Cell Lung Cancer

(NSCLC) patients. TLR are pattern recognition receptors for pathogen-associated molecular patterns (PAMP) and endogeneous molecules released from injured and necrotic cells (DAMP) (Kumar et al. 2009). Lungs are frequently exposed to viruses such as influenza or respiratory syncitia virus, that are mainly recognized by endogenous TLR3, 7 and 8 (Kumar et al. 2009). Among the 11 different TLR described to date, we thus focused our study on TLR7 and TLR8, receptors for ssRNA (Diebold et al. 2004; Heil et al. 2004) and to a minor extent on TLR3, receptor for dsRNA (Liu et al. 2008). The stimulation of TLR7, TLR8, and TLR3 that are commonly expressed by cells of the immune system leads to the activation of NFKB and the production of proinflammatory cytokines (Napolitani et al. 2005; Hart et al. 2005; Larangé et al. 2009). It induces a rapid antiviral response via the induction of type I and type II IFN which in turn enhance the adaptive immune response. Imiquimod, a TLR7 agonist is currently used topically to treat basal cell carcinoma (Tillman and Carroll 2008) or systemically in clinical trials in melanoma as immuno-stimulants and vaccine adjuvants (Dudek et al. 2007). We observed by immunohistochemistry that immune cells infiltrating NSCLC express TLR7 and TLR8 in situ, particularly within the TiBALT (Cherfils-Vicini et al. 2010).

An increasing body of evidence suggest that TLR are also expressed by nonimmune cells such as epithelial cells (Droemann et al. 2003; Tissari et al. 2005; Gribar et al. 2008) and therefore can maintain local inflammation during chronic infections. In agreement with these observations, we have detected that bronchial epithelial cells but not alveolar cells express TLR7 and TLR8 on nontumoral lung tissue sections (Cherfils-Vicini et al. 2010). Therefore, TLR7 and TLR8 may be one of the first line of defense against viruses in bronchial epithelium.

However, a close immuno-histochemical examination of tumor cells in NSCLC sections revealed that they expressed TLR7 and TLR8, at variable levels, regardless of their histological type, adenocarcinoma or squamous cell carcinoma. A first analysis of 13 tumors (8 adenocarcinoma and 5 squamous cell carcinoma) showed that all expressed TLR8 but in variable quantities; two-thirds of them were TLR7 positive, half being highly labeled. This heterogeneous expression of TLR7 and TLR8, receptors for single stranded RNA, suggested that high expressing and low expressing tumors may behave differently in the case of viral infections, or in the presence of endogenous ligands for these TLR, which could be released in the tumor microenvironment. To determine which effect could be induced by TLR7 and TLR8 triggering, we used two model cell-lines, A549 as a prototype of adenocarcinoma and SK-MES as prototypic of squamous cell carcinoma, that express TLR7 and 8. Triggering of both cell lines by Loxoribine (a TLR7 agonist), poly U (a TLR8 agonist), or gardiquimod (an agonist of both) resulted in better cell survival due to resistance to apoptosis, as assessed by a strong induction of expression of the antiapoptotic gene and protein, Bcl-2. Triggering of A549 or SK-MES by TLR7 and TLR8 agonists also induced the modulation of other genes (up regulation of CCR4 and down regulation of CD80, CD86, HLA-DR, and Fibronectin 1) which are often associated with an aggressive tumoral phenotype. The analysis of genes expressed in tumoral cells isolated from fresh tumor specimen showed that tumor cells had a transcription pattern similar to that of cell lines triggered through TLR7 and 8, suggesting that they were in an activated state in situ (Cherfils-Vicini et al. 2010).

Some patients with lung cancer are treated by neo-adjuvant polychemotherapy, consisting in platinum salts and often gemcitabine or navelbine. Both A549 and SK-MES cells stimulated by Loxoribin or Poly U were found to be resistant to chemotherapy-induced cell death. It is therefore tempting to postulate that tumoral cells which express TLR7 or TLR8 at high levels could be stimulated upon viral induced inflammation and become resistant to chemotherapy (Cherfils-Vicini et al. 2010). We are currently analyzing a cohort of lung cancer patients having received neo-adjuvant chemotherapy before surgical resection in order to assess whether high TLR7 or TLR8 expressors are less susceptible to chemotherapy than low expressors. If it were so, it would provide a novel mechanism by which tumor cells gain growth and spreading advantages, i.e., resistance to apoptosis, to chemotherapy, expression of chemokine receptors, loss of Fibronectin 1, etc. It also calls some warning on the use of TLR7 agonists as adjuvants in cancer treatment, prompting to characterize the expression of TLR7 on the tumor cells before treatment by TLR agonists. Several reports describe the expression of TLR 4 and TLR9 in lung carcinoma (Droemann et al. 2005; He et al. 2007; Ren et al. 2009). TLR expression by tumor cells of nonhematopoietic origin appears to be quite a general phenomenon as TLR2, TLR3, TLR4, TLR5, and/or TLR9 expressions have been documented in many cancer types (reviewed in Sato et al. 2009). In most cases TLR activation of cancer cells promotes survival, activates production of proinflammatory cytokines and chemokines, promotes angiogenesis, and therefore contributes to cancer progression. However, the response to TLR3 seems more complex and can induce opposite effects depending on the cell type. TLR3 ligation by Poly IC or Poly AU on breast cancer cells induces apoptosis in an IFNα dependent manner (Salaun et al. 2006; André 2005). In melanoma a proapoptotic response has been described in the presence of Poly IC as well as the induction of NFκB and production of proinflammatory cytokines (Salaun et al. 2007). We observed that the triggering of TLR3 induced apoptosis of A459 cells whereas it promoted survival of SK-MES cells. Moreover, in some cases the addition of Poly IC to chemotherapy increased sensitivity to chemotherapy-induced cell death. (Cherfils-Vicini et al. 2010).

The fact that TLR stimulation regulates cell survival and modulates their sensitivity to chemotherapy reinforces the importance of TLR expression status on tumor cells in patient's response to treatments.

5 "Paradoxical" Control of Inflammation Influences Clinical Outcome in Head and Neck Cancer

Head and neck cancers are a group of diseases affecting all sites of the upper respiratory tract, from the oral cavity to the larynx, through the oropharynx, the hypopharynx, and the epilarynx. Tobacco, synergized by alcohol, being the main causal factor, head and neck cancers have a higher incidence in males. Human papilloma viruses (HPV) have also been implicated in the genesis of these tumors. In any case, they develop in a context of chronic inflammation which usually persists during the clinical stage of the cancer. Classical treatment consists of surgical resection accompanied by radio/chemotherapy. However, despite new treatment modalities and their success in terms of organ preservation, survival rates have not improved over recent years.

Head and neck squamous cell carcinoma have quite intensively been investigated and the strong inflammatory component of these tumors is well established. In addition to macrophages, there exist, in some tumors, strong T lymphocyte infiltrates with all components of an adaptive immune reaction, i.e., CD3, CD4, and CD8 ; they are likely to control some aspects of tumor spreading, leading to recurrence and ultimately to death. In a first part of our studies, we tackled the question of cytokines that maintain and activate T cell functions. Two cytokines are major players in this prospect: IL-2 and IL-15 (Waldmann 2006). The latter appeared to be of particular interest in the context of head and neck tumors as it is not only critical for "*in vivo*" T cell survival and function but is also a strong inducer of inflammatory cytokines such as IL-6, TNFα, IL-17, etc. (Ohteki et al. 2006). We became interested by what appeared to be an IL-15 paradox: in mice models, IL-15 behaves as an antitumoral factor as it activates antitumoral CD8 and NK cells (Yajima et al. 2002; Kobayashi et al. 2005), rescues CD8 T cells from tolerance to leukemic cells (Teague et al. 2006), or improves the antitumoral activity of passively transferred CD8 T cells (Klebanoff et al. 2004). However, in humans, high intratumoral expression of IL-15 is associated with poor clinical outcome in lung (Seike et al. 2007) and head and neck (Nguyen et al. 2007) carcinomas.

IL-15 binds with high affinity to the IL-15 receptor (IL-15R)α chain, which associates with the IL-2 receptor (IL-2R)β and IL-2Rγ chains to tranduce IL-15 signaling. The trimeric receptor is therefore similar to the complex involved in IL-2 signaling where CD25 (IL-2Rα) would be the IL-2 specific counterpart of IL-15Rα. We had previously reported in a large cohort of 234 head and neck cancers that high serum levels of soluble IL-2R (sCD25) correlated with poor prognosis, both at the local regional level (control of recurrence) and for OS (Tartour et al. 2001). We measured levels of sIL-15R in the sera from 53 head and neck patients and compared them to that found in sera from 40 healthy individuals. We found significant quantities of circulating IL-15Rα in 66% of patients sera compared to very low levels, except one case, in sera from normal individuals. Interestingly, serum levels of sIL-15R had a clinical impact: patients with no circulating sIL-15Rα had a significantly longer recurrence free survival and OS than patients with circulating sIL-15R. What could be the underlying mechanisms by which sIL-15R exert its deleterious impact? To address this question, we analyzed IL-15Rα in head and neck tumors. Seventeen out of 48 tumors expressed IL-15Rα whereas normal epithelial cells did not. They also expressed ADAM-17 a protease that cleaves membrane associated IL-15Rα to produce soluble receptor. There was indeed a correlation between the expression of ADAM-17 by tumor cells and serum levels of

IL-15Rα. It is therefore likely that sIL-15Rα is produced by the tumor cells. Is it only a marker of tumor mass or does it perform biological functions that could explain its prognostic impact? We produced recombinant sIL-15Rα that we added to IL-15 to measure its effects on IL-15 mediated activities. To our surprise, sIL-15Rα did not act as a decoy receptor, but greatly synergized IL-15 induced production of IL-6, TNFα, and IL-17 by human peripheral blood mononuclear cells. It also increased IL-15, but not IL-2, induced CD8 proliferation. We propose that, with other pro-inflammatory components, the pro-inflammatory effect of the IL-15/sIL-15Rα complex dominates over that of the CD8 activation at the tumor site and entertains the bed for local tumor recurrence (Badoual et al. 2008).

Due to the high inflammatory content of head and neck tumors, it is possible that the lymphocytic infiltrates have no clinical impact, either because they are anergic or apoptotic or because they are overcome. We revisited various aspects of T cell infiltration in a cohort of 84 head and neck patients with squamous cell carcinoma in which the tumor had been resected. In contrast to colorectal cancer for example, we found no prognostic impact of the number of CD8 T cells. When infiltrating CD4 T cells were enumerated, we found large numbers in 60% of the tumors. In view of their heterogeneity, we counted CD4+CD25+, CD4+CD69+, and CD4 +Foxp3+ cells. Multivariate Cox analysis of histopathological (T stage) and immune (CD4+CD69+ and CD4+Foxp3+) markers revealed that CD4+Foxp3+ was associated with lack of local recurrence but not OS whereas CD4+CD69+ correlated with good survival but not local control (Badoual et al. 2006). This contrasts with a deleterious reported impact of the number of Foxp3+ cells (Curiel et al. 2004; Hiraoka et al. 2006; Fu et al. 2007).

Such a "paradoxical" beneficial effect of Treg (or at least Foxp3 positive T cells) has also been reported in colorectal cancer in man (Salama et al. 2009) and on the induction of colon cancer (Erdman et al. 2003, 2006) or spontaneous intestinal adenoma (Erdman et al. 2005) in mice. It is striking that the tumors in which Foxp3 positive T cells have been reported to be of favorable prognosis are highly inflammatory. We think that the overall interpretation of these data is that in inflammatory tumors, high numbers of infiltrating Treg are beneficial in terms of local control by their anti-inflammatory activities whereas activation of a tumor specific memory CD8 T cell response is necessary to control metastatic spread and OS (Badoual et al. 2009) (Fig. 4).

In fact, inflammation and immunosuppression are often associated in the tumor microenvironment. For example the proinflammatory cytokine IL-6 in conjunction with TGFβ permits the differentiation of Th17 cells (Wilson et al. 2007) which amplifies local recruitment of inflammatory cells (Ciree et al. 2004) and the production of other inflammatory mediators. However, IL-6 will also activate STAT3, a transcription factor overexpressed in 58.9% of head and neck tumors (Nagpal et al. 2002). Other factors, upregulated in head and neck cancer (IL-10, VEGF...), could also increase the expression of STAT3. Activation of STAT3 will be responsible for various immunosuppressive activities such as the blockade of DC maturation and the release of IL-10, which inhibits T cell and macrophage activation and downregulates HLA expression (Kortylewski and Yu 2008).

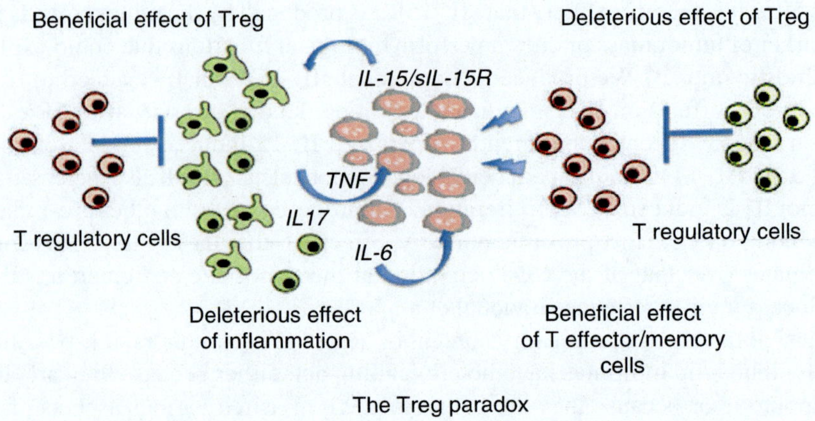

Fig. 4 Paradoxical effects of Treg: Treg are of good prognosis (on the *left*) in inflammatory tumors when they inhibit the protumoral effect of inflammation mediated by protumoral cytokines such as IL-6, IL-17, TNF, and IL-15/sIL-15R. Treg are of bad prognosis (on the *right*) when they inhibit the tumor specific memory CD8 T cells necessary to control metastatic spread and overall survival

Other inflammatory cytokines (TNFα, IL-1...) will induce cyclooxygenase 2 (COX-2) that converts arachidonic acids to PGE_2, a prostaglandin responsible for various immunosuppressive activities. Indeed, PGE_2 has been reported to enhance IL-10 production, down-regulate DC function and inhibit IL-12 production in DC (Harizi et al. 2002). PGE_2 facilitates the expansion of $FoxP3^{+}CD4^{+}CD25^{+}$ naturally occurring regulatory T (nTreg) cells (Baratelli et al. 2005) and the induction of IL-10 producing $CD4^{+}$ type 1 regulatory T (Tr1) cells in a COX-2–positive microenvironment (Akasaki et al. 2004; Bergmann et al. 2007). It is therefore tempting to postulate that the beneficial effects of anti-inflammatory compounds such as aspirin or Cox2 inhibitors in the prevention of human cancers, particularly colorectal cancer, may be not only the consequence of blockade of the well-known pro-tumoral effects of inflammation but also in part by "cooling" the tumor microenvironment, allowing a diluted or inhibited local immune reaction to control the tumor.

6 The Immune Reaction in a Tumor Developing in an Immuno-Priviledged Site: The Case of Primary Intraocular Lymphoma

The eye is considered to be an immunological sanctuary lacking any inflammatory and lymphocytic infiltration in its physiological state. In contrast, the vitreous cavity naturally contains immunosuppressive molecules such as TGFβ or VIP which are believed to suppress any attempt of potential immunological aggression. In pathology, the eye may be the site of an intense inflammation such as in uveitis, origin of which can be infectious or autoimmune (Bodaghi 2005; Mochizuki 2009).

Some tumors can develop in the eye, among which are retinoblastoma, choroïd ocular melanoma, and primary intraocular lymphoma (PIOL). PIOL is a rare disease from the group of Diffuse Large B-cell Lymphoma (DLCBL) and is usually called "uveitis masquerade syndrome" as it frequently displays misleading symptoms with forms of infectious uveitis. PIOL is genetically very similar to central nervous system lymphoma of other locations such as intra-cerebral, spinal cord, and lepto-meningeal lymphomas. Like other tumors developing in immune-privileged sites or in immune-compromised individuals, PIOLs are very aggressive with a 5-year survival rate of less than 5%. In addition, PIOLs have very peculiar invading characteristics with 85% developing cerebral lymphoma and 80% metastasing to the controlateral eye (Nussenblatt et al. 2006). The question therefore arose to the existence of immune surveillance toward PIOL in the eye. The presence of T cells in tumoral eyes has been reported and we confirmed this point. On measuring the cytokine levels in the vitreous humor from 17 PIOL patients, high levels of IL-10 were detected mainly produced by the B cell lymphomatous cells as previously reported since IL-10 levels are considered as a diagnostic marker for PIOL (Cassoux et al. 2007). We found low levels of IFNγ but no evidence for a local IL-2 and IL-4 production (Fig. 5). The presence of IFNγ and the lack of IL-2 support the hypothesis of an ongoing impaired Th1 reaction in the tumoral eye. In view of

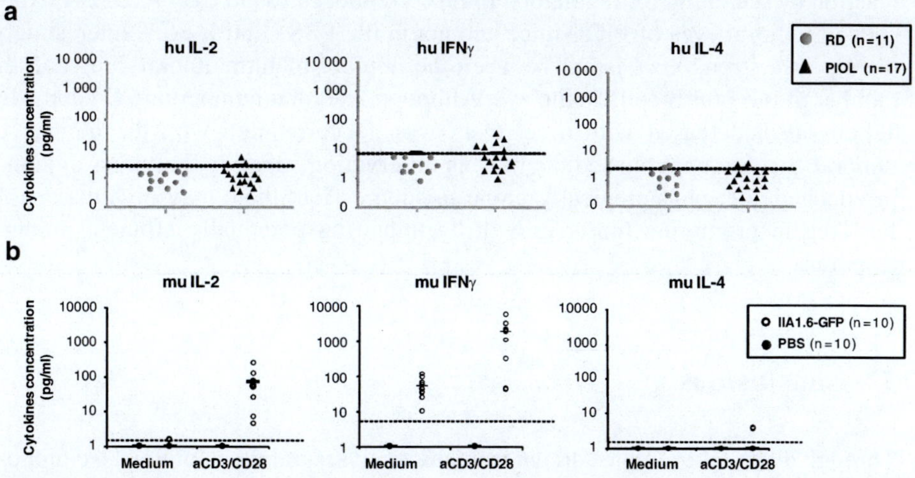

Fig. 5 Cytokine profile in eyes with intraocular lymphoma and influence of T-cell stimulation on cytokine secretion: (**a**) 25 μL of vitreous humor from patients with nonhaemorrhagic retinal detachment (RD) or primary intraocular lymphoma (PIOL) was subjected to IL-2, IFNγ and IL-4 measurement using a human (hu) Cytometric Bead Array Flex (BD Biosciences), according to the manufacturer's instructions. (**b**) 100,000 murine ocular cells obtained from PBS (*filled dots*) or IIA1.6-GFP (*open dots*) injected eyes were cultured in medium alone, or stimulated in vitro with anti-CD3ε and anti-CD28 mAbs (BD Biosciences). After 36 h, culture supernatants were assayed for IL-2, IFNγ, and IL-4 using a mouse (mu) Cytometric Bead Array Flex (BD Biosciences), according to the manufacturer's instructions. Each dot corresponds to the result of an individual eye and the horizontal black bars symbolize the mean of the respective results. The *dashed lines* represent the baseline of detection for each cytokine

the prognostic impact of a strong "in situ" Th1 infiltration in many tumors, as discussed above, we investigated more thoroughly the immune reaction in the eyes with PIOL. Owing to the scarce quantities obtained after surgical vitreous biopsy of human PIOL, we established a murine model of PIOL in which one eye of BALB/c mice was intravitreally injected with murine B lymphoma IIA1.6 cells (Touitou et al. 2007). As a control, PBS was injected in the eyes of naïve mice. The tumor cells progressively invaded and filled the whole posterior chamber. The tumoral and control eyes were surgically removed at day 19 and dissected for functional studies. Firstly, we observed a progressive increase of T cells, both CD4 and CD8 in the tumoral eyes. No T lymphocytes were found in the control eyes. Secondly, when living cells were incubated in medium for 36 h, IL-10 (produced by the lymphomatous cells; data not shown) and small amounts of IFNγ were detected, but no IL-2 or IL-4, mimicking the human situation (Fig. 5). Polyclonal T-cell stimulation using anti-CD3/CD28 antibodies resulted in the induction of IL-2 secretion, a high increase of IFNγ but did not allow IL-4 detection in the supernatants. Conversely, LPS had little effect on lymphocyte-produced cytokines, but highly increased the production of inflammatory (IL-6 and TNFα) cytokines (data not shown). Our mouse model confirmed the human situation showing that an impaired Th1 response is present in PIOL tumoral eyes, and can be rescued by proper T cell stimulation (anti-CD3/CD28). We question the possible reason for this impaired reaction by searching for regulatory T cells. We indeed found CD4+CD25+FoxP3+ cells in tumoral eyes of PIOL mice and not in the PBS control eyes. Interestingly, there was a strong correlation between the number of intratumoral Treg and the number of tumoral B cells in the eye. Although, the total number of CD4 and CD8 T cells also increased with time, there was no correlation with the number of tumoral B cells (unpublished data). This observation suggests that in an immunopriviledged site, physiologically prone to suppression, there may be a major role for Treg in promoting tumor growth by impairing potentially efficient immune reactions.

7 Conclusions

Through different examples drawn from our analyses of human tumors, we propose a few rules emerging to understand host–tumor interactions. We first believe that the microenvironmental immune reaction is essential in the natural history of a cancer. A strong Th1/cytotoxic memory T cell infiltrate, correctly located in tumoral territories is needed to control evading potential metastatic cells. The reaction needs to be coordinated and is influenced by other microenvironmental factors such as VEGF which induces a strong neovascularization but also acts as an immunosuppressive factor by blocking DC maturation thus favoring Treg production. A relevant adaptive immune reaction may be shaped in the draining lymph nodes but even more accurately in TLS adjacent to the tumor beds which behave as tertiary lymphoid organs. In these structures where mature DC interact with T cells and follicular DC with proliferating B cells, efficient memory T cells, both CD4 and CD8, are educated and may infiltrate the tumor to keep metastasis on hold. It is also possible that some educated memory T cells leave into the periphery where they control metastatic cells that have escaped the primary tumor, which explains the strong prognostic value of T memory cells and TLS on OS. In particular situations, such as highly inflammatory tumors or tumors developing in immunoprivileged sites, Treg may have a strong impact by diminishing inflammation or impairing immune responses. In case of inflammation decreased by Treg, one would expect a strong positive effect of Treg locally, rather than on distant metastasis, as is the case in head and neck cancer. Finally, a good knowledge of the complex tumor-immune cell interactions "in situ" provides excellent prognostic markers and therapeutic avenues. In this respect, it is of interest that efficient antiangiogenic therapy correlates with a decrease of Treg in responding patients (Adotevi et al., submitted). Tools now exist and time has come for a routinely adapted analysis of the intratumoral immune reaction, in addition to the classical tumor-associated markers, in clinical human cancers.

Acknowledgments This work was supported by grants from Association pour la Recherche sur le Cancer (ARC), National Cancer Institute (INCa), Canceropole Ile de France, Ville de Paris, Inserm, European Union (7FP, Geninca Consortium grant number 202230), Laboratoire Français de fractionnement et des Biotechnologies (LFB), and Pôle de Compétitivité Ile de France (Immucan). The authors wholeheartedly thank the doctoral and postdoctoral fellows, as well as the engineers and colleagues who performed the biological and statistical experiments: C. Badoual, G. Bindea, M. Camus, J. Cherfils, C. Daussy, L. de Chaisemartin, N. El Houda Afneznay, A. Gey, A. Kirilovski, C. Lagorce, L. Laurans, F. Marliot, B. Mlecnik, R. Molidor, F. Sandoval, M. Tosolini, V. Touitou, and Z. Trajanovski. They acknowledge the trustfull and enthusiastic collaboration with devoted and interactive clinicians and pathologists:M. Antoine, A. Berger, B. Bodaghi, D. Brasnu, P. Bruneval, J. Cadranel, N. Cassou, C. Danel, S. Hans, P. Le Hoang, H. Merle Béral, S. Oudart, P. Validire, P. Wind, and F. Zinzindouhé.

References

Akasaki Y, Liu G, Chung NH, Ehtesham M, Black KL, Yu JS (2004) Induction of a CD4+ T regulatory type 1 response by cyclooxygenase-2-overexpressing glioma. J Immunol 173:4352–4359

Badoual C, Hans S, Rodriguez J, Peyrard S, Klein C, Agueznay Nel H, Mosseri V, Laccourreye O, Bruneval P, Fridman WH, Brasnu DF, Tartour E (2006) Prognostic value of tumor-infiltrating CD4+ T-cell subpopulations in head and neck cancers. Clin Cancer Res 12:465–472

Badoual C, Bouchaud G, Agueznay Nel H, Mortier E, Hans S, Gey A, Fernani F, Peyrard S, -Puig PL, Bruneval P, Sastre X, Plet A, Garrigue-Antar L, Quintin-Colonna F, Fridman WH, Brasnu D, Jacques Y, Tartour E (2008) The soluble alpha chain of interleukin-15 receptor: a proinflammatory molecule associated with tumor progression in head and neck cancer. Cancer Res 68:3907–3914

Badoual C, Hans S, Fridman WH, Brasnu D, Erdman S, Tartour E (2009) Revisiting the prognostic value of regulatory T cells in patients with cancer. J Clin Oncol 27:e5–e6, author reply e7

Balkwill F, Mantovani A (2001) Inflammation and cancer: back to Virchow? Lancet 357:539–545, Review

Baratelli F, Lin Y, Zhu L, Yang SC, Heuze-Vourc'h N, Zeng G, Reckamp K, Dohadwala M, Sharma S, Dubinett SM (2005) Prostaglandin E2 induces FOXP3 gene expression and T regulatory cell function in human CD4+ T cells. J Immunol 175:1483–1490

Bergmann C, Strauss L, Zeidler R, Lang S, Whiteside TL (2007) Expansion of human T regulatory type 1 cells in the microenvironment of cyclooxygenase 2 overexpressing head and neck squamous cell carcinoma. Cancer Res 67:8865–8873

Bindea G, Mlecnik B, Hackl H, Charoentong P, Tosolini M, Kirilovsky A, Fridman WH, Pagès F, Trajanoski Z, Galon J (2009) ClueGO: a Cytoscape plug-in to decipher functionally grouped gene ontology and pathway annotation networks. Bioinformatics 25:1091–1093

Birkeland Sa, Hamilton-Dutoit S, Sandvej K, Andersen Hm, Bendtzen K, Møller B, Jørgensen Ka (1995) EBV-induced post-transplant lymphoproliferative disorder (PTLD). Transplant Proc 27:3467–3472

Bodaghi B (2005) New etiological concepts in uveitis. J Fr Ophtalmol 28:547–555

Burnet FM (1970) The concept of immunological surveillance. Prog Exp Tumor Res 13:1–27

Camus M, Tosolini M, Mlecnik B, Pages F, Kirilovsky A, Berger A, Costes A, Bindea G, Charoentong P, Bruneval P, Trajanoski Z, Fridman W-H, Galon J (2009) Coordination of intratumoral immune reaction and human colorectal cancer recurrence. Cancer Res 69:2685–2693

Cassoux N, Giron A, Bodaghi B, Tran TH, Baudet S, Davy F, Chan CC, Lehoang P, Merle-Béral H (2007) IL-10 measurement in aqueous humor for screening patients with suspicion of primary intraocular lymphoma. Invest Ophthalmol Vis Sci 48:3253–3259

Cherfils-Vicini J, Platonova S, Gillard M, Laurans L, Validire P, Caliandro R, Magdeleinat P, Mami-Chouaib F, Dieu-Nosjean MC, Fridman WH, Damotte D, Sautès-Fridman C, Cremer I (2010) Triggering of TLR7 and TLR8 expressed by human lung cancer cells induces cell survival and chemoresistance. J Clin Invest 120(4):1285–1297

Ciree A, Michel L, Camilleri-Broet S, Jean Louis F, Oster M, Flageul B, Senet P, Fossiez F, Fridman WH, Bachelez H, Tartour E (2004) Expression and activity of IL-17 in cutaneous T-cell lymphomas (mycosis fungoides and Sezary syndrome). Int J Cancer 112:113–120

Coussens LM, Werb Z (2002) Inflammation and cancer. Nature 420:860–867

Curiel TJ, Coukos G, Zou L, Alvarez X, Cheng P, Mottram P, Evdemon-Hogan M, Conejo-Garcia JR, Zhang L, Burow M, Zhu Y, Wei S, Kryczek I, Daniel B, Gordon A, Myers L, Lackner A, Disis ML, Knutson KL, Chen L, Zou W (2004) Specific recruitment of regulatory T cells in ovarian carcinoma fosters immune privilege and predicts reduced survival. Nat Med 10:942–949

Dalerba P, Maccalli C, Casati C, Castelli C, Parmiani G (2003) Immunology and immunotherapy of colorectal cancer. Crit Rev Oncol Hematol 46:33–57

Diebold SS, Kaisho T, Hemmi H, Akira S, Reis e Sousa C (2004) Innate antiviral responses by means of TLR7-mediated recognition of single-stranded RNA. Science 303:1529–1531

Dieu-Nosjean MC, Antoine M, Danel C, Heudes D, Wislez M, Poulot V, Rabbe N, Laurans L, Tartour E, De Chaisemartin L, Lebecque S, Fridman Wh, Cadranel J (2008) Long-term survival for patients with non-small-cell lung cancer with intratumoral lymphoid structures. J Clin Oncol 26:4410–4417

Droemann D, Goldmann T, Branscheid D, Clark R, Dalhoff K, Zabel P, Vollmer E (2003) Toll-like receptor 2 is expressed by alveolar epithelial cells type II and macrophages in the human lung. Histochem Cell Biol 119:103–108

Droemann D, Albrecht D, Gerdes J, Ulmer AJ, Branscheid D, Vollmer E, Dalhoff K, Zabel P, Goldmann T (2005) Human lung cancer cells express functionally active Toll-like receptor 9. Respir Res 6:1

Dudek AZ, Yunis C, Harrison LI, Kumar S, Hawkinson R, Cooley S, Vasilakos JP, Gorski KS, Miller JS (2007) First in human phase I trial of 852A, a novel systemic toll-like receptor 7 agonist, to activate innate immune responses in patients with advanced cancer. Clin Cancer Res 13:7119–7125

Dunn GP, Koebel CM, Schreiber RD (2006) Interferons, immunity and cancer immunoediting. Nat Rev Immunol 6:836–848

Erdman SE, Poutahidis T, Tomczak M, Rogers AB, Cormier K, Plank B, Horwitz BH, Fox JG (2003) CD4+ CD25+ regulatory T lymphocytes inhibit microbially induced colon cancer in Rag2-deficient mice. Am J Pathol 162:691–702

Erdman SE, Sohn JJ, Rao VP, Nambiar PR, Ge Z, Fox JG, Schauer DB (2005) CD4+CD25+ regulatory lymphocytes induce regression of intestinal tumors in ApcMin/+ mice. Cancer Res 65:3998–4004

Erdman SE, Rao VP, Poutahidis T, Ihrig MM, Ge Z, Feng Y, Tomczak M, Rogers AB, Horwitz BH, Fox JG (2006) CD4(+)CD25(+) regulatory lymphocytes require interleukin 10 to interrupt colon carcinogenesis in mice. Cancer Res 63:6042–6050

Fu J, Xu D, Liu Z, Shi M, Zhao P, Fu B, Zhang Z, Yang H, Zhang H, Zhou C, Yao J, Jin L, Wang H, Yang Y, Fu YX, Wang FS (2007) Increased regulatory T cells correlate with CD8 T-cell impairment and poor survival in hepatocellular carcinoma patients. Gastroenterology 132:2328–2339

Gajewska BU, Alvarez D, Vidric M, Goncharova S, Stämpfli MR, Coyle AJ, Gutierrez-Ramos JC, Jordana M (2001) Generation of experimental allergic airways inflammation in the absence of draining lymph nodes. J Clin Invest 108:577–583

Galon J, Costes A, Sanchez-Cabo F, Kirilovsky A, Berger A, Camus M, Mlecnik B, Bruneval P, Molidor R, Cugnenc P-H, Trajanoski Z, Fridman WH, Pagès F (2006) Type, density, and location of immune cells within human colorectal tumors predicts clinical outcome. Science 313:1960–1964

Galon J, Fridman WH, Pages F (2007) The adaptive immunologic microenvironment in colorectal cancer: a novel perspective. Cancer Res 67:1883–1886

Gould SJ, Isaacson PG (1993) Bronchus-associated lymphoid tissue (BALT) in human fetal and infant lung. J Pathol 169:229–234

Greene FL, Sobin LH (2009) A worldwide approach to the TNM staging system: collaborative efforts of the AJCC and UICC. J Surg Oncol 99:269–272

Gribar SC, Anand RJ, Sodhi CP, Hackam DJ (2008) The role of epithelial Toll-like receptor signaling in the pathogenesis of intestinal inflammation. J Leukoc Biol 83:493–498

Halle S, Dujardin HC, Bakocevic N, Fleige H, Danzer H, Willenzon S, Suezer Y, Hämmerling G, Garbi N, Sutter G, Worbs T, Förster R (2009) Induced bronchus-associated lymphoid tissue serves as a general priming site for T cells and is maintained by dendritic cells. J Exp Med 206:2593–2601

Harizi H, Juzan M, Pitard V, Moreau JF, Gualde N (2002) Cyclooxygenase-2-issued prostaglandin e(2) enhances the production of endogenous IL-10, which down-regulates dendritic cell functions. J Immunol 168:2255–2263

Hart OM, Athie-Morales V, O'Connor GM, Gardiner CM (2005) TLR7/8-mediated activation of human NK cells results in accessory cell-dependent IFN-gamma production. J Immunol 175:1636–1642

He W, Liu Q, Wang L, Chen W, Li N, Cao X (2007) TLR4 signaling promotes immune escape of human lung cancer cells by inducing immunosuppressive cytokines and apoptosis resistance. Mol Immunol 44:2850–2859

Heil F, Hemmi H, Hochrein H, Ampenberger F, Kirschning C, Akira S, Lipford G, Wagner H, Bauer S (2004) Species-specific recognition of single-stranded RNA via toll-like receptor 7 and 8. Science 303:1526–1529

Hiraoka N, Onozato K, Kosuge T, Hirohashi S (2006) Prevalence of FOXP3+ regulatory T cells increases during the progression of pancreatic ductal adenocarcinoma and its premalignant lesions. Clin Cancer Res 12:5423–5434

Johnson B, Osada T, Clay T, Lyerly H, Aorse M (2009) Physiology and therepeutics of vascular endothelial growth factor in tumor immuno-suppression. Curr nol ned 9:702–707

Kawamata N, Xu B, Nishijima H, Aoyama K, Kusumoto M, Takeuchi T, Tei C, Michie SA, Matsuyama T (2009) Expression of endothelia and lymphocyte adhesion molecules in bronchus-associated lymphoid tissue (BALT) in adult human lung. Respir Res 10:97

Klebanoff CA, Finkelstein SE, Surman DR, Lichtman MK, Gattinoni L, Theoret MR, Grewal N, Spiess PJ, Antony PA, Palmer DC, Tagaya Y, Rosenberg SA, Waldmann TA, Restifo NP (2004) IL-15 enhances the in vivo antitumor activity of tumor-reactive CD8+ T cells. Proc Natl Acad Sci USA 101:1969–1974

Kobayashi H, Dubois S, Sato N, Sabzevari H, Sakai Y, Waldmann TA, Tagaya Y (2005) Role of trans-cellular IL-15 presentation in the activation of NK cell-mediated killing, which leads to enhanced tumor immunosurveillance. Blood 105:721–727

Koebel CM, Vermi W, Swann JB, Zerafa N, Rodig SJ, Old LJ, Smyth MJ, Schreiber RD (2007) Adaptive immunity maintains occult cancer in an equilibrium state. Nature 450:903–907

Kortylewski M, Yu H (2008) Role of Stat3 in suppressing anti-tumor immunity. Curr Opin Immunol 20:228–233

Kumar H, Kawai T, Akira S (2009) Toll-like receptors and innate immunity. Biochem Biophys Res Commun 388:621–625

Lamm DL (1992) Long-term results of intravesical therapy for superficial bladder cancer. Urol Clin North Am 19:573–580

Larangé A, Antonios D, Pallardy M, Kerdine-Römer S (2009) TLR7 and TLR8 agonists trigger different signaling pathways for human dendritic cell maturation. J Leukoc Biol 85:673–683

Lebel-Binay S, Berger A, Zinzindohoué F, Cugnenc P, Thiounn N, Fridman WH, Pagès F (2000) Interleukin-18: biological properties and clinical implications. Eur Cytokine Netw 11:15–26

Liu L, Botos I, Wang Y, Leonard JN, Shiloach J, Segal DM, Davies DR (2008) Structural basis of toll-like receptor 3 signaling with double-stranded RNA. Science 320:379–381

Mlecnik B, Tosolini M, Charoentong P, Kirilovsky A, Bindea G, Berger A, Camus M, Gillard M, Bruneval P, Fridman Wh, Pagès F, Trajanoski Z, Galon J (2010) Biomolecular network reconstruction reveals mechanisms of immune reaction associated with improved prognosis in colorectal cancer. Gastroenterology 138:1429–1440

Mochizuki M (2009) Regional Immunity of the Eye. Acta Ophthalmol, Nov 7, Epub ahead of print

Moyron-Quiroz JE, Rangel-Moreno J, Kusser K, Hartson L, Sprague F, Goodrich S, Woodland DL, Lund FE, Randall TD (2004) Role of inducible bronchus associated lymphoid tissue (iBALT) in respiratory immunity. Nat Med 10:927–934

Nagpal JK, Mishra R, Das BR (2002) Activation of Stat-3 as one of the early events in tobacco chewing-mediated oral carcinogenesis. Cancer 94:2393–2400

Napolitani G, Rinaldi A, Bertoni F, Sallusto F, Lanzavecchia A (2005) Selected Toll-like receptor agonist combinations synergistically trigger a T helper type 1-polarizing program in dendritic cells. Nat Immunol 6:769–776

Nguyen ST, Hasegawa S, Tsuda H, Tomioka H, Ushijima M, Noda M, Omura K, Miki Y (2007) Identification of a predictive gene expression signature of cervical lymph node metastasis in oral squamous cell carcinoma. Cancer Sci 98:740–746

Nussenblatt RB, Chan CC, Wilson WH, Hochman J, Gottesman M and the CNS and Ocular Lymphoma Workshop Group (2006) International Central Nervous System and Ocular Lymphoma Workshop: recommendations for the future. Ocul Immunol Inflamm 14:139–144.

O'Connell JB, Maggard MA, Ko CY (2004) Colon cancer survival rates with the new American Joint Committee on Cancer sixth edition staging. J Natl Cancer Inst 96:1420–1425

Ohteki T, Tada H, Ishida K, Sato T, Maki C, Yamada T, Hamuro J, Koyasu S (2006) Essential roles of DC-derived IL-15 as a mediator of inflammatory responses in vivo. J Exp Med 203:2329–2338

Pagès F, Berger A, Henglein B, Piqueras B, Danel C, Zinzindohoue F, Thiounn N, Cugnenc PH, Fridman WH (1999) Modulation of interleukin-18 expression in human colon carcinoma: consequences for tumor immune surveillance. Int J Cancer 84:326–330

Pagès F, Berger A, Camus M, Sanchez-Cabo F, Costes A, Molidor R et al (2005) Effector memory T cells, early metastasis, and survival in colorectal cancer. N Engl J Med 353:2654–2666

Pagès F, Galon J, Fridman WH (2008) The essential role of the in situ immune reaction in human colorectal cancer. J Leukoc Biol 84:981–987

Pagès F, Galon J, Dieu-Nosjean MC, Tartour E, Sautes-Fridman C, Fridman WH (2010) Immune infiltration in human tumors, a prognostic factor that should not be ignored. Oncogene 29:1093–1102

Pagès F, Kirilovsky A, Mlecnik B, Asslaber M, Tosolini M, Bindea G, Lagorce C, Wind P, Bruneval P, Zatloukal K, Trajanoski Z, Berger A, Fridman Wh, Galon J (2009) In situ Cytotoxic and Memory T Cells Predict Outcome in Early-Stage Colorectal Cancer Patients. J Clin Oncol 35:5944–5951

Ren T, Xu L, Jiao S, Wang Y, Cai Y, Liang Y, Zhou Y, Zhou H, Wen Z (2009) TLR9 signaling promotes tumor progression of human lung cancer cell in vivo. Pathol Oncol Res 15:623–630

Salama P, Phillips M, Grieu F, Morris M, Zeps N, Joseph D, Platell C, Iacopetta B (2009) Tumor-infiltrating FOXP3+ T regulatory cells show strong prognostic significance in colorectal cancer. J Clin Oncol 27:186–192

Salaun B, Coste I, Rissoan MC, Lebecque SJ, Renno T (2006) TLR3 can directly trigger apoptosis in human cancer cells. J Immunol 176:4894–4901

Salaun B, Lebecque S, Matikainen S, Rimoldi D, Romero P (2007) Toll-like receptor 3 expressed by melanoma cells as a target for therapy? Clin Cancer Res 13:4565–4574

Sato Y, Goto Y, Narita N, Hoon DS (2009) Cancer Cells Expressing Toll-like Receptors and the Tumor Microenvironment. Cancer Microenviron 2(Suppl 1):205–214

Seike M, Yanaihara N, Bowman ED, Zanetti KA, Budhu A, Kumamoto K, Mechanic LE, Matsumoto S, Yokota J, Shibata T, Sugimura H, Gemma A, Kudoh S, Wang XW, Harris CC (2007) Use of a cytokine gene expression signature in lung adenocarcinoma and the surrounding tissue as a prognostic classifier. J Natl Cancer Inst 99:1257–1269

Shankaran V, Ikeda H, Bruce AT, White JM, Swanson PE, Old LJ, Schreiber RD (2001) IFNgamma and lymphocytes prevent primary tumour development and shape tumour immunogenicity. Nature 410:1107–1111

Smyth MJ, Dunn GP, Schreiber RD (2006) Cancer immunosurveillance and immunoediting: the roles of immunity in suppressing tumor development and shaping tumor immunogenicity. Adv Immunol 90:1–50

Tartour E, Gey A, Sastre-Garau X, Lombard Surin I, Mosseri V, Fridman WH (1998) Prognostic value of intratumoral interferon gamma messenger RNA expression in invasive cervical carcinomas. J Natl Cancer Inst 90:287–294

Tartour E, Mosseri V, Jouffroy T, Deneux L, Jaulerry C, Brunin F, Fridman WH, Rodriguez J (2001) Serum soluble interleukin-2 receptor concentrations as an independent prognostic marker in head and neck cancer. Lancet 357:1263–1264

Teague RM, Sather BD, Sacks JA, Huang MZ, Dossett ML, Morimoto J, Tan X, Sutton SE, Cooke MP, Ohlén C, Greenberg PD (2006) Interleukin-15 rescues tolerant CD8+ T cells for use in adoptive immunotherapy of established tumors. Nat Med 12:335–341

Tesar BM, Chalasani G, Smith-Diggs L, Baddoura FK, Lakkis FG, Goldstein DR (2004) Direct antigen presentation by a xenograft induces immunity independently of secondary lymphoid organs. J Immunol 173:4377–4386

Thaunat O, Hanf W, Dubois V, McGregor B, Perrat G, Chauvet C, Touraine JL, Morelon E (2009) Chronic humoral rejection mediated by anti-HLA-DP alloantibodies: insights into the role of epitope sharing in donor-specific and non-donor specific alloantibodies generation. Transpl Immunol 20:209–211

Tillman DK Jr, Carroll MT (2008) A 36-month clinical experience of the effectiveness of curettage and imiquimod 5% cream in the treatment of basal cell carcinoma. J Drugs Dermatol 7:s7–s14

Tissari J, Sirén J, Meri S, Julkunen I, Matikainen S (2005) IFN-alpha enhances TLR3-mediated antiviral cytokine expression in human endothelial and epithelial cells by up-regulating TLR3 expression. J Immunol 174:4289–4294

Touitou V, Daussy C, Bodaghi B, Camelo S, de Kozak Y, Lehoang P, Naud MC, Varin A, Thillaye-Goldenberg B, Merle-Béral H, Fridman WH, Sautès-Fridman C, Fisson S (2007)

Impaired th1/tc1 cytokine production of tumor-infiltrating lymphocytes in a model of primary intraocular B-cell lymphoma. Invest Ophthalmol Vis Sci 48:3223–3229

Tschernig T, Pabst R (2000) Bronchus-associated lymphoid tissue (BALT) is not present in the normal adult lung but in different diseases. Pathobiology 68:1–8, Review

Van der Meer JW, Weening RS, Schellekens PT, van Munster IP, Nagengast FM (1993) Colorectal cancer in patients with X-linked agammaglobulinaemia. Lancet 341:1439–1440

Waldmann TA (2006) The biology of interleukin-2 and interleukin-15: implications for cancer therapy and vaccine design. Nat Rev Immunol 6:595–601, Review

Wilson NJ, Boniface K, Chan JR, McKenzie BS, Blumenschein WM, Mattson JD, Basham B, Smith K, Chen T, Morel F, Lecron JC, Kastelein RA, Cua DJ, McClanahan TK, Bowman EP, de Waal Malefyt R (2007) Development, cytokine profile and function of human interleukin 17-producing helper T cells. Nat Immunol 8:950–957

Yajima T, Nishimura H, Wajjwalku W, Harada M, Kuwano H, Yoshikai Y (2002) Overexpression of interleukin-15 *in vivo* enhances antitumor activity against MHC class I-negative and -positive malignant melanoma through augmented NK activity and cytotoxic T-cell response. Int J Cancer 99:573–578

Subversion and Coercion: The Art of Redirecting Tumor Immune Surveillance

John B. Mumm and Martin Oft

Contents

1 Introduction 26
2 The Inflammatory Trio: TNF-α, TGF-β, IL-6 28
3 The Local Trigger: IL-23 and IL-12 Balance in the Tumor Microenvironment 30
4 Feeding the Inflammatory Niche: Adaptive T Cell Responses Fostering the Tumor 31
5 Turning Foes into Friends, CD8+ T Cells Lose Their Teeth 32
6 Inflammatory Control at the Tumor Site 33
7 Conclusions 35
References 36

Abstract Tumor immune surveillance and CD8+ T cells in particular appear capable of recognizing the antigenic properties of human tumor cells. However, those antigen specific T cells are often excluded from tumor tissue or are functionally limited in their cytotoxic capacity. Instead, the immune response provides proinflammatory cytokines and proteases promoting tumor growth and progression while subverting cytotoxic anti-tumor immunity. The cytokines and the inflammatory mechanisms driving tumor associated inflammation resemble tissue remodeling processes during wound healing and chronic inflammatory diseases. In this chapter, we summarize the current knowledge of how inflammatory cytokines may promote the deviation of anti-tumor immunity toward a tumor promoting, noncytotoxic inflammation.

M. Oft (✉) and J.B. Mumm
Merck Research Labs (formerly DNAX) 901 California Avenue, Palo Alto, CA 94303, USA
e-mail: martin.oft@spcorp.com

G. Dranoff (ed.), *Cancer Immunology and Immunotherapy*,
Current Topics in Microbiology and Immunology 344, DOI 10.1007/82_2010_47

1 Introduction

After decades of research, it has become clear that the human immune system recognizes the antigenic profile of tumors and amplifies tumor specific T and B cell populations (Jager et al. 2003; Van Der Bruggen et al. 2002). While cytotoxic T cells directly recognize the antigenic properties of human tumor cells (Knuth et al. 1984; van der Bruggen et al. 1991), their infiltration into tumor tissue is very limited. The presence of IFN-γ+ CD8+ T cells correlates with an improved patient prognosis (Galon et al. 2006; Naito et al. 1998). Antigen presentation to CD8+ T cells is also negatively regulated in tumors, and major histocompatibility complex (MHC) molecules are expressed at low levels in the majority of cancers (Seliger et al. 2002). Moreover, low expression MHC molecules have been correlated with reduced survival of cancer patients (Han et al. 2008). However, human tumors occur more often in sites of chronic inflammation, and the chronic use of nonsteroidal anti inflammatory drugs conveys a lower incidence of cancer (Coussens and Werb 2002; Koehne and Dubois 2004; Lin and Karin 2007). In addition, survival of cancer patients appears to be negatively associated with an abundance of immune stimulatory and proinflammatory cytokines in systemic circulation. The significant upregulation of proinflammatory cytokines is particularly evident during tumor cachexia and metastasis associated with late stage cancer (Balkwill et al. 2005; Loberg et al. 2007) (Fig. 1). These data raise the question whether the failure of the adaptive immune system to eliminate disseminated tumor burden in late stage cancer patients is caused by a failure to mount the right type of response rather

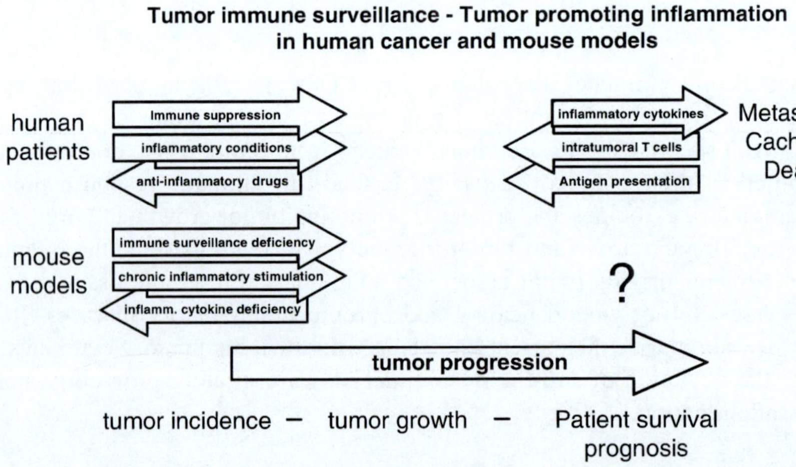

Fig. 1 *The polarization of the immune response control cancer incidence and death.* Chronic tissue damage and inflammation is not only associated with tumor incidence in human patients and mouse models but cytokines triggering inflammation are also predictors of a decreased life expectancy in human cancer patients. In sharp contrast, presence of mediators of the adaptive immune surveillance – CD8+ T cells and antigen presenting molecules – convey a favorable prognosis to cancer patients and control tumor incidence in mice and men

than a failure to detect the antigenic properties of the tumor. More specifically, do cancer patients suffer from a misguided immune response against their cancer cells, dominated by systemic immune stimulatory and proinflammatory cytokines that inhibit the intratumoral cytotoxic-immune response?

We have recently reported that the very regulation of tissue regenerating inflammation might directly inhibit the ability of cytotoxic T cell to destroy tumor cells within the inflamed tissue (Langowski et al. 2007). As a consequence, immune surveillance against tumors is largely prevented in the local microenvironment by proinflammatory mediators such as IL-23 (Langowski et al. 2006).

As described above, a solid body of evidence associates chronic inflammation with increased tumor incidence. Additionally, clinical and experimental findings also show to the up-regulation of proinflammatory molecules during tumor progression, particularly during late stages of cancer progression and during tumor cachexia (Balkwill et al. 2005). The same cytokines upregulated in tumor promoting inflammation are essential for the development of proinflammatory CD4+ and CD8+ T cells, essential for inflammatory diseases.

We outline the players in the tumor centric cytokine network and describe their simultaneous influence on effector cells of the tumor-associated inflammatory responses and on tumor immune surveillance (Fig. 2).

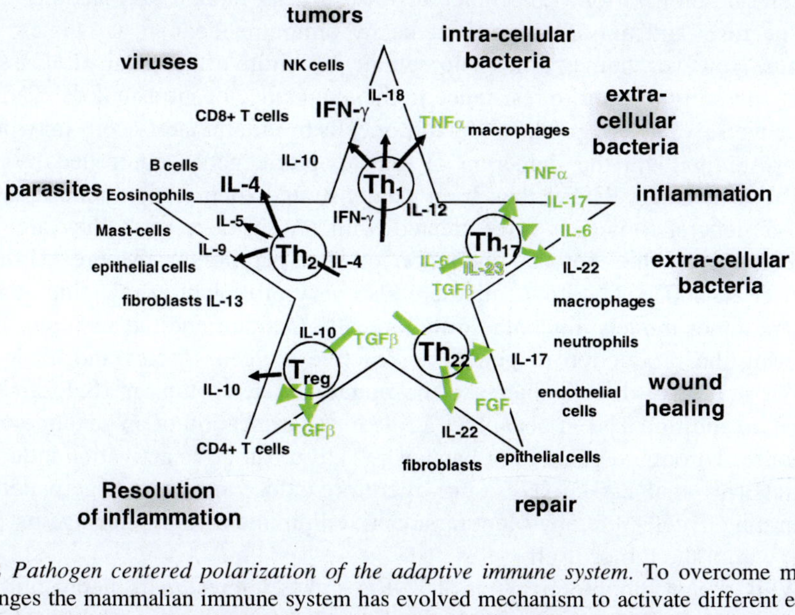

Fig. 2 *Pathogen centered polarization of the adaptive immune system.* To overcome multiple challenges the mammalian immune system has evolved mechanism to activate different effector populations. Closing a wound typically requires antibacterial effectors, myeloid and stromal cells, but not primarily the adaptive or cytotoxic responses required for anti-viral mechanisms. The immune response to tumors often replicates wound healing like immune reactions, inherently less capable of eliminating malignant cells. *Green*: Cytokines activated in human cancer tumors, associated with decreased prognosis or short survival of human patients. *Circle*: polarized CD4+ T cells

2 The Inflammatory Trio: TNF-α, TGF-β, IL-6

TNF-α is an essential effector cytokine for the initiation and maintenance of chronic inflammation as shown in mouse models of immune mediated disorders such as rheumatoid arthritis (Williams et al. 2000). The relevance of the TNF-α pathway for human disease is best exemplified in the success of anti-TNF-α therapies in inflammatory diseases (Feldmann and Maini 2001). Elevated concentrations of TNF-α are also found in the serum of cancer patients and correlate with a poor patient prognosis (Szlosarek and Balkwill 2003). TNF-α is closely associated with metastasis, tumor induced cachexia, an inflammation mediated multiorgan failure in late stage cancer patients and inflammatory paraneoplastic syndromes (Loberg et al. 2007). Genetic polymorphisms conferring higher TNF-α production are associated with increased risk of a variety of human cancers (Szlosarek et al. 2006).

In providing inhibitory and stimulatory signals to tumor growth, TNF-α exemplifies the conundrum of the inflammatory cytokine milieu within the tumor microenvironment. TNF-α is produced by Th1 and Th17 CD4+ T cells and macrophages. TNF-α promotes the maturation of dendritic cells but also inhibits the expression of type I interferons (Caux et al. 1992; Palucka et al. 2005; Zhou and Tedder 1996). Induction of high local concentrations of TNF-α promote tumor vascular destabilization (Lejeune et al. 1998; Ruegg et al. 1999) leading to tumor cell necrosis and tumor antigen uptake by tumor resident or associated macrophages. However, human tumors upregulate inhibitors of apoptosis (LaCasse et al. 2008), possibly to acquire resistance to the abundance of intra-tumoral TNF-α.

Conversely, TNF-α produced by tumor cells or inflammatory cells may promote tumor survival via the induction of anti-apoptotic genes controlled by NF-kB activation. Indeed, TNF-α has been demonstrated to promote tumorigenesis as TNF-α deficient mice or mice treated with anti-TNF-α antibodies are largely protected from the chemical induction of skin papillomas (Moore et al. 1999; Scott et al. 2003). TNF-α -/- mice are also very proficient at rejecting syngeneic murine tumor models implanted orthotopically (Mumm and Oft unpublished). By fostering the production of genotoxic reactive oxygen species and nitric oxide, TNF-α may also directly increase the mutation rate in tumors (Szlosarek et al. 2006). In addition TNF-α also plays a role in the truncation of an adaptive immune response. Through regulation of Fas/FasL, TNF-α can drive activation induced cell death (Elzey et al. 2001). TNF-α may therefore induce apoptosis of activated tumor infiltrating T cells, thereby blunting adaptive immune surveillance against tumors from within the tumor itself.

While the pro-apoptotic effects of TNF-α spiked interest in its therapeutic utility, the concentrations necessary to achieve therapeutic response are too high (Mocellin et al. 2005). Moreover, elevated TNF-α levels in the serum associate with a poor prognosis of cancer patients which suggests that the microenvironment of the tumor is already desensitized to high intra-tumoral levels of TNF-α. Attempting to increase the TNF-α level further may be deleterious to the host rather than eliciting a de novo immune response. Most endogenous mouse tumor models and clinical studies indeed underline the pro-neoplastic functions of TNF-α rather than its pro-apoptotic functions on tumor cells.

Another key regulator of inflammatory processes tightly associated with chronic inflammation and cancer is transforming the growth factor β (TGF-β). TGF-β contributes to tumorigenesis by local suppression of the immune surveillance, in particular of antigen specific cytotoxic CD8+ T cells. Only recently it became clear that TGF-β is equally important for proinflammatory CD4 T cells (see below).

TGF-β inhibits the maturation, antigen presentation and costimulation by both macrophages and dendritic cells (Li et al. 2006). Immature dendritic cells produce large amounts of TGF-β and might efficiently prime regulatory CD4+ T cells (Treg). TGF-β is required for the development of Tregs and TGF-β expression by Tregs is essential for their proliferation and function. Regulatory T cells are found in human tumors and their presence correlates again with a poorer prognosis (Curiel et al. 2004). TGF-β also plays a role in the development of the proinflammatory murine IL-17 producing Th17 which share a common path with regulatory T cells.

Similar to helper T cells, TGF-β inhibits the proliferation and differentiation of CD8+ cytotoxic T cells. (Wrzesinski et al. 2007). TGF-β inhibits the expression of Interferon-γ (IFN-γ), the cytotoxic effector molecule Perforin, and the exocytosis of the cytotoxic granules (Li et al. 2006). Moreover, CD8+ T cells stimulated with both IL-6 and TGF-β, cease expression of IFN-γ, lose their cytotoxicity and secrete IL-17 (Liu et al. 2007). IFN-γ induces major histocompatibility complex (MHCI) in both dendritic cells and tumor cells. Replacing intratumoral IFN-γ expressing T cells by Th17 might severely compromise tumor immune recognition and surveillance.

IL-6 activates STAT3 and induces survival and proliferation of tumor cells in numerous experimental systems (Aggarwal et al. 2006; Naugler and Karin 2008; Rose-John et al. 2006). IL-6Rα is highly expressed on tumor cells, and soluble sIL-6Rα stimulates trans-signaling in cells not expressing IL-6Rα (Becker et al. 2004; Rose-John et al. 2006). IL-6 protects tumor cells from apoptosis and serves as an autocrine growth factor (Baffet et al. 1991). IL-6 is also essential in the initiation and maintenance of chronic inflammation of the colon (Atreya et al. 2000) and the development of inflammation induced colon tumors (Becker et al. 2004).

IL-6 levels are typically elevated in the serum and tissue of cancer patients and correlate with a negative prognosis (Smith et al. 2001). Increased IL-6 expression due to IL-6 promoter polymorphisms may be a cancer predisposing genetic risk factor in colon cancer patients (Landi et al. 2003).

Recently, however, it has become clear that IL-6 acts with TGF-β, which is crucial to induce the IL-17 producing Th17 helper cell lineages (Mangan et al. 2006; Wilson et al. 2007). It remains to be tested how many of the effects of IL-6 in the regulation of tissue inflammation and cancer are dependent on the induction and subsequent control of this T cell lineage. Importantly, it has been shown that the proinflammatory T helper cells continue to express both IL-17 and IL-6 (Becker et al. 2004; Langrish et al. 2005).

3 The Local Trigger: IL-23 and IL-12 Balance in the Tumor Microenvironment

IL-12 and IL-23 are hetrodimeric cytokines sharing the common p40 subunit, with receptors expressed on T, NK and NKT cells but low levels are present also on myeloid cells. Both cytokines are produced primarily by activated antigen presenting cells in response to toll like receptor stimulation (Gerosa et al. 2008; Trinchieri et al. 2003). For immune responses against most of bacterial pathogens, IL-12 is essential, while the IL-23 mediated induction of IL-17 might be essential for the rapid release of granulocytes in high pathogen infections (Christopher and Link 2007; Happel et al. 2005). In contrast, humans deficient for IL-12p40 or IL12Rb1 suffer exclusively from mycobacterial and salmonella infection but show normal resistance to most other pathogens, including viruses (Novelli and Casanova 2004).

IL-12 promotes IFN-γ-producing Th1 cells and the proliferation and cytotoxic activity of CD8+ T cells and NK cells. In preclinical tumor models, IL-12 induced IFN-γ promotes immune surveillance against transplanted syngeneic tumors. IFN-g is not only rate limiting for T cell activity but also required for intratumoral expression of MHCI thereby increasing recognition of tumor antigens (Wong et al. 1984). Tumor immune surveillance in mouse models is largely dependent on IFN-γ expressing T cells (Kaplan et al. 1998). Experiments using IL-23 or IL-12 expressed in transplanted tumor cell or systemically were equally efficient in rejecting syngeneic transplanted tumors, however the mechanisms of IL-23 mediated anti-tumor activity are not clearly understood (Lo et al. 2003).

Cancer patients have been treated with recombinant IL-12 in several clinical studies, but dose limiting toxicities were observed before clinical benefits were achieved (Atkins et al. 1997). The toxicities were most likely manifestations of a systemic immune response brought about by high systemic IFN-γ expression. Subsequent attempts to combine IL-12 therapy with peptide vaccines have not yet revealed clearly enhanced clinical benefits (Cebon et al. 2003).

Despite the similarities between Il-12 and IL-23, IL-12 or IL-23 deficient animals have striking differences in tumor immune regulation. IL-12 deficiency in mice increases tumor incidence and allows for more rapid tumor growth. In contrast, deficiency in IL-23 or the IL-23 receptor dramatically reduces tumor incidence, and profoundly reduces established tumor growth (Langowski et al. 2006). IL-23 deficiency reduced anti-tumor immunosurveillance by locally increasing the presence of intratumoral CD8+ T cells. More importantly, the hallmarks of chronic inflammation such as metalloproteases, angiogenesis and macrophage infiltration were largely dependent on the presence and the amount of IL-23 in the host. The absence of IL-12 leads to exacerbation of the myeloid driven inflammation but with a coincident lack of CD8+ T cells (Langowski et al. 2006).

This proinflammatory function of IL-23 appears to orchestrate inflammatory tissue remodeling by the adaptive immune system. IL-23 controls IL-17 expression in T cells and other cell types. IL-17 can directly promote angiogenesis and matrix metalloproteinases (MMPs), two events that potentiate tumor growth

(Numasaki et al. 2003). In addition, IL-17 controls neutrophil chemotaxis, proliferation and maturation further fueling innate immune activation (Kolls and Linden 2004). Moreover, IL-17 producing CD8+ and CD4+ T cells have recently been reported to be widely present in human and mouse tumor microenvironments (Kryczek et al. 2007). The importance of IL-17 itself in the control of tumor growth however, is still debated and depends on the experimental setting (Kryczek et al. 2009b; Wang et al. 2009). In this context, it is noteworthy that IL-23 can induce, independent of IL-17, angiogenic erythema, inflammation and keratinocyte hyperproliferation and phenocopying aspects of human psoriatic lesions (Chan et al. 2006). Similarly, experimental encephalitis depends on IL-23 expression in the host (Cua et al. 2003) but IL17 or IL17F or both are dispensable (Haak et al. 2009).

In human cancers, IL-23p19 and IL12p40 are found to be over expressed in the majority of tumors, with IL-12p35 to be un-altered. IL-17 can be concomitantly upregulated in tumors or even lost in tumor progression (Kryczek et al. 2009a). It will be very important to understand the bifurcation of this pathway in cancer patients.

4 Feeding the Inflammatory Niche: Adaptive T Cell Responses Fostering the Tumor

How the adaptive immune system responds to perceived injury or infection is regulated on various levels, most intriguingly exemplified in the differential polarization of CD4+ helper cells (Reiner 2007 and Fig. 2). Cytokines such as IL-4, IL-12 and IL-23 regulate the initiation or activity of those divergent immunological pathways (McKenzie et al. 2006). IL-12 and IFN-γ prime and maintain the development of Th1 cells which produce IFN-γ and TNF-α and enhance antimicrobial and cytotoxic responses. IL-23 is essential in the proinflammatory function of a memory T cell subset characterized by the production of the cytokine IL-17, named therefore Th_{17} (Aggarwal et al. 2003; Langrish et al. 2005). Through the attraction and activation of granulocytes and other innate myeloid cells, Th17 cells are thought to safeguard against extracellular bacteria. IL-17 engages its receptor, commonly found on stromal, epithelial, endothelial cells and monocytes – resulting in the release of additional inflammatory factors (such as IL-1, IL-6, IL-8, TNF-α, ProstaglandinE2, ICAM and several chemokines) to further the inflammatory cascade (Fossiez et al. 1998; Kolls and Linden 2004). Indeed, the IL-23/IL-17 inflammatory pathway, rather than the IL-12/IFN-γ pathway, has been highlighted by various recent reports as being central to inflammatory conditions exhibited in psoriasis, ischemic injury, inflammatory bowel disease (Yen et al. 2006), and autoimmune inflammation of the joint and brain (McKenzie et al. 2006). In those mouse models of inflammatory diseases Th_{17} cells have been identified as the major pathogenic population (Langrish et al. 2005). Murine Th_{17} cells develop from naïve

T cells under the influence of TGF-β and IL-6 (Mangan et al. 2006; Veldhoen et al. 2006). Th17 T cells express also IL-6, TNF-α and IL-22 a cytokine of the IL-10 family predominantly activating nonhematopoietic cell types. Recently, proinflammatory Th22 cells have been described from human blood, expressing a cytokine profile similar to Th17 but expressing different FGF isoforms instead of TNF-α (Eyerich et al. 2009). It is unclear if Th22 cells represent a separate helper cell lineage or a further polarization of the Th17 fate.

One important role for IL-23 was recently uncovered in its suppression of TGF-β mediated induction of the anti-inflammatory cytokine IL-10 (McGeachy et al. 2007). TGF-β stimulation increases the up-regulation of the Foxp3 transcription factor, inducing differentiation into regulatory T cells (Treg). Simultaneous stimulation with TGF-β and IL-6 diverted the CD4+ T cell toward the proinflammatory Th_{17} cell (Bettelli et al. 2006). Since then numerous groups have confirmed the close relationship and the convertibility of regulatory T cells into proinflammatory Th17 cells (Yang et al. 2008).

The cytokines polarizing T cells towards Th17 or possibly Th22 such as IL-6, TGF-β, TNF-α, and IL-23 are also known to be present at high levels in the tumor environment and are typically associated with an unfavorable prognosis for human patient. IL-23 appears to be crucial for the function, survival and propagation of this important T cell population in the inflamed environment.

5 Turning Foes into Friends, CD8+ T Cells Lose Their Teeth

While most of the attention has been concentrated on IL-17 production by CD4+ T cells, there is more and more evidence that NK, γδ T cells, and CD8+ T cells express IL-17 and are even in some instances the dominant source of this proinflammatory cytokine (He et al. 2006; Lockhart et al. 2006). Importantly, CD8+ T cells expressing IL-17 largely lack cytotoxic capacity (Liu et al. 2007).

CD8+ T cells deficient in the key transcription factors Eomes and Tbet fail to differentiate into functional cytotoxic T cells, do not control virus infection but induce multiorgan inflammation and death of the host in response to virus infection (Intlekofer et al. 2008). Those CD8+ T cells fail to express IFN-γ but up-regulate the transcription factor FOXp3, RORγT, the inflammatory cytokines IL-17 and IL-22 along with the IL-23 receptor. Most importantly, however, those Tc17 CD8+ T cells have a strongly reduced cytotoxic activity against antigen specific targets (Intlekofer et al. 2008). Recently, it has been shown that normal CD8+ T cells polarized in the combined presence of IL-6, TGF-β and IL-23 and the absence of IL-4 and IFN-γ differentiate into very similar Tc17 cells (Yen et al. 2009). Under those conditions CD8+ T cells gain the expression of Foxp3 and RORγt, IL-17 and IL-22, but have reduced levels of Eomes, Tbet and IFN-γ. Again, such polarized cells fail to produce cytotoxic enzymes and also fail to kill cognate target cells. However, when transferred into mice Tc17 cells reverted rapidly into IFN-γ and TNF-α expressing Tc1 cells demonstrating that the phenotypic plasticity might be determined by the local cytokine milieus. Unexpectedly, extraction of IFN-γ producing Tc1 like CD8+ T cells was more efficient when Tc17 were transferred, than after transfer of bona fide Tc1 cells, indicating that the IL-17 producing population displayed a marked increase in the capability of in vivo expansion (Yen et al. 2009). Interestingly, CD8+ T cells with a very similar differentiation pattern have been described to promote tumor progression in carcinogen induced skin tumors in mice (Kwong et al. 2009). Here, tumor infiltrating CD8+ T cells fail to express cytotoxic characteristics but express all the hallmarks of an inflammatory T cell in vivo, such and IL-17 and IL-22. Importantly, deficiency of CD8+ T cells in this model of skin carcinogenesis lead not to increased tumor formation but to a decreased progression rate from benign tumors to carcinomas (Roberts et al. 2007).

Taken together, the recent data suggest that both CD4+ and CD8+ T cells can not only fail to support the elimination of malignant cells but they may significantly contribute to tumor progression. Such noncytotoxic cells may possibly drive the physiological changes seen in late stage cancer patients, such as inflammatory multi organ failure.

6 Inflammatory Control at the Tumor Site

There is considerable controversy concerning the volatility of the polarization of an adaptive immune response. As it pertains to the regulation of tumor immunity, one has to note that immunization protocols and adaptive T cell transfers typically result in Th1 or Tc1 polarized T cell responses. Despite strong antigen specific in vitro activities of such induced or transferred cells, their therapeutic effectiveness does not, in most cases satisfy expectations. In the tumor microenvironment, the same T cells appear to lose their function or fail to infiltrate the tumor altogether. An attractive explanation for this phenomenon is the induction of energy or functional depolarization in the local environment.

In inflammatory models, where Th17 polarized cells are pathogenic through the activation and attraction of myeloid cells and neutrophils, it had been shown that the pathogenic effect of the transferred IL-17 producing T cells was stable and still dependent upon IL-17 in vivo (Langrish et al. 2005). Th17 cells can however swiftly repolarize into Th1 cells when transferred in the appropriate host (Bending et al. 2009).

Adoptive transfer of tumor specific Th17 into mice harboring primary irradiated tumors or experimental lung nodules of B16 melanoma cells reduced their tumor burden. The anti-tumor effects appeared to depend on the presence of host IFN-γR, but antibody mediated depletion of IFN-γ did not change the outcome (Martin-Orozco et al. 2009; Muranski et al. 2008). It is therefore not clear if in the anti-tumor function of proinflammatory Th17 induced anti-tumor effects by attracting myeloid cells, or if the transferred cells reverted to a Th1 profile *in vivo*.

CD8+ T cells polarized and sorted for the IL-17+ population revert very efficiently in lung tissue expressing the cognate antigen from IL-17 to IFN-γ production

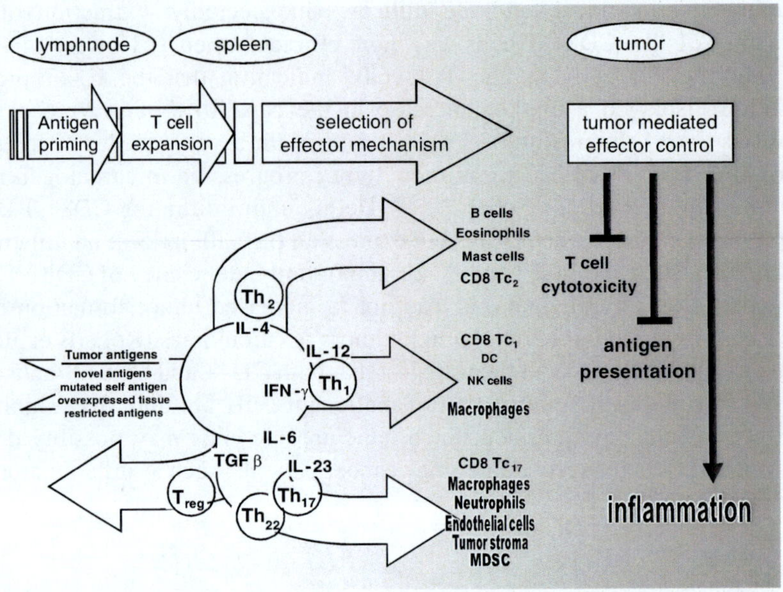

Fig. 3 *Location – Location – Location*. Cancer patients can have systemic tumor specific responses, but the frequency of cytotoxic memory T cells in the tumor tissue is typically low and their presence correlates positively with clinical outcome. While priming and expansion of tumor antigen specific T cells in secondary lymphoid organs might not be abrogated, the resulting immune response is blunted and altered in the local, immune deviating microenvironment of the tumor

(Yen et al. 2009). Importantly, Foxp3+ regulatory T cells express inflammatory Th17 polarization when isolated from intestinal polyps of APC-Min mice (Gounaris et al. 2009). Similarly, the transition form a Treg to a Th17 cell has been observed by several groups and is influenced by IL-6 or IL-1 and stabilized by IL-23, the same cytokines influencing the differentiation of naïve cells (Yang et al. 2008 and Fig. 3).

Inflammatory cytokines like IFN-γ and IL-12 or TGF-β, IL-6 and IL-23 appear to control the bifurcation of tumor infiltrating immune cells into tumor immune surveillance or tumor associated inflammation respectively. In the local tumor microenvironment, IL-23 induces the hallmarks of chronic inflammation such as metalloproteases, angiogenesis and macrophage infiltration, but it also reduces anti-tumor immunosurveillance by locally suppressing the presence of CD8+ T cells. The absence of IL-12 lead to an exacerbation of the myeloid driven inflammation with a coincident lack of CD8+ T cells (Langowski et al. 2006). Increased CD8+ T cell infiltration and enhanced tumor immune surveillance was observed when IL-12 dominated IL-23, either in the absence of IL-23 or upon injection of IL-12. IL-12 and IL-23 induce differential chemokine patterns (MO unpublished), but it is not clear if differential chemoattraction causes the local immune polarization. Also, it remains to be shown if other tumor associated proinflammatory cytokines reduce the local CD8+ T cell response in similar ways.

Moreover, Il-12 and IL-23 can regulate inflammation independently of T cells. Rag deficient mice treated with an activating anti-CD40 antibody developed an IL-23

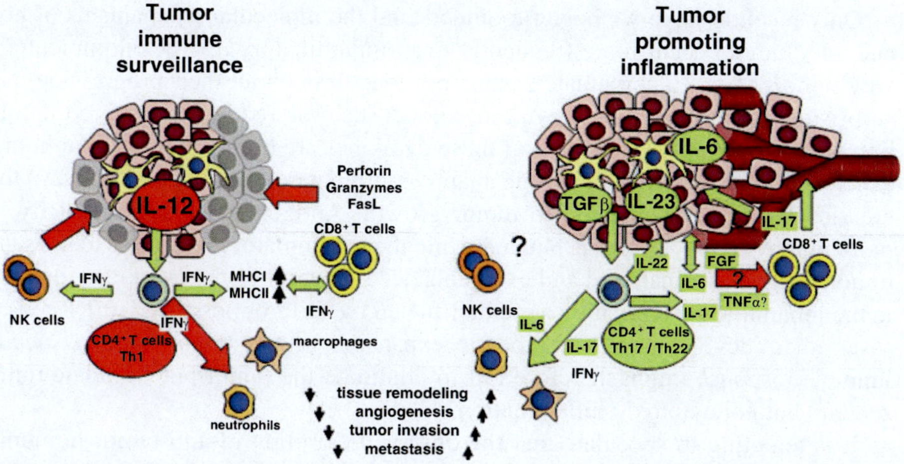

Fig. 4 *IL-23 mediated deviation from a cytotoxic immune response*. Exposure to novel antigens in an inflammatory milieu stimulates antigen specific immune responses. However the composition of the local cytokine milieu regulates which effector molecules and cells are deemed appropriate to eliminate the challenge, The activation of inappropriate cytokine cascades, might not only inhibit efficient elimination of tumor cells but might also contribute to immune pathologies, promoting tumor growth by providing an essential growth environment. *Green arrow*: stimulation, *red arrow*: inhibition. *Green highlight*: tumor promoting or tumor associated mechanism

dependent colitis while the wasting syndrome observed in wt mice was dependent on the systemic function of IL-12 (Uhlig et al. 2006). This observation might have some importance for human cancer patients where systemic inflammatory responses including elevated levels of IFN-γ in the serum are thought to underlie weight loss in cancer associated cachexia.

In preclinical tumor models, IL-12 and INF-γ promote immune surveillance against endogenous and transplanted syngeneic tumors (Koebel et al. 2007). IFN-γ is not only rate limiting for T cell activity but required for the expression of intratumoral MHCI thereby enabling the recognition of tumor antigens (Wong et al. 1984). In many human tumors, MHCI is expressed only at very low levels, unless induced by IFN-γ (Seliger et al. 2002). In the absence of IL-12, or in a local cytokine milieu preventing Th1 differentiation and IFN-γ expression, MHCI expression might be limited and the recognition of the tumor specific epitopes by $CD8^+$ T cells might be far less efficient (Fig. 4).

7 Conclusions

For centuries, increased cancer incidence has been observed in locations of chronically inflamed, damaged tissue, and there exists a correlation between high serum concentrations of immune stimulating inflammatory cytokines and detrimental prognosis for human cancer patients.

Only recently have we begun to understand the molecular mechanisms of how and why tumors occur more frequently in an inflammatory microenvironment and why tumors seem to perpetuate such conditions throughout their progression. Not surprisingly proinflammatory cytokines are at the crossroad of this altered regulation. As described above several of these cytokines are highly expressed in human cancers (Figs. 2 and 4) and alter the adaptive immune response in several ways that are simultaneously beneficial to tumor growth. Antigen specific cytotoxicity, in particular by CD8+ T cells, is blunted while the inflammatory responses to the same tumor antigen are unaltered and even enhanced. Several of the cytokines involved in the inflammatory regulation are either fueled by Th17 or possibly Tc17 T cells or foster their development. Therapeutic expansion of the tumor antigen specific immune response might therefore fail to eliminate the tumor but stimulate tumor specific but noncytotoxic inflammation.

It is tempting to speculate that the observed derailing of anti-tumor immunity into an inflammatory response is at its core a defensive strategy of the tumor, selected for independently of the tumor cell transformation. Expression of the inflammatory cytokines such as IL-23 by the tumor cell can be seen as evidence for this model. At first the presence of mutant cell clones in an inflamed and regenerating tissue could simply be an unfortunate coincidence. Tumor cells fostering this cytokine milieu may be preferentially selected due to improved cytokine mediated growth conditions for the nascent tumor while the same cytokines such as IL-23 may inhibit the immune mediated tumor surveillance elimination.

Alternatively, inflammation induction might be the mere result of, and the default reaction to the expression of transforming oncogenes within the tumor cell. The observation that necrosis, often seen as a consequence of oncogene activation or chemo-therapeutic intervention, fosters inflammation provide support for the latter explanation (Fonseca and Dranoff 2008).

It remains to be seen if selective therapeutic blockade of inflammation can deliver benefits to patients suffering from large tumors, rather than merely serving a prophylactic role potentially preventing cancer occurrence and inhibiting early cancer growth. The simultaneous inhibition of inflammation and the induction of cytotoxicity may be necessary to eliminate tumor cells in the tumor and in micrometastatic sites.

References

Aggarwal S, Ghilardi N, Xie MH, de Sauvage FJ, Gurney AL (2003) J Biol Chem 278:1910–1914

Aggarwal BB, Sethi G, Ahn KS, Sandur SK, Pandey MK, Kunnumakkara AB, Sung B, Ichikawa H (2006) Ann N Y Acad Sci 1091:151–169

Atkins MB, Robertson MJ, Gordon M, Lotze MT, DeCoste M, DuBois JS, Ritz J, Sandler AB, Edington HD, Garzone PD, Mier JW, Canning CM, Battiato L, Tahara H, Sherman ML (1997) Clin Cancer Res 3:409–417

Atreya R, Mudter J, Finotto S, Mullberg J, Jostock T, Wirtz S, Schutz M, Bartsch B, Holtmann M, Becker C, Strand D, Czaja J, Schlaak JF, Lehr HA, Autschbach F, Schurmann G, Nishimoto N, Yoshizaki K, Ito H, Kishimoto T, Galle PR, Rose-John S, Neurath MF (2000) Nat Med 6:583–588

Baffet G, Braciak TA, Fletcher RG, Gauldie J, Fey GH, Northemann W (1991) Mol Biol Med 8:141–156
Balkwill F, Charles KA, Mantovani A (2005) Cancer Cell 7:211–217
Becker C, Fantini MC, Schramm C, Lehr HA, Wirtz S, Nikolaev A, Burg J, Strand S, Kiesslich R, Huber S, Ito H, Nishimoto N, Yoshizaki K, Kishimoto T, Galle PR, Blessing M, Rose-John S, Neurath MF (2004) Immunity 21:491–501
Bending D, De La Pena H, Veldhoen M, Phillips JM, Uyttenhove C, Stockinger B, Cooke A (2009) J Clin Invest 119:565–572
Bettelli E, Carrier Y, Gao W, Korn T, Strom TB, Oukka M, Weiner HL, Kuchroo VK (2006) Nature 441:235–238
Caux C, Dezutter-Dambuyant C, Schmitt D, Banchereau J (1992) Nature 360:258–261
Cebon J, Jager E, Shackleton MJ, Gibbs P, Davis ID, Hopkins W, Gibbs S, Chen Q, Karbach J, Jackson H, MacGregor DP, Sturrock S, Vaughan H, Maraskovsky E, Neumann A, Hoffman E, Sherman ML, Knuth A (2003) Cancer Immun 3:7
Chan JR, Blumenschein W, Murphy E, Diveu C, Wiekowski M, Abbondanzo S, Lucian L, Geissler R, Brodie S, Kimball AB, Gorman DM, Smith K, de Waal Malefyt R, Kastelein RA, McClanahan TK, Bowman EP (2006) J Exp Med 203(12):2577–2587
Christopher MJ, Link DC (2007) Curr Opin Hematol 14:3–8
Coussens LM, Werb Z (2002) Nature 420:860–867
Cua DJ, Sherlock J, Chen Y, Murphy CA, Joyce B, Seymour B, Lucian L, To W, Kwan S, Churakova T, Zurawski S, Wiekowski M, Lira SA, Gorman D, Kastelein RA, Sedgwick JD (2003) Nature 421:744–748
Curiel TJ, Coukos G, Zou L, Alvarez X, Cheng P, Mottram P, Evdemon-Hogan M, Conejo-Garcia JR, Zhang L, Burow M, Zhu Y, Wei S, Kryczek I, Daniel B, Gordon A, Myers L, Lackner A, Disis ML, Knutson KL, Chen L, Zou W (2004) Nat Med 10:942–949
Elzey BD, Griffith TS, Herndon JM, Barreiro R, Tschopp J, Ferguson TA (2001) J Immunol 167:3049–3056
Eyerich S, Eyerich K, Pennino D, Carbone T, Nasorri F, Pallotta S, Cianfarani F, Odorisio T, Traidl-Hoffmann C, Behrendt H, Durham SR, Schmidt-Weber CB, Cavani A (2009) J Clin Invest 119:3573–3585
Feldmann M, Maini RN (2001) Annu Rev Immunol 19:163–196
Fonseca C, Dranoff G (2008) Clin Cancer Res 14:1603–1608
Fossiez F, Banchereau J, Murray R, Van Kooten C, Garrone P, Lebecque S (1998) Int Rev Immunol 16:541–551
Galon J, Costes A, Sanchez-Cabo F, Kirilovsky A, Mlecnik B, Lagorce-Pages C, Tosolini M, Camus M, Berger A, Wind P, Zinzindohoue F, Bruneval P, Cugnenc PH, Trajanoski Z, Fridman WH, Pages F (2006) Science 313:1960–1964
Gerosa F, Baldani-Guerra B, Lyakh LA, Batoni G, Esin S, Winkler-Pickett RT, Consolaro MR, De Marchi M, Giachino D, Robbiano A, Astegiano M, Sambataro A, Kastelein RA, Carra G, Trinchieri G (2008) J Exp Med 205:1447–1461
Gounaris E, Blatner NR, Dennis K, Magnusson F, Gurish MF, Strom TB, Beckhove P, Gounari F, Khazaie K (2009) Cancer Res 69:5490–5497
Haak S, Croxford AL, Kreymborg K, Heppner FL, Pouly S, Becher B, Waisman A (2009) J Clin Invest 119:61–69
Han LY, Fletcher MS, Urbauer DL, Mueller P, Landen CN, Kamat AA, Lin YG, Merritt WM, Spannuth WA, Deavers MT, De Geest K, Gershenson DM, Lutgendorf SK, Ferrone S, Sood AK (2008) Clin Cancer Res 14:3372–3379
Happel KI, Dubin PJ, Zheng M, Ghilardi N, Lockhart C, Quinton LJ, Odden AR, Shellito JE, Bagby GJ, Nelson S, Kolls JK (2005) J Exp Med 202:761–769
He D, Wu L, Kim HK, Li H, Elmets CA, Xu H (2006) J Immunol 177:6852–6858
Intlekofer AM, Banerjee A, Takemoto N, Gordon SM, Dejong CS, Shin H, Hunter CA, Wherry EJ, Lindsten T, Reiner SL (2008) Science 321:408–411
Jager E, Jager D, Knuth A (2003) Int J Cancer 106:817–820

Kaplan DH, Shankaran V, Dighe AS, Stockert E, Aguet M, Old LJ, Schreiber RD (1998) Proc Natl Acad Sci USA 95:7556–7561
Knuth A, Danowski B, Oettgen HF, Old LJ (1984) Proc Natl Acad Sci USA 81:3511–3515
Koebel CM, Vermi W, Swann JB, Zerafa N, Rodig SJ, Old LJ, Smyth MJ, Schreiber RD (2007) Nature 450:903–907
Koehne CH, Dubois RN (2004) Semin Oncol 31:12–21
Kolls JK, Linden A (2004) Immunity 21:467–476
Kryczek I, Wei S, Zou L, Altuwaijri S, Szeliga W, Kolls J, Chang A, Zou W (2007) J Immunol 178:6730–6733
Kryczek I, Banerjee M, Cheng P, Vatan L, Szeliga W, Wei S, Huang E, Finlayson E, Simeone D, Welling TH, Chang A, Coukos G, Liu R, Zou W (2009a) Blood 114:1141–1149
Kryczek I, Wei S, Szeliga W, Vatan L, Zou W (2009b) Blood 114:357–359
Kwong BY, Roberts SJ, Silberzahn T, Filler RB, Neustadter JH, Galan A, Reddy S, Lin WM, Ellis PD, Langford CF, Hayday AC and Girardi M (2009) J Invest Dermatol Doi: 10.1038/jid.2009.362
LaCasse EC, Mahoney DJ, Cheung HH, Plenchette S, Baird S, Korneluk RG (2008) Oncogene 27:6252–6275
Landi S, Moreno V, Gioia-Patricola L, Guino E, Navarro M, de Oca J, Capella G, Canzian F (2003) Cancer Res 63:3560–3566
Langowski JL, Zhang X, Wu L, Mattson JD, Chen T, Smith K, Basham B, McClanahan T, Kastelein RA, Oft M (2006) Nature 442:461–465
Langowski JL, Kastelein RA, Oft M (2007) Trends Immunol 28:207–212
Langrish CL, Chen Y, Blumenschein WM, Mattson J, Basham B, Sedgwick JD, McClanahan T, Kastelein RA, Cua DJ (2005) J Exp Med 201:233–240
Lejeune FJ, Ruegg C, Lienard D (1998) Curr Opin Immunol 10:573–580
Li MO, Wan YY, Sanjabi S, Robertson AK, Flavell RA (2006) Annu Rev Immunol 24:99–146
Lin WW, Karin M (2007) J Clin Invest 117:1175–1183
Liu SJ, Tsai JP, Shen CR, Sher YP, Hsieh CL, Yeh YC, Chou AH, Chang SR, Hsiao KN, Yu FW, Chen HW (2007) J Leukoc Biol 82:354–360
Lo CH, Lee SC, Wu PY, Pan WY, Su J, Cheng CW, Roffler SR, Chiang BL, Lee CN, Wu CW, Tao MH (2003) J Immunol 171:600–607
Loberg RD, Bradley DA, Tomlins SA, Chinnaiyan AM, Pienta KJ (2007) CA Cancer J Clin 57:225–241
Lockhart E, Green AM, Flynn JL (2006) J Immunol 177:4662–4669
Mangan PR, Harrington LE, O'Quinn DB, Helms WS, Bullard DC, Elson CO, Hatton RD, Wahl SM, Schoeb TR, Weaver CT (2006) Nature 441:231–234
Martin-Orozco N, Muranski P, Chung Y, Yang XO, Yamazaki T, Lu S, Hwu P, Restifo NP, Overwijk WW, Dong C (2009) Immunity 31:787–798
McGeachy MJ, Bak-Jensen KS, Chen Y, Tato CM, Blumenschein W, McClanahan T, Cua DJ (2007) Nat Immunol 8:1390–1397
McKenzie BS, Kastelein RA, Cua DJ (2006) Trends Immunol 27:17–23
Mocellin S, Rossi CR, Pilati P, Nitti D (2005) Cytokine Growth Factor Rev 16:35–53
Moore RJ, Owens DM, Stamp G, Arnott C, Burke F, East N, Holdsworth H, Turner L, Rollins B, Pasparakis M, Kollias G, Balkwill F (1999) Nat Med 5:828–831
Muranski P, Boni A, Antony PA, Cassard L, Irvine KR, Kaiser A, Paulos CM, Palmer DC, Touloukian CE, Ptak K, Gattinoni L, Wrzesinski C, Hinrichs CS, Kerstann K, Feigenbaum L, Chan CC, Restifo NP (2008) Blood 112(2):362–373
Naito Y, Saito K, Shiiba K, Ohuchi A, Saigenji K, Nagura H, Ohtani H (1998) Cancer Res 58:3491–3494
Naugler WE, Karin M (2008) Trends Mol Med 14:109–119
Novelli F, Casanova JL (2004) Cytokine Growth Factor Rev 15:367–377
Numasaki M, Fukushi J, Ono M, Narula SK, Zavodny PJ, Kudo T, Robbins PD, Tahara H, Lotze MT (2003) Blood 101:2620–2627

Palucka AK, Blanck JP, Bennett L, Pascual V, Banchereau J (2005) Proc Natl Acad Sci USA 102:3372–3377
Reiner SL (2007) Cell 129:33–36
Roberts SJ, Ng BY, Filler RB, Lewis J, Glusac EJ, Hayday AC, Tigelaar RE, Girardi M (2007) Proc Natl Acad Sci USA 104:6770–6775
Rose-John S, Scheller J, Elson G, Jones SA (2006) J Leukoc Biol 80:227–236
Ruegg C, Oguey D, Lejeune F (1999) Melanoma Res 9:2–3
Scott KA, Moore RJ, Arnott CH, East N, Thompson RG, Scallon BJ, Shealy DJ, Balkwill FR (2003) Mol Cancer Ther 2:445–451
Seliger B, Cabrera T, Garrido F, Ferrone S (2002) Semin Cancer Biol 12:3–13
Smith PC, Hobisch A, Lin DL, Culig Z, Keller ET (2001) Cytokine Growth Factor Rev 12:33–40
Szlosarek PW, Balkwill FR (2003) Lancet Oncol 4:565–573
Szlosarek P, Charles KA, Balkwill FR (2006) Eur J Cancer 42:745–750
Trinchieri G, Pflanz S, Kastelein RA (2003) Immunity 19:641–644
Uhlig HH, McKenzie BS, Hue S, Thompson C, Joyce-Shaikh B, Stepankova R, Robinson N, Buonocore S, Tlaskalova-Hogenova H, Cua DJ, Powrie F (2006) Immunity 25:309–318
van der Bruggen P, Traversari C, Chomez P, Lurquin C, De Plaen E, Van den Eynde B, Knuth A, Boon T (1991) Science 254:1643–1647
Van Der Bruggen P, Zhang Y, Chaux P, Stroobant V, Panichelli C, Schultz ES, Chapiro J, Van Den Eynde BJ, Brasseur F, Boon T (2002) Immunol Rev 188:51–64
Veldhoen M, Hocking RJ, Atkins CJ, Locksley RM, Stockinger B (2006) Immunity 24:179–189
Wang L, Yi T, Kortylewski M, Pardoll DM, Zeng D, Yu H (2009) J Exp Med 206:1457–1464
Williams RO, Marinova-Mutafchieva L, Feldmann M, Maini RN (2000) J Immunol 165:7240–7245
Wilson NJ, Boniface K, Chan JR, McKenzie BS, Blumenschein WM, Mattson JD, Basham B, Smith K, Chen T, Morel F, Lecron JC, Kastelein RA, Cua DJ, McClanahan TK (2007) Bowman EP and de Waal Malefyt R. Nat Immunol 8:950–957
Wong GH, Bartlett PF, Clark-Lewis I, Battye F, Schrader JW (1984) Nature 310:688–691
Wrzesinski SH, Wan YY, Flavell RA (2007) Clin Cancer Res 13:5262–5270
Yang XO, Nurieva R, Martinez GJ, Kang HS, Chung Y, Pappu BP, Shah B, Chang SH, Schluns KS, Watowich SS, Feng XH, Jetten AM, Dong C (2008) Immunity 29:44–56
Yen D, Cheung J, Scheerens H, Poulet F, McClanahan T, McKenzie B, Kleinschek MA, Owyang A, Mattson J, Blumenschein W, Murphy E, Sathe M, Cua DJ, Kastelein RA, Rennick D (2006) J Clin Invest 116:1310–1316
Yen HR, Harris TJ, Wada S, Grosso JF, Getnet D, Goldberg MV, Liang KL, Bruno TC, Pyle KJ, Chan SL, Anders RA, Trimble CL, Adler AJ, Lin TY, Pardoll DM, Huang CT, Drake CG (2009) J Immunol 183:7161–7168
Zhou LJ, Tedder TF (1996) Proc Natl Acad Sci USA 93:2588–2592

STAT3: A Target to Enhance Antitumor Immune Response

Heehyoung Lee, Sumanta Kumar Pal, Karen Reckamp, Robert A. Figlin, and Hua Yu

Contents

1 Introduction 42
2 Stat3-Mediated Immune Suppression 43
2.1 Inhibition of the Th1 Immune Response 43
2.2 Relevant Immunologic Signaling Pathways 45
2.3 Role in Myeloid Derived Suppressor Cells 46
2.4 Role in Regulatory T-Cells 47
3 Therapeutic Relevance 48
3.1 Genetic Evidence and Potential Toxicity 49
3.2 JAK Inhibitors 49
3.3 Other Oncogenic Kinase Inhibitors 50
3.4 RTK Inhibitors 51
3.5 siRNA 52
4 Concluding Remarks 53
References 53

H. Lee
Beckman Research Institute, City of Hope Comprehensive Cancer Center, 1500 East Duarte Road, Duarte, CA 91010, USA

S.K. Pal
Division of Genitourinary Malignancies, Department of Medical Oncology and Experimental Therapeutics, City of Hope Comprehensive Cancer Center, 1500 East Duarte Road, Duarte, CA 91010, USA

K. Reckamp
Division of Thoracic Malignancies, Department of Medical Oncology and Experimental Therapeutics, City of Hope Comprehensive Cancer Center, 1500 East Duarte Road, Duarte, CA 91010, USA

R.A. Figlin
Department of Medical Oncology and Experimental Therapeutics, City of Hope Comprehensive Cancer Center, 1500 East Duarte Road, Duarte, CA 91010, USA

H. Yu (✉)
Cancer Immunotherapeutics and Tumor Immunology, City of Hope Comprehensive Cancer Center, 1500 East Duarte Road, Duarte, CA 91010, USA
e-mail: hyu@coh.org

G. Dranoff (ed.), *Cancer Immunology and Immunotherapy*,
Current Topics in Microbiology and Immunology 344, DOI 10.1007/82_2010_51

Abstract Signal transducer and activator of transcription 3 (Stat3) has emerged as a critical regulator for tumor-associated inflammation. Activation of Stat3 negatively regulates the Th1-type immune response and promotes expansion of myeloid-derived suppressor cells (MDSCs) and regulatory T-cell functions in the tumor microenvironment. Mounting evidence suggests that Stat3 and related pathways may serve as a target for changing the tumor immunologic microenvironment to benefit cancer immunotherapies. Many recent studies support the use of certain tyrosine kinase inhibitors, through inhibition of Stat3, in decreasing immunosuppression in the tumor microenvironment. Other potential therapeutic avenues include the use of targeted delivery of Stat3 siRNA into immune cells. Here, we describe the role of Stat3 in regulating the immunologic properties of tumors as a background for Stat3-based therapeutic interventions.

1 Introduction

The ability of tumors to evade immune surveillance plays a central role in tumor progression (Dunn et al. 2002; Yu et al. 2007). Studies performed in our laboratory, supported by work at other institutions, have suggested an important role of signal transducer and activator of transcription 3 (Stat3), an important oncogenic transcriptional factor, in mediating tumor-induced immune suppression at various levels (Yu et al. 2007, 2009). In the setting of malignancy, Stat3 is activated by many cytokine signaling pathways, which is highlighted by interleukin-6 (IL-6). As a point of convergence for numerous oncogenic signaling pathways, Stat3 is also persistently activated by abnormal signaling of various growth factor receptors, including epidermal growth factor receptor (EGFR) and vascular growth factor receptor (VEGFR), along with oncoproteins such as Src and BCR-ABL. Activated Stat3 not only downregulates Th1 cytokines and other mediators critical for potent anti-tumor immune responses, but also activates many genes involved in immune suppression. Many Stat3 driven tumor-derived factors, including IL-6, IL-10, and VEGF, ensure persistent Stat3 activation in the tumor microenvironment through a crosstalk between tumor cells and tumor-associated immune cells, thereby creating "feed-forward loop" (Kortylewski et al. 2005; Wang et al. 2004; Yu et al. 2007, 2009). Activated Stat3 in tumor-associated immune cells further promotes expression of growth factors and angiogenic factors (Kujawski et al. 2008). As such, Stat3 limits the antitumor effects from host immune system and accelerates tumor growth and metastasis (Kortylewski et al. 2005; Wang et al. 2004; Yu et al. 2007, 2009).

Inhibiting Stat3 using various means induces robust anti-tumor innate and adaptive immune responses in the tumor microenvironment (Kortylewski et al. 2005; Wang et al. 2004; Yu et al. 2007, 2009). Considering the critical role of Stat3 in both tumor cells as well as in tumor-associated immune cells in inducing immune suppression, a more detailed understanding of the mechanism underlying

Stat3-mediated immune suppression may lead to advances in cancer therapy. In this review, we will summarize recent findings related to the role of Stat3 in tumor-induced immune suppression and discuss different therapeutic approaches involving abrogation of Stat3 signaling and enhancement of immunotherapy.

2 Stat3-Mediated Immune Suppression

2.1 *Inhibition of the Th1 Immune Response*

The first study demonstrating Stat3 as a negative regulator of Th1-type immune responses reported that ablation of *Stat3* in neutrophils and macrophages increased production of Th1 cytokines, such as IFNγ, TNFα, and IL-1, after LPS stimulation (Takeda et al. 1999). A role of Stat3 in inhibiting immunostimulatory Th1 cytokines and other mediators in tumors was subsequently shown (Nabarro et al. 2005; Sumimoto et al. 2006; Wang et al. 2004). Because of Stat3 is a critical oncogenic molecule, a direct link between oncogenesis and tumor immune evasion was thus substantiated. Further studies revealed that Stat3 activation in immune cells is in part mediated by tumor-derived factors, such as VEGF, IL-10, and IL-6 (Sumimoto et al. 2006; Wang et al. 2004). Conversely, *Stat3* ablation in immune cells leads to induction of Th1 mediators involved in both innate and T-cell-mediated adaptive immunity. In turn, this causes increased anti-tumor activity of immune cells that impedes tumor progression (Kortylewski et al. 2005) (Fig. 1).

Many of the Th1 mediators produced in tumors upon *Stat3* ablation are typical targets of other immune regulators, such as NF-κB and/or Stat1, whose role is pivotal in Th1-mediated immune responses (Yu et al. 2009). Deletion of *Stat3* facilitates activation of NF-κB (Welte et al. 2003) and Stat1 (Takeda et al. 1999), leading to increased production of Th1 type immune mediators required for anti-tumor immunity (Kortylewski et al. 2009c; Yu et al. 2009). Although various mechanisms have been suggested, how Stat3 antagonizes NF-κB and Stat1 remains to be further defined. It has been implicated from several studies that Stat3 negatively regulates IκB kinase β (IKKβ), which is required for phosphorylation of IκBα and its subsequent degradation (Lee et al. 2009; Welte et al. 2003). This may render NF-κB in a suppressed state, keeping it from activating downstream genes involved in Th1 type immune responses. However, a synergistic interaction between Stat3 and NF-κB is also documented during tumor progression through autocrine/parcrine signaling of IL-6 and IL-10 (Bollrath et al. 2009; Grivennikov et al. 2009; Lam et al. 2008; Lee et al. 2009). Distinct from the interaction between Stat3 and NF-κB, Stat3 and Stat1 often oppose each other in cancer models – if Stat3 is highly activated, Stat1 is downregulated. In the setting of melanoma, it has been noted that increased expression of activated Stat1 is an important predictor of therapeutic responsiveness to interferon-α (IFNα) (Lesinski et al. 2007; Wang

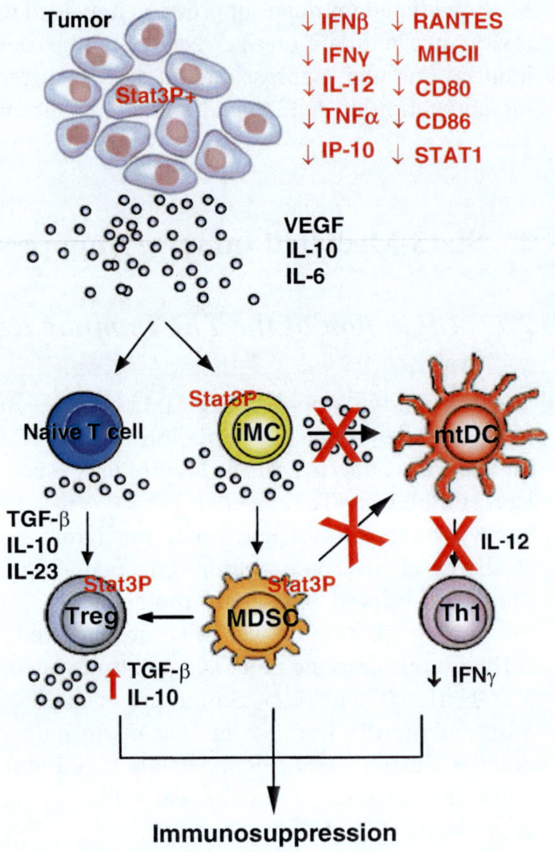

Fig. 1 Multifaceted role of Stat3 in anti-tumor immunity. Stat3 is persistently activated in tumors and the tumor microenvironment, inducing production of many tumor-derived factors such as VEGF, IL-10, and IL-6. Increased Stat3 activity in tumor-associated immune cells promotes immunosuppressive environment, by mediating the generation of immune suppressor cells, including MDSC and T regs. The expression of MDSC and Treg effector molecules, such as TGF-β, IL-10, and IL-23, is in part mediated by Stat3. Activated Stat3 in tumor-associated immune cells also inhibits DC maturation as well as the production of Th1-type cytokines such as IL-12 and IFN-γ. As such, Stat3 activity in tumor impairs both adaptive and innate immune responses against tumor

et al. 2007; Zimmerer et al. 2007) and correlates with longer overall survival (Wang et al. 2007). These studies suggest that the balance between Stat1 and Stat3 may determine the therapeutic outcome of cancer immunotherapy and targeting Stat3 may shift cellular balance more favorable toward host. It has recently been noted that single nucleotide polymorphism associated with Stat3 expression may be a significant predictor of IFNα response. In a study of 174 patients with chronic myelogenous leukemia (CML), the single nucleotide polymorphism (SNP) rs6503691 was tightly correlated with the level of STAT3 mRNA, and could further reliably distinguish responders and non-responders to IFN-α (Kreil et al. 2010). In a separate assessment of 75 patients with metastatic renal cell carcinoma (mRCC) treated with IFN-α, it was documented that the rs4796793 polymorphism in the 5′ region of *Stat3* was a significant predictor of clinical response (odds ratio [OR] = 2.73, 95% CI 1.38–5.78) (Ito et al. 2007). The enhanced growth inhibitory effects of IFNα upon Stat3 suppression in renal cell carcinoma also supports the notion that Stat3 inhibition is a useful tool to boost the efficacy of IFNα therapy in patients with renal cell carcinoma.

2.2 Relevant Immunologic Signaling Pathways

Tumors produce various factors that in turn activate Stat3 by forming feed-forward loops with signaling pathways (Yu et al. 2007, 2009). Persistent Stat3 activation can be propagated from tumor cells to diverse immune cells through factors such as IL-6, IL-10, and VEGF (Kortylewski et al. 2005; Kujawski et al. 2008; Lee et al. 2009; Sumimoto et al. 2006; Wang et al. 2004; Yu et al. 2007, 2009). These factors impede appropriate immune cell functioning in both innate and adaptive immunity. Specifically, release of IL-10, VEGF, and IL-6 prevents immature dendritic cells (DCs) from maturing into antigen-presenting cells (Gabrilovich 2004; Gabrilovich et al. 1996; Ohm et al. 2003; Park et al. 2004). Expression levels of MHC class II, co-stimulatory molecule CD86 and IL-12, all of which are required for proper DC-mediated immune function, are decreased by IL-10-induced Stat3 activation, leading to the generation of tolerogenic DCs (Li et al. 2006; Liang et al. 2008). Moreover, the constitutive activation of Stat3 by IL-10, VEGF, and IL-6 impedes functional maturation of tumor-associated DCs (Bharadwaj et al. 2007; Gabrilovich 2004; Nabarro et al. 2005; Yang et al. 2009), leading to increased tumor growth and metastasis (Kortylewski et al. 2005; Wang et al. 2004). Demonstrating cross-talk amongst these pathways, IL-6 is shown to upregulate production of IL-10 in both colon cancer cell lines and T cells through Stat3 activation (Herbeuval et al. 2004; Stumhofer et al. 2007).

Interplays between tumor cells and immune cells are mainly regulated by cytokines, which can stimulate either tumorigenic or anti-tumorigenic effects. For example, IL-23 was first identified as a proinflammatory cytokine, sharing a common p40 subunit with IL-12 (Oppmann et al. 2000). IL-12 has a critical role in regulating Th1 cells that are essential for tumor suppression. Unlike IL-12, IL-23 does not promote IFN-γ-producing Th1 cells, but is one of the essential factors required for the expansion of a pathogenic memory T cell population, which is characterized by the production of IL-17, IL-6, and tumor necrosis factor (TNF) (Langrish et al. 2005). The production of IL-17 and IL-6 is mediated through Stat3 (Chen et al. 2006; Cho et al. 2006). In addition, IL-23 receptor is shown to be engaged with the Jak2/Stat3 pathway (Parham et al. 2002) and is required for the terminal differentiation of Th17 cell into effector cells in a Stat3-dependent fashion (McGeachy et al. 2009). Impaired Th17 function causes immune deficiencies such as hyper-IgE syndrome (HIES), which harbors dominant-negative Stat3 mutation (Ma et al. 2008; Milner et al. 2008; Minegishi 2009; Minegishi et al. 2007).

In contrast to its role in promoting inflammatory responses, IL-23 has been implicated in tumor-mediated immunosuppression (Kortylewski et al. 2009c; Langowski et al. 2006). While suppressing NF-κB activation is required for IL-12 mediated anti-tumor immune responses, Stat3 markedly upregulates transcriptional activity of IL-23p19 subunit in tumor-associated macrophages (Kortylewski et al. 2009c), thereby promoting IL-23 mediated pro-tumorigenic immune responses. Given that Stat3 inhibits IL-12 expression (Hoentjen et al. 2005;

Wang et al. 2004) and that enhanced IL-12 production upon IL-23 blockade intensifies Th1 type immune responses (Uemura et al. 2009), targeting Stat3 may be a relevant approach to shift IL-12/IL-23 balance towards Th1-mediated anti-tumor immune responses. It is noteworthy that IL-17 expression is concomitantly increased in tumors driven by IL-23 (Langrish et al. 2005). IL-17 also enhances tumor angiogenesis and growth (Numasaki et al. 2003) through Stat3 activation in various tumors (Charles et al. 2009; He et al. 2010; Wang et al. 2009). Since both cytokines share regulatory network through Stat3 (Kortylewski et al. 2009c; Wang et al. 2009; Yu et al. 2009), it is possible that IL-23-mediated Th17 response to tumors promote tumor progression. This notion is supported by *in vivo* studies assessing the link between enterotoxigenic *Bacteroides fragilies* (ETBF), a common gastrointestinal pathogen linked to colon carcinogenesis. These studies suggested that Stat3 is required for ETBF-mediated IL-17 production. Dual blockade of the receptors for IL-17 and IL-23 resulted in decreased formation of colonic tumors (Wu et al. 2009). Nevertheless, IL-17 may also play an antitumor role (Kryczek et al. 2009), and further studies are required to clarify why IL-17 can both promote and inhibit tumor development.

2.3 Role in Myeloid Derived Suppressor Cells

Tumor myeloid-derived suppressor cells (MDSCs) inhibit $CD4^+$ and $CD8^+$ T cell activation as well as innate immune responses (Gabrilovich and Nagaraj 2009; Sinha et al. 2007). In addition to its role in regulating immunosuppressive cytokines, Stat3 also promotes expansion of MDSCs (Yu et al. 2007, 2009). Several factors regulate tumor MDSC accumulation. These include IL-1β, IL-6 (Bunt et al. 2007), VEGF (Melani et al. 2003), COX2 (Xiang et al. 2009) and GM-CSF (Serafini et al. 2004), all of which trigger signaling pathways activating Stat3 (Yu et al. 2007, 2009). Exposure of myeloid cells to tumor cell conditioned medium upregulates Stat3 activity and triggers MDSC expansion (Nefedova et al. 2004). Moreover, Stat3 is persistently elevated in MDSCs from tumor-bearing mice (Nefedova et al. 2005), indicating that Stat3 activation in MDSCs may result from tumor-derived factors. Conversely, ablation of the *Stat3* gene using conditional knockout mice or Stat3 blockade by tyrosine kinase inhibitor significantly reduces the number of tumor-associated MDSCs and consequently elicits robust anti-tumor immune responses (Kortylewski et al. 2005; Xin et al. 2009).

A recent study suggests an integral role of S100A9 in MDSC accumulation in tumors (Cheng et al. 2008). MDSC accumulation appears to result from impaired DC differentiation, caused by overexpressed S100A9 protein. Stat3 serves as transcriptional activator of S100A9, inducing its expression by directly binding to its promoter region (Cheng et al. 2008). S100A9 expression is reduced in myeloid cells isolated from mice with *Stat3* deletion in hematopoietic cells compared to wild-type counterpart, further confirming the critical role of Stat3 in regulating S100A9 expression. Mice lacking Stat3-inducible *S100A9* mount potent anti-tumor immune responses, leading to the rejection of implanted tumors. A separate series of experiments suggests that mice with a dominant-negative Stat3 mutation have markedly reduced S100A9 expression (Li et al. 2004).

One of the main characteristics of tumor MDSCs is high production of reactive oxygen species (ROS), which is essential for the suppressive function of cells (Gabrilovich and Nagaraj 2009). The increased ROS production by MDSCs is mediated by up-regulated activity of NADPH oxidase (NOX2). Owing to the fact that S100A9 upregulates ROS production by NADPH oxidase (Cheng et al. 2008), it is plausible to speculate that Stat3 may involve the suppressive function of MDSCs. Indeed, MDSCs from tumor-bearing mice had significantly higher expression of NOX2 subunits, primarily p47(phox) and gp91 (phox), as compared to immature myeloid cells from tumor-free mice. Furthermore, Stat3 directly controls transcriptional activity of p47(phox) subunit of NOX2 (Corzo et al. 2009). Treatment of MDSCs with a Stat3 inhibitor dramatically reduces the level of ROS in these cells accompanied by reduction in NOX2 expression (Corzo et al. 2009). In the absence of NOX2 activity, MDSCs lost the ability to suppress T cell responses and quickly differentiated into mature DCs (Corzo et al. 2009). Therefore, Stat3 plays a diverse role in MDSC-mediated immune suppression. Constitutive activation of Stat3 results in expansion of MDSCs that contain a high level of NOX2 components. This drives MDSCs in tumor-bearing mice to release ROS, leading to immunosuppressive activity of these cells.

2.4 Role in Regulatory T-Cells

Regulatory T-cells (Tregs) are critical in the induction of T-cell tolerance to tumor antigens by suppressing immune responses mediated by $CD8^+$ T cells (Curiel et al. 2004; Liyanage et al. 2002; Viguier et al. 2004; Yang et al. 2006). Tregs release several immunosuppressive mediators including TGF-β and IL-10, both of which are activated and upregulated by Stat3 in tumors (Dercamp et al. 2005; Yu et al. 2007). Tumors with *Stat3* ablation in hematopoietic cells markedly decrease the number of infiltrating $CD4^+CD25^+Foxp3^+$ Tregs when compared to tumors with intact Stat3 activity (Kortylewski et al. 2005). This is further associated with a proliferation of $CD8^+$ T cells, leading to potent anti-tumor immune responses (Kortylewski et al. 2005). Moreover, recent findings demonstrate that tumor-associated Tregs maintain constitutive Stat3 activity through IL-23 receptor expression (Kortylewski et al. 2009c). The contribution of constitutive Stat3 activation may be enhanced in Tregs by tumor-derived factors such as IL-23. How constitutive Stat3 activity in tumors contribute to Treg expansion is further illustrated in several studies. Constitutive activation of tumor Stat3 by oncogenes, such as nucleophosmin/anaplastic lymphoma kinase (NPM/ALK), promotes Treg expansion and expression of the Treg specific transcription factor Foxp3 as well (Kasprzycka et al. 2006). Stat3 binds to the promoter of

Foxp3, although to a lesser extent compared to Stat5 (Yao et al. 2007; Zorn et al. 2006), and physically interacts with Foxp3 protein (Chaudhry et al. 2009). Conversely, inhibition of Stat3 using either siRNA or upstream tyrosine kinase inhibitor abrogates Foxp3 expression and suppressive function of Tregs. Thus, Stat3 is important for the functional maintenance of Tregs (Kong et al. 2009; Larmonier et al. 2008; Pallandre et al. 2007). Of interest, co-culturing MDSCs with T cells induces the $Foxp3^{+}$ Treg phenotype in both mouse and human tumor models, leading to tumor-induced T cell tolerance (Hoechst et al. 2008; Serafini et al. 2008).

3 Therapeutic Relevance

As a point of convergence for numerous oncogenic signaling pathways, Stat3 is continuously activated in various human cancers. Numerous genetic studies validate Stat3 as one of the most promising target for cancer immunotherapy. Moreover, new approaches directly targeting Stat3, either alone or in conjunction with other therapeutic modalities, elicit robust anti-tumor immune responses that are highly efficacious in the treatment of cancer (Table 1).

Table 1 Therapeutic strategies under investigation with the intent of abrogating Stat3-mediated signaling

Approaches	Mechanism	References
Stat3 ablation	Preclinical *in vivo* studies suggest that ablation of Stat3 in tumor cells or tumor-associated immune cells decreases tumor progression	Kortylewski et al. (2005), Wang et al. (2004), Yu and Jove (2004), and Yu et al. (2007, 2009)
JAK inhibitors	Use of these agents (i.e., AG490, WP1066, AZD1480) decreases Stat3 activation and augments the tumor-associated immune response in preclinical models of both hematologic and solid tumors	Burdelya et al. (2002), Fujita et al. (2008), Hussain et al. (2007), Kong et al. (2008), Kong et al. (2009), and Nefedova et al. (2005)
Other tyrosine kinase inhibitors	Inhibitors of fusion proteins (i.e., products of NPM/ALK or BCR-ABL) Both directly and indirectly inhibit activation of Stat3 Agents such as sunitinib decrease recruitment of Tregs and MDSC to sites of tumor in a Stat3-dependent fashion	Kasprzycka et al. (2006), Larmonier et al. (2008), Ozao-Choy et al. (2009), and Xin et al. (2009)
CpG-siRNA	Stat3 siRNA linked to the Toll-like receptor agonist 9 (TLR9), CpG, both silences genes in TLR9(+) myeloid cells and decreases the Stat3-mediated immune response; in preclinical models, a marked antitumor effect is observed	Kortylewski et al. (2009a, b)

3.1 Genetic Evidence and Potential Toxicity

Mouse studies using knockout mice demonstrate that ablation of *Stat3* in either tumor cells or tumor-associated immune cells prevent tumor progression (Bollrath et al. 2009; Chiarle et al. 2005; Kortylewski et al. 2005). Potent anti-tumor immune responses can also be achieved from reconstitution of mice with *Stat3*-deficient immune cells (Kortylewski et al. 2005). Although long-term ablation of *Stat3* in hematopoietic cells can lead to severe inflammatory disease (Welte et al. 2003), there appears to be a therapeutic window for inducing antitumor immune responses (Kortylewski et al. 2009a,b,c). Recent genetic studies in patients afflicted by HIES reveal that dominant-negative mutations in *STAT3* are strongly associated with the disease (Minegishi et al. 2007). All mutations are located in the Stat3 DNA-binding domain and as a result, signaling responses to cytokines, including IL-6 and IL-23, are defective (Milner et al. 2008; Minegishi 2009; Minegishi et al. 2007). These studies in individuals with HIES suggest that short term STAT3 blockade may not lead to severe side effects and that STAT3 may be exploited as a molecular target for therapeutic development.

3.2 JAK Inhibitors

Aberrant Stat3 activity in cancer, to a large degree, is the result of overactivation of upstream tyrosine kinases. Owing to the fact that Jak tyrosine kinase is an important activator of Stat3 both in tumor and immune cells in the tumor microenvironment, much effort has been devoted to studying Jak kinase inhibitors in various tumor models. The prototype Jak inhibitor, AG490, prevents Stat3 phosphorylation and activation of its downstream pro-survival genes (Rahaman et al. 2002). The opportunity to use AG490 was shown to enhance immunotherapy by several studies. For examples, *in vivo* administration of AG490 in conjunction to IL-12 results in better anti-tumor effects than either one alone (Burdelya et al. 2002). A structurally related compound, WP1066, also disrupts Jak/Stat3 activation and reduces the malignant tumor growth (Ferrajoli et al. 2007; Iwamaru et al. 2007). WP1066 has the capacity to penetrate blood–brain barrier and has demonstrated activity in preclinical glioma models (Hussain et al. 2007). Consistent with the role of Stat3 in inducing and maintaining tumor-associated Tregs is the observation that tumors treated with WP1066 show a marked reduction in number of Tregs. This, in turn, results in reversal of immune tolerance elicited by Tregs (Kong et al. 2009). Tumor growth in mice with subcutaneously established syngeneic melanoma was markedly inhibited by WP1066 (Kong et al. 2008).

Another Jak2/Stat3 inhibitor shown to induce anti-tumor immune responses is JSI-124, a member of curcubitacin compounds (Blaskovich et al. 2003). Treatment of tumors with JSI-124 limits the number of tumor-infiltrating MDSCs, inhibits DC differentiation, and thereby inhibits tumor growth (Fujita et al. 2008; Nefedova et al. 2005). Improved anti-tumor immune responses achieved by JSI-124 are associated with prolonged survival in murine glioma models. Tumor response appears to be dependent upon host immunity (Fujita et al. 2008). Importantly, combined use of JSI-124 with DC vaccines for the treatment of mouse sarcoma induces IFNγ production by $CD8^+$ T cells and synergistic eradication of tumors (Nefedova et al. 2005).

As with the previously noted compounds, the novel JAK2 inhibitor AZD1480 also caused growth arrest in solid tumor cell lines with cytokine-induced Stat3 activation (Hedvat et al. 2009). In these studies, JAK2 inhibition resulted in decreased nuclear translocation of Stat3 and proliferation. Studies are underway to evaluate this compound in modulating the tumor immunologic environment. The agent is currently undergoing clinical evaluation in the setting of myelofibrosis (NCT00910728), and further studies in solid tumors are highly anticipated. Collectively, these studies indicate that targeting of Stat3 using Jak2 inhibitors have the potential to revert tumor mediated-immune suppression and generate anti-tumor immune responses.

3.3 Other Oncogenic Kinase Inhibitors

Numerous oncoproteins (including NPM/ALK, Src and BCR-ABL) possess intrinsic kinase activity and may regulate Stat3 activity. For example, chromosomal translocations that juxtapose NPM and ALK lead to ALK overexpression and concomitant Stat3 activation in anaplastic large cell lymphoma (ALCL) (Chiarle et al. 2005). Persistent Stat3 activation by NPM/ALK facilitates induction of Treg-like phenotypes in ALCLs by promoting secretion of IL-10 and TGF-β as well as expression of Foxp3 (Kasprzycka et al. 2006). Moreover, Stat3 activation by NPM/ALK negatively modulates immune responses by activating gene transcription of immunosuppressive cell surface protein CD274 (B7-H1) in T cell lymphoma, where Stat3 directly binds to the promoter region of CD274 (Marzec et al. 2008). Given that antibody-mediated blockade of CD274 in conjunction with T cell depletion therapy leads to complete tumor regression (Webster et al. 2007), targeting NPM/ALK-mediated STAT3 activity may offer therapeutic advantages for the treatment of T cell lymphoma. Two small molecular inhibitors, WHI-131 and 154, effectively inhibit Stat3 phosphorylation by blocking enzymatic activity of NPM/ALK (Marzec et al. 2005). More detailed investigation is required to identify whether desirable anti-tumor immune responses are elicited by these compounds.

Targeting BCR-ABL also reverses Stat3-mediated immune suppression in tumors. The most widely studied BCR-ABL kinase inhibitors, imatinib mesylate is applied as standard therapy for the treatment of Philadelphia chromosome-positive CML and gastrointestinal stromal tumor (GIST), where it has demonstrated significant clinical activity (Blanke et al. 2008; Druker et al. 2001). Intriguing findings related to the immune responses associated with imatinib treatment have been reported. However, treatment with imatinib induces both suppressive as well as stimulating effects on $CD4^+$ and $CD8^+$ T cells or DCs, suggesting the exact nature of imatinib effect on immune cells remains to be further explored. Nonetheless, used at clinically achievable concentrations, imatinib reduces suppressive activity of Tregs as well as Foxp3 expression in Tregs through inhibition of Stat3 (Larmonier et al. 2008). Also, the quantity of tumor-infiltrating Tregs is diminished with imatinib therapy (Larmonier et al. 2008). Similar to Jak inhibitors, treatment of tumor with imatinib significantly enhances the efficacy of DC vaccine against lymphoma, lessening tumor metastasis in conjunction with effective IFNγ production by splenocytes (Larmonier et al. 2008). All of these studies indicate that there is a significant opportunity to advance immunotherapy using imatinib. Although imatinib does have substantial activity in CML, a proportion of patients do become resistance to this agent. Presumably, the bone marrow (which harbors multiple soluble factors that activate Stat3) is an ideal environment for the development of resistance CML clones (Bewry et al. 2008). While Stat3 activity may be downregulated to some extent by imatinib-mediated Abl inhibition, other kinases, such as Jak kinase, may continue to drive Stat3 activation (Sen et al. 2009). Using direct Stat3 inhibitors in conjunction with imatinib may prevent Stat3 reactivation by pleiotropic Stat3 activators present in the tumor microenvironment.

3.4 RTK Inhibitors

In addition to cytokines and oncoproteins, Stat3 is constitutively activated in cancers by many growth factors including EGF, PDGF, and VEGF. Receptors for these growth factors are transmembrane receptor tyrosine kinases (RTKs), which trigger downstream signaling through a number of distinct cascades. Targeting RTKs can be a clinically effective strategy across a wide variety of malignancies, including lung cancer, hepatocellular carcinoma (HCC) and mRCC (Llovet et al. 2008; Motzer et al. 2009; Shepherd et al. 2005). However, a multitude of escape mechanisms exist to circumvent RTK inhibitors. Given that Stat3 represents a point of convergence for numerous growth factor signaling pathways in tumors, targeting Stat3 activation may be a useful strategy.

Sunitinib is a multi-targeted growth factor inhibitor that is widely used in the treatment of mRCC (Motzer et al. 2009). The inhibitory effect of sunitinib on a variety of kinases impairs Stat3 activation in tumors, thereby inducing tumor cell apoptosis (Xin et al. 2009; Yang et al. 2010). Treatment with sunitinib intensifies the anti-tumor immune response by limiting the number of tumor-associated MDSCs and Tregs in mouse tumor models (Xin et al. 2009). mRCC patients show elevated levels of $CD33^+HLA\text{-}DR^-$ and $CD15^+CD14^-$ MDSCs in peripheral blood (Ko et al. 2009). While treatment with sunitinib results in inhibition of Treg mediators such as IL-10, TGF-β, and Foxp3, it also elevates Th1 cytokine and IFNγ in murine models (Ozao-Choy et al. 2009). Moreover, treatment of tumors with sunitinib increases efficacy of IL-12 based immune activation therapy (Ozao-Choy et al. 2009). Therefore, sunitinib-based therapy has great potential to modulate anti-tumor immunity as an adjunct for the treatment of certain human cancers including RCC.

It is important to note that the effects of sunitinib may not extend across this class of agents. As one example, the small molecule RTK inhibitor sorafenib is also widely used in the treatment of mRCC (Escudier et al. 2007). In contrast to sunitinib, recent studies suggest that sorafenib inhibits the function of DCs and decreases induction of antigen-specific T-cells (Hipp et al. 2008). Thus, the immunologic phenomena triggered by RTK inhibitors should be separately considered in tailoring clinical strategies.

3.5 siRNA

Combined use of kinase-targeted Stat3 inhibitors with other immunotherapeutic approaches such as tumor vaccines may augment efficacy of cancer immunotherapy. For example, combination of DC-based vaccine together with RTK inhibitors leads to a greater therapeutic efficacy in preclinical models, suggesting various levels of Stat3 inhibition facilitate immune cell mediated anti-tumor effect (Larmonier et al. 2008; Nefedova et al. 2005). Alternatively, these inhibitors can synergize with different immune modulators that elicit innate immunity, such as the Toll-like receptor agonist CpG. Given that Stat3 downregulates CpG-mediated innate immune responses, ablation of *Stat3* has been shown to enhance and prolong a potent anti-tumor immune responses elicited by CpG in a murine melanoma xenograft model (Kortylewski et al. 2009a). Furthermore, conjugation of CpG to siRNA targeting *Stat3* activates various populations of immune cells including DCs and macrophages and ultimately induces robust anti-tumor immune responses (Kortylewski et al. 2009b). Therefore, CpG-coupled siRNA can maximize therapeutic efficacy by inducing anti-tumor responses through CpG while knocking down *Stat3*.

As previously noted, a major hurdle in the clinical use of RTK inhibitors is the development of resistance mechanisms. This concept is supported by a recent study demonstrating that long-term sunitinib treatment increases tumor cell invasiveness and metastasis (Paez-Ribes et al. 2009). Accelerated tumor progression upon prolonged sunitinib treatment is in part mediated by intense hypoxia during metastatic processes (Paez-Ribes et al. 2009). The role of Stat3 in regulating the expression of hypoxia-inducible factor-1α (HIF-1α), which is a critical regulator of hypoxic response in tumors, has been previously shown (Niu et al. 2008). Directly targeting Stat3 using gene-specific approaches, such as CpG-*Stat3* siRNA, may thus overcome undesirable effects of sunitinib by reducing tumor hypoxia. Using CpG-*Stat3* siRNA and sunitinib in combination therefore may have clinical merit.

4 Concluding Remarks

Stat3 is persistently activated in diverse cancers, promoting tumor cell survival, proliferation, angiogenesis/metastasis, and immune escape. Targeting Stat3 has the potential to not only directly inhibit tumor growth but also alter the tumor immunologic environment in favor of immunotherapy. Stat3 therefore represents a promising target for cancer therapy. With the emergence of Stat3 inhibitors, both indirect and direct, we are entering a new era of cancer immunotherapy.

References

Bewry NN, Nair RR, Emmons MF, Boulware D, Pinilla-Ibarz J, Hazlehurst LA (2008) Stat3 contributes to resistance toward BCR-ABL inhibitors in a bone marrow microenvironment model of drug resistance. Mol Cancer Ther 7:3169–3175

Bharadwaj U, Li M, Zhang R, Chen C, Yao Q (2007) Elevated interleukin-6 and G-CSF in human pancreatic cancer cell conditioned medium suppress dendritic cell differentiation and activation. Cancer Res 67:5479–5488

Blanke CD, Rankin C, Demetri GD, Ryan CW, von Mehren M, Benjamin RS, Raymond AK, Bramwell VHC, Baker LH, Maki RG et al (2008) Phase III Randomized, Intergroup Trial Assessing Imatinib Mesylate At Two Dose Levels in Patients With Unresectable or Metastatic Gastrointestinal Stromal Tumors Expressing the Kit Receptor Tyrosine Kinase: S0033. J Clin Oncol 26:626–632

Blaskovich MA, Sun J, Cantor A, Turkson J, Jove R, Sebti SM (2003) Discovery of JSI-124 (cucurbitacin I), a selective Janus kinase/signal transducer and activator of transcription 3 signaling pathway inhibitor with potent antitumor activity against human and murine cancer cells in mice. Cancer Res 63:1270–1279

Bollrath J, Phesse TJ, von Burstin VA, Putoczki T, Bennecke M, Bateman T, Nebelsiek T, Lundgren-May T, Canli O, Schwitalla S et al (2009) gp130-mediated Stat3 activation in enterocytes regulates cell survival and cell-cycle progression during colitis-associated tumorigenesis. Cancer Cell 15:91–102

Bunt SK, Yang L, Sinha P, Clements VK, Leips J, Ostrand-Rosenberg S (2007) Reduced inflammation in the tumor microenvironment delays the accumulation of myeloid-derived suppressor cells and limits tumor progression. Cancer Res 67:10019–10026

Burdelya L, Catlett-Falcone R, Levitzki A, Cheng F, Mora LB, Sotomayor E, Coppola D, Sun J, Sebti S, Dalton WS et al (2002) Combination therapy with AG-490 and interleukin 12 achieves greater antitumor effects than either agent alone. Mol Cancer Ther 1:893–899

Charles KA, Kulbe H, Soper R, Escorcio-Correia M, Lawrence T, Schultheis A, Chakravarty P, Thompson RG, Kollias G, Smyth JF et al (2009) The tumor-promoting actions of TNF-alpha involve TNFR1 and IL-17 in ovarian cancer in mice and humans. J Clin Invest 119:3011–3023

Chaudhry A, Rudra D, Treuting P, Samstein RM, Liang Y, Kas A, Rudensky AY (2009) CD4+ Regulatory T Cells Control TH17 Responses in a Stat3-Dependent Manner. Science 326 (5955):986–991

Chen Z, Laurence A, Kanno Y, Pacher-Zavisin M, Zhu BM, Tato C, Yoshimura A, Hennighausen L, O'Shea JJ (2006) Selective regulatory function of Socs3 in the formation of IL-17-secreting T cells. Proc Natl Acad Sci USA 103:8137–8142

Cheng P, Corzo CA, Luetteke N, Yu B, Nagaraj S, Bui MM, Ortiz M, Nacken W, Sorg C, Vogl T et al (2008) Inhibition of dendritic cell differentiation and accumulation of myeloid-derived suppressor cells in cancer is regulated by S100A9 protein. J Exp Med 205:2235–2249

Chiarle R, Simmons WJ, Cai H, Dhall G, Zamo A, Raz R, Karras JG, Levy DE, Inghirami G (2005) Stat3 is required for ALK-mediated lymphomagenesis and provides a possible therapeutic target. Nat Med 11:623–629

Cho ML, Kang JW, Moon YM, Nam HJ, Jhun JY, Heo SB, Jin HT, Min SY, Ju JH, Park KS et al (2006) STAT3 and NF-kappaB signal pathway is required for IL-23-mediated IL-17 production in spontaneous arthritis animal model IL-1 receptor antagonist-deficient mice. J Immunol 176:5652–5661

Corzo CA, Cotter MJ, Cheng P, Cheng F, Kusmartsev S, Sotomayor E, Padhya T, McCaffrey TV, McCaffrey JC, Gabrilovich DI (2009) Mechanism regulating reactive oxygen species in tumor-induced myeloid-derived suppressor cells. J Immunol 182:5693–5701

Curiel TJ, Coukos G, Zou L, Alvarez X, Cheng P, Mottram P, Evdemon-Hogan M, Conejo-Garcia JR, Zhang L, Burow M et al (2004) Specific recruitment of regulatory T cells in ovarian carcinoma fosters immune privilege and predicts reduced survival. Nat Med 10:942–949

Dercamp C, Chemin K, Caux C, Trinchieri G, Vicari AP (2005) Distinct and overlapping roles of interleukin-10 and CD25+ regulatory T cells in the inhibition of antitumor CD8 T-cell responses. Cancer Res 65:8479–8486

Druker BJ, Sawyers CL, Kantarjian H, Resta DJ, Reese SF, Ford JM, Capdeville R, Talpaz M (2001) Activity of a Specific Inhibitor of the BCR-ABL Tyrosine Kinase in the Blast Crisis of Chronic Myeloid Leukemia and Acute Lymphoblastic Leukemia with the Philadelphia Chromosome. N Engl J Med 344:1038–1042

Dunn GP, Bruce AT, Ikeda H, Old LJ, Schreiber RD (2002) Cancer immunoediting: from immunosurveillance to tumor escape. Nat Immunol 3:991–998

Escudier B, Eisen T, Stadler WM, Szczylik C, Oudard S, Siebels M, Negrier S, Chevreau C, Solska E, Desai AA et al (2007) Sorafenib in Advanced Clear-Cell Renal-Cell Carcinoma. N Engl J Med 356:125–134

Ferrajoli A, Faderl S, Van Q, Koch P, Harris D, Liu Z, Hazan-Halevy I, Wang Y, Kantarjian HM, Priebe W et al (2007) WP1066 disrupts Janus kinase-2 and induces caspase-dependent apoptosis in acute myelogenous leukemia cells. Cancer Res 67:11291–11299

Fujita M, Zhu X, Sasaki K, Ueda R, Low KL, Pollack IF, Okada H (2008) Inhibition of STAT3 promotes the efficacy of adoptive transfer therapy using type-1 CTLs by modulation of the immunological microenvironment in a murine intracranial glioma. J Immunol 180:2089–2098

Gabrilovich D (2004) Mechanisms and functional significance of tumour-induced dendritic-cell defects. Nat Rev Immunol 4:941–952

Gabrilovich DI, Nagaraj S (2009) Myeloid-derived suppressor cells as regulators of the immune system. Nat Rev Immunol 9:162–174

Gabrilovich DI, Chen HL, Girgis KR, Cunningham HT, Meny GM, Nadaf S, Kavanaugh D, Carbone DP (1996) Production of vascular endothelial growth factor by human tumors inhibits the functional maturation of dendritic cells. Nat Med 2:1096–1103

Grivennikov S, Karin E, Terzic J, Mucida D, Yu GY, Vallabhapurapu S, Scheller J, Rose-John S, Cheroutre H, Eckmann L et al (2009) IL-6 and stat3 are required for survival of intestinal epithelial cells and development of colitis-associated cancer. Cancer Cell 15:103–113

He D, Li H, Yusuf N, Elmets CA, Li J, Mountz JD, Xu H (2010) IL-17 Promotes Tumor Development through the Induction of Tumor Promoting Microenvironments at Tumor Sites and Myeloid-Derived Suppressor Cells. J Immunol 184:2281–2288

Hedvat M, Huszar D, Herrmann A, Gozgit JM, Schroeder A, Sheehy A, Buettner R, Proia D, Kowolik CM, Xin H et al (2009) The JAK2 Inhibitor AZD1480 Potently Blocks Stat3 Signaling and Oncogenesis in Solid Tumors. Cancer Cell 16:487–497

Herbeuval JP, Lelievre E, Lambert C, Dy M, Genin C (2004) Recruitment of STAT3 for production of IL-10 by colon carcinoma cells induced by macrophage-derived IL-6. J Immunol 172:4630–4636

Hipp MM, Hilf N, Walter S, Werth D, Brauer KM, Radsak MP, Weinschenk T, Singh-Jasuja H, Brossart P (2008) Sorafenib, but not sunitinib, affects function of dendritic cells and induction of primary immune responses. Blood 111:5610–5620

Hoechst B, Ormandy LA, Ballmaier M, Lehner F, Kruger C, Manns MP, Greten TF, Korangy F (2008) A new population of myeloid-derived suppressor cells in hepatocellular carcinoma patients induces CD4(+)CD25(+)Foxp3(+) T cells. Gastroenterology 135:234–243

Hoentjen F, Sartor RB, Ozaki M, Jobin C (2005) STAT3 regulates NF-kappaB recruitment to the IL-12p40 promoter in dendritic cells. Blood 105:689–696

Hussain SF, Kong LY, Jordan J, Conrad C, Madden T, Fokt I, Priebe W, Heimberger AB (2007) A novel small molecule inhibitor of signal transducers and activators of transcription 3 reverses immune tolerance in malignant glioma patients. Cancer Res 67:9630–9636

Ito N, Eto M, Nakamura E, Takahashi A, Tsukamoto T, Toma H, Nakazawa H, Hirao Y, Uemura H, Kagawa S et al (2007) STAT3 Polymorphism Predicts Interferon-Alfa Response in Patients With Metastatic Renal Cell Carcinoma. J Clin Oncol 25:2785–2791

Iwamaru A, Szymanski S, Iwado E, Aoki H, Yokoyama T, Fokt I, Hess K, Conrad C, Madden T, Sawaya R et al (2007) A novel inhibitor of the STAT3 pathway induces apoptosis in malignant glioma cells both *in vitro* and *in vivo*. Oncogene 26:2435–2444

Kasprzycka M, Marzec M, Liu X, Zhang Q, Wasik MA (2006) Nucleophosmin/anaplastic lymphoma kinase (NPM/ALK) oncoprotein induces the T regulatory cell phenotype by activating STAT3. Proc Natl Acad Sci USA 103:9964–9969

Ko JS, Zea AH, Rini BI, Ireland JL, Elson P, Cohen P, Golshayan A, Rayman PA, Wood L, Garcia J et al (2009) Sunitinib mediates reversal of myeloid-derived suppressor cell accumulation in renal cell carcinoma patients. Clin Cancer Res 15:2148–2157

Kong LY, Abou-Ghazal MK, Wei J, Chakraborty A, Sun W, Qiao W, Fuller GN, Fokt I, Grimm EA, Schmittling RJ et al (2008) A novel inhibitor of signal transducers and activators of transcription 3 activation is efficacious against established central nervous system melanoma and inhibits regulatory T cells. Clin Cancer Res 14:5759–5768

Kong LY, Wei J, Sharma AK, Barr J, Abou-Ghazal MK, Fokt I, Weinberg J, Rao G, Grimm E, Priebe W et al (2009) A novel phosphorylated STAT3 inhibitor enhances T cell cytotoxicity against melanoma through inhibition of regulatory T cells. Cancer Immunol Immunother 58:1023–1032

Kortylewski M, Kujawski M, Wang T, Wei S, Zhang S, Pilon-Thomas S, Niu G, Kay H, Mule J, Kerr WG et al (2005) Inhibiting Stat3 signaling in the hematopoietic system elicits multicomponent antitumor immunity. Nat Med 11:1314–1321

Kortylewski M, Kujawski M, Herrmann A, Yang C, Wang L, Liu Y, Salcedo R, Yu H (2009a) Toll-like receptor 9 activation of signal transducer and activator of transcription 3 constrains its agonist-based immunotherapy. Cancer Res 69:2497–2505

Kortylewski M, Swiderski P, Herrmann A, Wang L, Kowolik C, Kujawski M, Lee H, Scuto A, Liu Y, Yang C et al (2009b) *In vivo* delivery of siRNA to immune cells by conjugation to a TLR9 agonist enhances antitumor immune responses. Nat Biotechnol 27(10):925–932

Kortylewski M, Xin H, Kujawski M, Lee H, Liu Y, Harris T, Drake C, Pardoll D, Yu H (2009c) Regulation of the IL-23 and IL-12 balance by Stat3 signaling in the tumor microenvironment. Cancer Cell 15:114–123

Kreil S, Waghorn K, Ernst T, Chase A, White H, Hehlmann R, Reiter A, Hochhaus A, Cross NC (2010) A polymorphism associated with STAT3 expression and response of chronic myeloid leukemia to interferon alpha. Haematologica 95:148–152

Kryczek I, Wei S, Szeliga W, Vatan L, Zou W (2009) Endogenous IL-17 contributes to reduced tumor growth and metastasis. Blood 114:357–359

Kujawski M, Kortylewski M, Lee H, Herrmann A, Kay H, Yu H (2008) Stat3 mediates myeloid cell-dependent tumor angiogenesis in mice. J Clin Invest 118:3367–3377

Lam LT, Wright G, Davis RE, Lenz G, Farinha P, Dang L, Chan JW, Rosenwald A, Gascoyne RD, Staudt LM (2008) Cooperative signaling through the signal transducer and activator of transcription 3 and nuclear factor-{kappa}B pathways in subtypes of diffuse large B-cell lymphoma. Blood 111:3701–3713

Langowski JL, Zhang X, Wu L, Mattson JD, Chen T, Smith K, Basham B, McClanahan T, Kastelein RA, Oft M (2006) IL-23 promotes tumour incidence and growth. Nature 442:461–465

Langrish CL, Chen Y, Blumenschein WM, Mattson J, Basham B, Sedgwick JD, McClanahan T, Kastelein RA, Cua DJ (2005) IL-23 drives a pathogenic T cell population that induces autoimmune inflammation. J Exp Med 201:233–240

Larmonier N, Janikashvili N, LaCasse CJ, Larmonier CB, Cantrell J, Situ E, Lundeen T, Bonnotte B, Katsanis E (2008) Imatinib mesylate inhibits CD4+ CD25+ regulatory T cell activity and enhances active immunotherapy against BCR-ABL- tumors. J Immunol 181:6955–6963

Lee H, Herrmann A, Deng JH, Kujawski M, Niu G, Li Z, Forman S, Jove R, Pardoll DM, Yu H (2009) Persistently activated Stat3 maintains constitutive NF-kappaB activity in tumors. Cancer Cell 15:283–293

Lesinski GB, Trefry J, Brasdovich M, Kondadasula SV, Sackey K, Zimmerer JM, Chaudhury AR, Yu L, Zhang X, Crespin TR et al (2007) Melanoma cells exhibit variable signal transducer and activator of transcription 1 phosphorylation and a reduced response to IFN-alpha compared with immune effector cells. Clin Cancer Res 13:5010–5019

Li C, Zhang F, Lin M, Liu J (2004) Induction of S100A9 Gene Expression by Cytokine Oncostatin M in Breast Cancer Cells Through the STAT3 Signaling Cascade. Breast Cancer Research and Treatment 87:123–134

Li Y, Chu N, Rostami A, Zhang GX (2006) Dendritic cells transduced with SOCS-3 exhibit a tolerogenic/DC2 phenotype that directs type 2 Th cell differentiation *in vitro* and *in vivo*. J Immunol 177:1679–1688

Liang S, Ristich V, Arase H, Dausset J, Carosella ED, Horuzsko A (2008) Modulation of dendritic cell differentiation by HLA-G and ILT4 requires the IL-6–STAT3 signaling pathway. Proc Natl Acad Sci USA 105:8357–8362

Liyanage UK, Moore TT, Joo HG, Tanaka Y, Herrmann V, Doherty G, Drebin JA, Strasberg SM, Eberlein TJ, Goedegebuure PS et al (2002) Prevalence of regulatory T cells is increased in peripheral blood and tumor microenvironment of patients with pancreas or breast adenocarcinoma. J Immunol 169:2756–2761

Llovet JM, Ricci S, Mazzaferro V, Hilgard P, Gane E, Blanc J-F, de Oliveira AC, Santoro A, Raoul J-L, Forner A et al (2008) Sorafenib in Advanced Hepatocellular Carcinoma. N Engl J Med 359:378–390

Ma CS, Chew GY, Simpson N, Priyadarshi A, Wong M, Grimbacher B, Fulcher DA, Tangye SG, Cook MC (2008) Deficiency of Th17 cells in hyper IgE syndrome due to mutations in STAT3. J Exp Med 205:1551–1557

Marzec M, Kasprzycka M, Ptasznik A, Wlodarski P, Zhang Q, Odum N, Wasik MA (2005) Inhibition of ALK enzymatic activity in T-cell lymphoma cells induces apoptosis and suppresses proliferation and STAT3 phosphorylation independently of Jak3. Lab Invest 85:1544–1554

Marzec M, Zhang Q, Goradia A, Raghunath PN, Liu X, Paessler M, Wang HY, Wysocka M, Cheng M, Ruggeri BA et al (2008) Oncogenic kinase NPM/ALK induces through STAT3 expression of immunosuppressive protein CD274 (PD-L1, B7-H1). Proc Natl Acad Sci USA 105:20852–20857

McGeachy MJ, Chen Y, Tato CM, Laurence A, Joyce-Shaikh B, Blumenschein WM, McClanahan TK, O'Shea JJ, Cua DJ (2009) The interleukin 23 receptor is essential for the terminal differentiation of interleukin 17-producing effector T helper cells *in vivo*. Nat Immunol 10:314–324

Melani C, Chiodoni C, Forni G, Colombo MP (2003) Myeloid cell expansion elicited by the progression of spontaneous mammary carcinomas in c-erbB-2 transgenic BALB/c mice suppresses immune reactivity. Blood 102:2138–2145

Milner JD, Brenchley JM, Laurence A, Freeman AF, Hill BJ, Elias KM, Kanno Y, Spalding C, Elloumi HZ, Paulson ML et al (2008) Impaired T(H)17 cell differentiation in subjects with autosomal dominant hyper-IgE syndrome. Nature 452:773–776

Minegishi Y (2009) Hyper-IgE syndrome. Curr Opin Immunol 21:487–492

Minegishi Y, Saito M, Tsuchiya S, Tsuge I, Takada H, Hara T, Kawamura N, Ariga T, Pasic S, Stojkovic O et al (2007) Dominant-negative mutations in the DNA-binding domain of STAT3 cause hyper-IgE syndrome. Nature 448:1058–1062

Motzer RJ, Hutson TE, Tomczak P, Michaelson MD, Bukowski RM, Oudard S, Negrier S, Szczylik C, Pili R, Bjarnason GA et al (2009) Overall Survival and Updated Results for Sunitinib Compared With Interferon Alfa in Patients With Metastatic Renal Cell Carcinoma. J Clin Oncol 27:3584–3590

Nabarro S, Himoudi N, Papanastasiou A, Gilmour K, Gibson S, Sebire N, Thrasher A, Blundell MP, Hubank M, Canderan G et al (2005) Coordinated oncogenic transformation and inhibition of host immune responses by the PAX3-FKHR fusion oncoprotein. J Exp Med 202:1399–1410

NCT00910728 (2010) A PhaseI/II, Open label multi-centre study to assess the safety, tolerability, pharmacokinetics and preliminary efficacy of the JAK2 inhibitor AZD1480 administered orally to patients with primary myelofibrosis (PMF) and post-polycythaemia vera/essential thrombocythaemia myelofibrosis (post-PV/ET MF). http://www.clinicaltrials.gov. Accessed 17 Feb 2010

Nefedova Y, Huang M, Kusmartsev S, Bhattacharya R, Cheng P, Salup R, Jove R, Gabrilovich D (2004) Hyperactivation of STAT3 is involved in abnormal differentiation of dendritic cells in cancer. J Immunol 172:464–474

Nefedova Y, Nagaraj S, Rosenbauer A, Muro-Cacho C, Sebti SM, Gabrilovich DI (2005) Regulation of dendritic cell differentiation and antitumor immune response in cancer by pharmacologic-selective inhibition of the janus-activated kinase 2/signal transducers and activators of transcription 3 pathway. Cancer Res 65:9525–9535

Niu G, Briggs J, Deng J, Ma Y, Lee H, Kortylewski M, Kujawski M, Kay H, Cress WD, Jove R et al (2008) Signal transducer and activator of transcription 3 is required for hypoxia-inducible factor-1alpha RNA expression in both tumor cells and tumor-associated myeloid cells. Mol Cancer Res 6:1099–1105

Numasaki M, Fukushi J, Ono M, Narula SK, Zavodny PJ, Kudo T, Robbins PD, Tahara H, Lotze MT (2003) Interleukin-17 promotes angiogenesis and tumor growth. Blood 101: 2620–2627

Ohm JE, Gabrilovich DI, Sempowski GD, Kisseleva E, Parman KS, Nadaf S, Carbone DP (2003) VEGF inhibits T-cell development and may contribute to tumor-induced immune suppression. Blood 101:4878–4886

Oppmann B, Lesley R, Blom B, Timans JC, Xu Y, Hunte B, Vega F, Yu N, Wang J, Singh K et al (2000) Novel p19 protein engages IL-12p40 to form a cytokine, IL-23, with biological activities similar as well as distinct from IL-12. Immunity 13:715–725

Ozao-Choy J, Ma G, Kao J, Wang GX, Meseck M, Sung M, Schwartz M, Divino CM, Pan PY, Chen SH (2009) The novel role of tyrosine kinase inhibitor in the reversal of immune suppression and modulation of tumor microenvironment for immune-based cancer therapies. Cancer Res 69:2514–2522

Paez-Ribes M, Allen E, Hudock J, Takeda T, Okuyama H, Vinals F, Inoue M, Bergers G, Hanahan D, Casanovas O (2009) Antiangiogenic therapy elicits malignant progression of tumors to increased local invasion and distant metastasis. Cancer Cell 15:220–231

Pallandre JR, Brillard E, Crehange G, Radlovic A, Remy-Martin JP, Saas P, Rohrlich PS, Pivot X, Ling X, Tiberghien P et al (2007) Role of STAT3 in CD4+CD25+FOXP3+ regulatory lymphocyte generation: implications in graft-versus-host disease and antitumor immunity. J Immunol 179:7593–7604

Parham C, Chirica M, Timans J, Vaisberg E, Travis M, Cheung J, Pflanz S, Zhang R, Singh KP, Vega F et al (2002) A receptor for the heterodimeric cytokine IL-23 is composed of IL-12Rbeta1 and a novel cytokine receptor subunit, IL-23R. J Immunol 168:5699–5708

Park SJ, Nakagawa T, Kitamura H, Atsumi T, Kamon H, Sawa S, Kamimura D, Ueda N, Iwakura Y, Ishihara K et al (2004) IL-6 regulates *in vivo* dendritic cell differentiation through STAT3 activation. J Immunol 173:3844–3854

Rahaman SO, Harbor PC, Chernova O, Barnett GH, Vogelbaum MA, Haque SJ (2002) Inhibition of constitutively active Stat3 suppresses proliferation and induces apoptosis in glioblastoma multiforme cells. Oncogene 21:8404–8413

Sen B, Saigal B, Parikh N, Gallick G, Johnson FM (2009) Sustained Src inhibition results in signal transducer and activator of transcription 3 (STAT3) activation and cancer cell survival via altered Janus-activated kinase-STAT3 binding. Cancer Res 69:1958–1965

Serafini P, Carbley R, Noonan KA, Tan G, Bronte V, Borrello I (2004) High-dose granulocyte-macrophage colony-stimulating factor-producing vaccines impair the immune response through the recruitment of myeloid suppressor cells. Cancer Res 64:6337–6343

Serafini P, Mgebroff S, Noonan K, Borrello I (2008) Myeloid-derived suppressor cells promote cross-tolerance in B-cell lymphoma by expanding regulatory T cells. Cancer Res 68:5439–5449

Shepherd FA, Rodrigues Pereira J, Ciuleanu T, Tan EH, Hirsh V, Thongprasert S, Campos D, Maoleekoonpiroj S, Smylie M, Martins R et al (2005) Erlotinib in Previously Treated Non-Small-Cell Lung Cancer. N Engl J Med 353:123–132

Sinha P, Clements VK, Bunt SK, Albelda SM, Ostrand-Rosenberg S (2007) Cross-talk between myeloid-derived suppressor cells and macrophages subverts tumor immunity toward a type 2 response. J Immunol 179:977–983

Stumhofer JS, Silver JS, Laurence A, Porrett PM, Harris TH, Turka LA, Ernst M, Saris CJ, O'Shea JJ, Hunter CA (2007) Interleukins 27 and 6 induce STAT3-mediated T cell production of interleukin 10. Nat Immunol 8:1363–1371

Sumimoto H, Imabayashi F, Iwata T, Kawakami Y (2006) The BRAF-MAPK signaling pathway is essential for cancer-immune evasion in human melanoma cells. J Exp Med 203: 1651–1656

Takeda K, Clausen BE, Kaisho T, Tsujimura T, Terada N, Forster I, Akira S (1999) Enhanced Th1 activity and development of chronic enterocolitis in mice devoid of Stat3 in macrophages and neutrophils. Immunity 10:39–49

Uemura Y, Liu TY, Narita Y, Suzuki M, Nakatsuka R, Araki T, Matsumoto M, Iwai LK, Hirosawa N, Matsuoka Y et al (2009) Cytokine-dependent modification of IL-12p70 and IL-23 balance in dendritic cells by ligand activation of Valpha24 invariant NKT cells. J Immunol 183:201–208

Viguier M, Lemaitre F, Verola O, Cho MS, Gorochov G, Dubertret L, Bachelez H, Kourilsky P, Ferradini L (2004) Foxp3 expressing CD4+CD25(high) regulatory T cells are overrepresented in human metastatic melanoma lymph nodes and inhibit the function of infiltrating T cells. J Immunol 173:1444–1453

Wang T, Niu G, Kortylewski M, Burdelya L, Shain K, Zhang S, Bhattacharya R, Gabrilovich D, Heller R, Coppola D et al (2004) Regulation of the innate and adaptive immune responses by Stat-3 signaling in tumor cells. Nat Med 10:48–54

Wang W, Edington HD, Rao UN, Jukic DM, Land SR, Ferrone S, Kirkwood JM (2007) Modulation of signal transducers and activators of transcription 1 and 3 signaling in melanoma by high-dose IFNalpha2b. Clin Cancer Res 13:1523–1531

Wang L, Yi T, Kortylewski M, Pardoll DM, Zeng D, Yu H (2009) IL-17 can promote tumor growth through an IL-6-Stat3 signaling pathway. J Exp Med 206:1457–1464

Webster WS, Thompson RH, Harris KJ, Frigola X, Kuntz S, Inman BA, Dong H (2007) Targeting molecular and cellular inhibitory mechanisms for improvement of antitumor memory responses reactivated by tumor cell vaccine. J Immunol 179:2860–2869

Welte T, Zhang SS, Wang T, Zhang Z, Hesslein DG, Yin Z, Kano A, Iwamoto Y, Li E, Craft JE et al (2003) STAT3 deletion during hematopoiesis causes Crohn's disease-like pathogenesis and lethality: a critical role of STAT3 in innate immunity. Proc Natl Acad Sci USA 100:1879–1884

Wu S, Rhee K-J, Albesiano E, Rabizadeh S, Wu X, Yen H-R, Huso DL, Brancati FL, Wick E, McAllister F et al (2009) A human colonic commensal promotes colon tumorigenesis via activation of T helper type 17 T cell responses. Nat Med 15:1016–1022

Xiang X, Poliakov A, Liu C, Liu Y, Deng ZB, Wang J, Cheng Z, Shah SV, Wang GJ, Zhang L et al (2009) Induction of myeloid-derived suppressor cells by tumor exosomes. Int J Cancer 124:2621–2633

Xin H, Zhang C, Herrmann A, Du Y, Figlin R, Yu H (2009) Sunitinib inhibition of Stat3 induces renal cell carcinoma tumor cell apoptosis and reduces immunosuppressive cells. Cancer Res 69:2506–2513

Yang ZZ, Novak AJ, Stenson MJ, Witzig TE, Ansell SM (2006) Intratumoral CD4+CD25+ regulatory T-cell-mediated suppression of infiltrating CD4+ T cells in B-cell non-Hodgkin lymphoma. Blood 107:3639–3646

Yang DH, Park JS, Jin CJ, Kang HK, Nam JH, Rhee JH, Kim YK, Chung SY, Choi SJ, Kim HJ et al (2009) The dysfunction and abnormal signaling pathway of dendritic cells loaded by tumor antigen can be overcome by neutralizing VEGF in multiple myeloma. Leuk Res 33:665–670

Yang F, Jove V, Xin H, Hedvat M, Van Meter TE, Yu H (2010) Sunitinib induces apoptosis and growth arrest of medulloblastoma tumor cells by inhibiting STAT3 and AKT signaling pathways. Mol Cancer Res 8:35–45

Yao Z, Kanno Y, Kerenyi M, Stephens G, Durant L, Watford WT, Laurence A, Robinson GW, Shevach EM, Moriggl R et al (2007) Nonredundant roles for Stat5a/b in directly regulating Foxp3. Blood 109:4368–4375

Yu H, Jove R (2004) The STATs of cancer–new molecular targets come of age. Nat Rev Cancer 4:97–105

Yu H, Kortylewski M, Pardoll D (2007) Crosstalk between cancer and immune cells: role of STAT3 in the tumour microenvironment. Nat Rev Immunol 7:41–51

Yu H, Pardoll D, Jove R (2009) STATs in cancer inflammation and immunity: a leading role for STAT3. Nat Rev Cancer 9:798–809

Zimmerer JM, Lesinski GB, Kondadasula SV, Karpa VI, Lehman A, Raychaudhury A, Becknell B, Carson WE 3rd (2007) IFN-alpha-induced signal transduction, gene expression, and antitumor activity of immune effector cells are negatively regulated by suppressor of cytokine signaling proteins. J Immunol 178:4832–4845

Zorn E, Nelson EA, Mohseni M, Porcheray F, Kim H, Litsa D, Bellucci R, Raderschall E, Canning C, Soiffer RJ et al (2006) IL-2 regulates FOXP3 expression in human CD4+CD25+ regulatory T cells through a STAT-dependent mechanism and induces the expansion of these cells *in vivo*. Blood 108:1571–1579

Biology and Clinical Observations of Regulatory T Cells in Cancer Immunology

Michele W.L. Teng, David S. Ritchie, Paul Neeson, and Mark J. Smyth

Contents

1 Introduction 63
2 Treg Lineage and Development 63
3 Treg Subsets 64
3.1 Cell Surface Markers of Mouse Tregs 64
3.2 Cell Surface Markers of Human Tregs 65
3.3 Toll Like Receptors Expressed by Tregs 66
3.4 Functional Subsets of Tregs 66
3.5 Treg-Derived Malignancies 67
4 Mechanisms of Treg-Mediated Immune Suppression in Cancer 67
4.1 Immunosuppressive Cytokines and Factors 68
4.2 Suppression by Direct Cell–Cell Contact 68
4.3 Treg-Mediated Cytotoxicity 69
5 Clinical Observations of the Association of Tregs with Cancer 69
6 Modification of Treg Biology as Cancer Immunotherapy 77
6.1 The Cellular Microenvironment 77
6.2 Strategies to Modulate Treg Number and Function 79
6.3 Attenuating Treg Function 80
7 Conclusions 83
References 83

M.W.L. Teng and M.J. Smyth (✉)
Cancer Immunology Program, Peter MacCallum Cancer Centre, East Melbourne 3002, VIC, Australia

Department of Pathology, University of Melbourne, Parkville 3010, VIC, Australia

D.S. Ritchie
Division of Haematology and Medical Oncology, Peter MacCallum Cancer Centre, Locked Bag 1, A'Beckett St., East Melbourne 3002, VIC, Australia

Department of Health Sciences, University of Melbourne, Parkville 3010, VIC, Australia

P. Neeson
Cancer Immunology Program, Peter MacCallum Cancer Centre, East Melbourne 3002, VIC, Australia

G. Dranoff (ed.), *Cancer Immunology and Immunotherapy*,
Current Topics in Microbiology and Immunology 344, DOI 10.1007/82_2010_50

Abstract This review specifically examines the role of regulatory T cells (Tregs) in cancer in both mice and the clinic. Due to the rapid refinement of the definition of Tregs and their heterogeneity, emphasis is given to research findings over the past three years. For clarity, this review is broadly divided into three short sections that outline the basic biology of Tregs – (1) Treg lineage and development, (2) Treg subsets, and (3) mechanisms of Treg-mediated immune suppression; followed by two more comprehensive sections that cover; (4) clinical observations of Tregs and cancer, and (5) modifications of Treg biology as cancer immunotherapies. The latter two sections discuss the measurement of function and frequency of Treg in model systems and clinical trials and possible ways to interfere with Treg-mediated immune suppression with the focus on recent pre-clinical and clinical findings.

Abbreviations

AML	Acute myeloid leukemia
CTL	Cytotoxic T lymphocyte
CTLA-4	Cytotoxic T-lymphocyte antigen 4
DLBCL	Diffuse large B cell lymphoma
FNHL	Follicular non-Hodgkin lymphoma
Foxp3	Forkhead box P3
FR4	Folate receptor 4
GITR	Glucocorticoid-induced tumor necrosis factor receptor
GrzB	Granzyme B
Gvax	Granulocyte/macrophage-colony stimulating factor–secreting cellular vaccine
HCC	Hepatocellular carcinoma
HL	Hodgkin lymphoma
ICOS	Inducible costimulatory molecule
iTreg	Induced Treg
LAG3	Late activation gene 3
LN	Lymph node
mAb	Monoclonal antibody
NRP-1	Neuropilin-1
nTregs	Natural Tregs
SP	Single positive
TCC	Urinary transitional cell carcinoma
TDSR	Treg cell-specific demethylated region
Teff	Effector T cells
TGFβ	Transforming growth factor β
Th1	Thelper1
Th2	Thelper 2
Th17	T helper17
TLR	Toll-like receptor
Tregs	Regulatory T cells

1 Introduction

Regulatory T cells (Tregs) constitute 5–10% of peripheral $CD4^+$ T cells in normal mice and humans, play a key role in maintaining immune tolerance to self, and regulate the immune response to pathogens, commensal organisms, and tumors. Tregs are found in both lymphoid and non-lymphoid tissues with studies demonstrating that preferential accumulation of Tregs over effector T cells (Teff) at sites of disease may be driven by differences in trafficking signals (reviewed by Huehn and Hamann 2005). However, a decrease in Treg numbers and/or function can result in loss of protection against non-tolerant immune responses resulting in autoimmune diseases and conversely, excessive Treg activity may contribute to the suppression of endogenous anti-tumor immune responses and allow the progression of malignancy.

2 Treg Lineage and Development

In mice, Tregs were first described as population of T cells that were capable of suppressing immune responses in a variety of experimental models and were defined by the surface markers CD4 and the IL-2R receptor alpha chain (CD25) (Sakaguchi et al. 1995). The discovery that the X chromosome-encoded gene forkhead box P3 (Foxp3) was the genetic basis for the autoimmune disorder in human patients suffering from IPEX (immune dysregulation, polyendocrinopathy, enteropathy, X-linked) syndrome and in the spontaneous mouse mutant scurfy allowed for the further understanding of Treg biology (Bennett et al. 2001; Brunkow et al. 2001; Hori et al. 2003; Wildin et al. 2001). Foxp3 is critical for the development of thymic derived Tregs (also called natural Tregs) (Fontenot et al. 2003) and sustained high expression of Foxp3 is required to maintain the suppressor function and phenotypic characteristics of peripheral nTregs (Wan and Flavell 2007; Williams and Rudensky 2007). In a recent review, Josefowicz and Rudensky (2009) discuss in detail the requisites of nTreg cell differentiation as defined by induction of Foxp3. While the thymus is a critical organ for the generation of nTregs, naïve $CD4^+$ T cells in the periphery can be induced in several experimental settings either in vitro or in vivo to express Foxp3 and consequently acquire Treg function (Sakaguchi et al. 2008). These peripheral $Foxp3^+$ expressing cells have been called adaptive, induced, or converted Tregs (iTregs) (Curotto de Lafaille and Lafaille 2009; Feuerer et al. 2009; Shevach 2006), and transforming growth factor β (TGF-β) receptor signaling appears to be required for most, if not all, of the induction of Foxp3 among peripheral naive $CD4^+$ T cells (Josefowicz and Rudensky 2009). Interestingly, there is ongoing debate regarding whether Foxp3 is the only transcription factor required to define the Treg lineage (see Feuerer et al. 2009) for detailed review and discussion). Nevertheless, Foxp3 is currently accepted as the most specific marker to define Tregs and most studies now define

Tregs derived from the thymus as $CD4^+CD25^+Foxp3^+$. In this regard, it is a caveat to keep in mind when analyzing prior work on Tregs defined as $CD4^+CD25^+$ T cells without regard to Foxp3 status.

In addition to nTregs and iTregs, two regulatory subsets of $CD4^+$ T cells termed Th3 and Tr1 have also been described in the Treg literature. Th3 cells are induced following oral administration of antigens (Chen et al. 1994) whereas Tr1 cells are antigen-specific T cells induced in the presence of IL-10 (Groux et al. 1997). Tr1 cells generally do not express Foxp3 (Shevach 2006) and not all Th3 cells express Foxp3 (Carrier et al. 2007). While iTregs, Tr1, and Th3 cells have been shown to have suppressive capabilities similar to nTregs in vitro (Hori et al. 2003; Sakaguchi et al. 2008), they do not have the same transcriptional profile as nTregs and as yet there are no definitive surface markers to distinguish between nTregs and iTregs (Feuerer et al. 2009). iTregs, together with other immune cells play an important role in the maintaining homeostasis of gut-associated lymphoid tissue (Weaver and Hatton 2009). There is accumulating evidence that the difference in stability of FoxP3 expression between nTreg and iTreg cells is due to epigenetic changes at the Treg cell-specific demethylated region (TDSR) in the FoxP3 locus (Huehn et al. 2009; Baron et al. 2007; Floess et al. 2007; Kim and Leonard 2007; Nagar et al. 2008; Polansky et al. 2008). Key questions are whether Tregs induced from naive T cells in the periphery are functionally stable in vivo and to what extent do iTregs contribute to the peripheral pool of $Foxp3^+$ Tregs and in suppressing anti-tumor immunity (Josefowicz and Rudensky 2009; Sakaguchi et al. 2008). In the remainder of this review, we will focus on the role of thymic derived $Foxp3^+$ nTregs (which we will just refer to as Tregs henceforth) and cancer, but we will discuss iTregs where appropriate.

3 Treg Subsets

3.1 *Cell Surface Markers of Mouse Tregs*

In both mice and humans, nTregs are a heterogeneous population and can be categorized into several subsets based on their differential expression of surface markers for activation/memory, adhesion molecules, and chemokine receptors. In mice, nTregs express surface markers characteristic of an activated T cell such as CTLA-4 (cytotoxic T-lymphocyte antigen 4) and GITR (glucocorticoid-induced tumor necrosis factor receptor) (Sakaguchi et al. 2008). Although neuropilin-1 (NRP-1) (Bruder et al. 2004; Sarris et al. 2008) and folate receptor 4 (FR4) (Yamaguchi et al. 2007) are highly expressed on Tregs, there are currently no surface markers that are exclusively expressed by Tregs. In addition, co-stimulatory molecules such as 4-1BB (CD137) and OX40 (CD134) are constitutively expressed on Tregs (Burmeister et al. 2008; Vu et al. 2007) while a proportion of Tregs express ICOS (inducible costimulatory molecule, CD278) (Gotsman et al. 2006).

Studies have reported that ligating both OX40 and 4-1BB on Treg can strongly influence their responsiveness to self or non-self antigen, both in positive and negative manners (reviewed in So et al. 2008).

3.2 *Cell Surface Markers of Human Tregs*

Human Tregs were originally defined as $CD4^{+}CD25^{hi}$ and while this phenotype included cells with suppressor function, this proved to be an inaccurate definition as $CD4^{+}CD25^{hi}$ included activated $CD4^{+}$ T cells (Jonuleit et al. 2001; Seddiki et al. 2006a, b). Thus, interpretation of human Treg frequency and functional suppressor studies was difficult, as the results were likely skewed by a contaminating population of activated non-Treg $CD4^{+}$ T cells. As in mice, Foxp3 was revealed as the hallmark transcription factor for human Treg (Roncador et al. 2005; Yagi et al. 2004). More recently, Tregs have been also shown to express CD127 (IL-7Rα) at low levels, due to CD127 transcriptional down regulation by Foxp3 (Liu et al. 2006b). Currently, the multi-parameter phenotype $CD3^{+}CD4^{+}Foxp3^{+}CD127^{lo}$ defines human peripheral blood Treg cells (Hartigan-O'Connor et al. 2007; Seddiki et al. 2006a). These Tregs have functional suppressor function in T cell proliferation assays. The expression of CD25 is no longer a defining phenotype for Treg as the $CD3^{+}CD4^{+}Foxp3^{+}CD127^{lo}CD25^{-}$ T cell population also shows potent suppressor function (Seddiki et al. 2006a). Finally, in an elegant study by Sakaguchi et al. (Miyara et al. 2009), human $CD4^{+}$ T cells with suppressor function (in vitro) were shown to have two main phenotypes, including $Foxp3^{lo}CD45RA^{+}$ resting Tregs (rTregs) and $CD45RA^{-}Foxp3^{hi}$ activated Tregs (aTregs). Interestingly, they described a third population of cells that were $CD45RA^{-}/Foxp3^{lo}$ cytokine-secreting non-suppressive cells. Terminally differentiated aTregs died rapidly while rTregs proliferated rapidly and converted into aTregs both in vitro and in vivo (Miyara et al. 2009).

In addition, to $CD4^{+}Foxp3^{+}$ Tregs, $CD8^{+}CD25^{+}$ Tregs have recently been identified and are present within the human tumor microenvironment (Joosten et al. 2007; Kiniwa et al. 2007). These $CD8^{+}$ Tregs express CD122, Foxp3, and GITR, markers associated with $CD4^{+}$ Treg (Cosmi et al. 2003; Kiniwa et al. 2007). The $CD8^{+}$ Tregs suppress antigen-specific $CD4^{+}$ and $CD8^{+}$ T cell responses (proliferation and cytokine release) through a cell–cell contact dependent pathway or cytokines, e.g., IL-10 (Endharti et al. 2005; Kiniwa et al. 2007). Thus, $CD8^{+}$ $CD25^{+}$ Tregs resemble $CD4^{+}$ Treg in function and phenotype. $CD8^{+}$ Tregs are not detectable in the peripheral blood and are restricted to the tumor microenvironment, and this suggests that they are induced within the tumor or a cytokine environment favorable to Treg induction (Kiniwa et al. 2007). Human $CD8^{+}$ Tregs have been detected in many types of cancer including gastrointestinal, breast, lung, head and neck, cervical, prostate, ovarian, melanoma, and liver (Beyer and Schultze 2006; Jarnicki et al. 2006; Joosten et al. 2007; Kiniwa et al. 2007; Piersma et al. 2008; Wang and Wang 2007; Wei et al. 2005).

3.3 Toll Like Receptors Expressed by Tregs

TLRs which recognize conserved molecular products derived from various classes of pathogens are expressed by mouse Tregs (Dai et al. 2009); however, many of the current studies assessing TLR expression on mouse or human Tregs have not used Foxp3 to define Tregs and TLR expression was often assessed by mRNA expression rather than by flow cytometry. Nevertheless, mouse nTregs ($Foxp3^+$) have been shown to express TLR2 intracellularly and on their surface following activation (Liu et al. 2006a), while human Tregs (defined by $CD4^+CD25^{hi}$) have also been shown to express TLR2, TLR4 (Rajashree and Das 2008), TLR5 (defined by Foxp3) (Crellin et al. 2005), and TLR8 (mRNA expression of Foxp3) (Peng et al. 2005). Interestingly, $CD4^+$ Tregs were reported to express higher levels of TLR4, TLR5, TLR7, and TLR8 compared with effector T cells (Kabelitz 2007; Sutmuller et al. 2006b). Peng et al. (2005) demonstrated that triggering of human TLR8 with synthetic (poly G10) and natural TLR8 ligands inhibited human $CD4^+$ Treg suppressive function, but not effector T cell function.

3.4 Functional Subsets of Tregs

A number of studies have demonstrated that certain homing receptors such as selectin ligands and chemokine receptors on Treg subsets critically influence their suppressive capacity in vivo suggesting that appropriate localization is indispensable for Treg function (Siegmund et al. 2005; Siewert et al. 2007). A definitive role for CCR4 in the recruitment of $CCR4^+$ Tregs to tumor sites has been reported in mice (Mailloux and Young 2009; Olkhanud et al. 2009) and in humans (Gobert et al. 2009; Mizukami et al. 2008; Takegawa et al. 2008). In addition to CCR4, a recent study reported an increased infiltration of $CCR5^+$ Tregs into the pancreas in a mouse model of pancreatic cancer (Tan et al. 2009).

A proportion of Tregs have an activated/memory phenotype, characterized by a higher expression of CD103, CD44, GITR, and CTLA4, and are thought to be involved in the permanent suppression of immune responses against self antigens (Huehn et al. 2004; Stephens et al. 2007). A recent study demonstrated that these self-specific activated/memory Tregs (amTregs) were able to immediately sense tumors that were either implanted or induced in-situ (Darrasse-Jeze et al. 2009). Such a rapid response by these amTregs prevented naïve anti-tumor T cells to be activated. In addition, another study showed that amTregs played an important role in the suppression of concomitant immunity in the mouse (BALB/c) colon cancer cell line, CT26 and suggested that loss of this immunity may contribute to tumor metastasis (Lin et al. 2009). Chen et al. described that amTregs expressing TNFR2 had even greater suppressive effects than $CD103^+$ expressing Tregs (Chen et al. 2008).

Although Tregs can be phenotyped by their differential expression of surface markers as discussed above, very recent studies have demonstrated that Tregs can express different transcription factors such as Tbet, IRF-4, or STAT3, which allows them to mediate specific suppression on Th1, Th2, or Th17 cells, respectively (Chaudhry et al. 2009; Koch et al. 2009; Zheng et al. 2009). Very elegantly, Koch et al. demonstrated that Tregs from Tbet-deficient mice were unable to express CXCR3 and thus were not able to traffic to sites of inflammation induced by Th1 cells. In addition, this study also demonstrated that in vivo, Tregs upregulate their Tbet expression when exposed to a Th1 cytokine milieu and that IFN-γR plays a key role in the induction of Tbet expression in Tregs. Thus, by being able to express similar patterns of homing receptors as effector T cells, Tregs can selectively traffic and localize to different lymphoid organs and tissues to mediate their immune suppression.

3.5 Treg-Derived Malignancies

An intriguing recent realization is that Tregs may also be a source population from which malignancy develops or alternatively, that $CD4^+$ T cell malignancies may mimic Treg function. These malignancies include a proportion of patients with adult T cell leukemia/lymphoma (Abe et al. 2008; Karube et al. 2004) or the $CD4^+$ T cell malignancy Sezary Syndrome (Krejsgaard et al. 2008; Marzano et al. 2009). While the Treg-like phenotype of these tumors has largely relied on the demonstration of either wild type or splice variant form of Foxp3, the functional suppressor function of Sezary Syndrome mediated by IL-10 and TGF-β production has also recently been demonstrated, strongly suggesting that this malignant T cell lymphoma has a true Treg origin (Krejsgaard et al. 2008).

4 Mechanisms of Treg-Mediated Immune Suppression in Cancer

Tregs suppress the proliferation of naïve T cells and their differentiation to Teff in vivo. They have also been shown to mediate suppression on innate and adaptive immune cells such as suppression of the effector function of differentiated $CD4^+$ and $CD8^+$ T cells and of the function of NK cells, NKT cells, B cells, macrophages, osteoclasts, and DCs (reviewed in Sakaguchi et al. 2008). From a functional perspective, there are three major mechanisms of Treg-mediated suppression: immunosuppressive cytokines and factors, suppression by direct cell–cell contact, and cytolysis, (previously reviewed in Shevach 2009; Vignali et al. 2008). It should be noted that most of the studies ascribing a molecule or a process utilized by Tregs to mediate their suppressive activities derive from in vitro studies and a limited number of in vivo disease models (Tang and Bluestone 2008). We will only briefly describe these here in the context of recent work.

4.1 *Immunosuppressive Cytokines and Factors*

These include TGF-β (Wrzesinski et al. 2007), interleukin-10 (IL-10) (Maynard et al. 2007), and the newly discovered IL-12 family member IL-35 (Collison et al. 2007). Although the general importance of IL-10 and TGF-β as mediators of immunoregulation and inflammation is undisputed, their role as suppressor molecules remains controversial (Chen et al. 2005; Ghiringhelli et al. 2005; Larmonier et al. 2007; Loser et al. 2007; Petrausch et al. 2009; Ralainirina et al. 2007; Rubtsov et al. 2008; Shevach 2006; Smyth et al. 2006). Further analysis of the contribution of IL-35 to Treg-mediated suppression will require the development of neutralizing monoclonal antibodies (mAbs) and characterization of its receptor (Shevach 2009). In addition to immunosuppressive cytokines, Tregs can produce suppressive factors such as adenosine (Deaglio et al. 2007; Kobie et al. 2006) and cAMP (Bopp et al. 2007) to mediate suppression. Pericellular adenosine is generated by the degradation of extracellular nucleotide by two ectoenzymes, CD39 and CD73 which are expressed on ~80% of Foxp3^{+} Treg cells (Deaglio et al. 2007). Although these mechanisms represent interesting additions to the arsenal of Tregs, further studies will be required to corroborate these findings and assess their relative use by Tregs in different disease settings including cancer.

4.2 *Suppression by Direct Cell–Cell Contact*

Tregs can mediate suppression through direct modulation of immune cells by cell–cell contact using different cell surface molecules such as CTLA-4, lymphocyte activation gene 3 (LAG-3), and Nrp-1. The critical role for CTLA-4 in Treg suppression was recently clarified by the generation of mice lacking CTLA-4 only in Foxp3^{+} Tregs (Wing et al. 2008). Other surface molecules that may play a role in Treg suppression or modulation of DC function are LAG-3 (Liang et al. 2008) and Nrp-1 (Sarris et al. 2008). LAG-3 is a CD4 homolog that binds MHC class II molecules with very high affinity and has been shown to suppress DC maturation and immunostimulatory capacity, while Nrp-1 is thought to promote long interactions between Tregs and immature DCs, which may potentially give Tregs a lead kinetically over naïve responder T cells under conditions in which antigen is limiting (reviewed in Shevach et al. 2008). However, it is not known whether these molecules are employed by Tregs during suppression of tumor immunity.

4.3 *Treg-Mediated Cytotoxicity*

Cytotoxicity of target cells has been proposed as another suppressive mechanism used by Tregs (Gondek et al. 2005; Zhao et al. 2006). Although both studies were interesting, Tregs in these studies were defined only as $CD4^{+}CD25^{+}$ and the role of Tregs lacking Granzyme B (GrzB) or perforin in suppression of anti-tumor immunity was not directly demonstrated. To address this issue, Cao et al., attempted to determine whether Treg utilized GrzB and/or perforin to suppress immune responses in a number tumor models in vivo (Cao et al. 2007). The authors reported that Tregs suppressed the ability of NK cells and cytotoxic T lymphocytes (CTLs) to clear tumors by killing these cells in a GrzB- and perforin-dependent manner. However, their study did not directly assess if there was a reduction in survival of tumor bearing GrzB-deficient mice following transfer of wild-type Tregs. Indeed, in five different tumor models where tumor rejection was stringently dependent upon perforin, including some of those used above, GrzA and B clusters were not essential for CTL- and NK cell-mediated rejection of spontaneous and experimental tumors (Davis et al. 2001; Smyth et al. 2003). To definitively assess if Tregs do utilize GrzB or perforin to mediate suppression of tumor immunity, it will be necessary to create mice specifically lacking GrzB or perforin in $Foxp3^{+}$ Tregs.

Overall, results from in vitro and in vivo studies suggested that Tregs use multiple mechanisms to suppress immune responses. However, the relative dominance of each mechanism in the suppression of anti-tumor immunity, and whether there are differential requirements for distinct suppressive functions of Tregs at different tissues or against different tumor types, still need to be assessed. Generating Tregs deficient in individual molecules and testing them in various tumor models will be useful. Such work will further our understanding of Treg suppressor mechanism and offer us insight into how we can attenuate Treg function in vivo to enhance anti-tumor immunity.

5 Clinical Observations of the Association of Tregs with Cancer

The main clinical observations are summarized for hematological malignancies and solid organ malignancies in Tables 1 and 2, respectively. The clearest functional association of Tregs in hematological malignancy is with the B cell-derived lymphomas, follicular non-Hodgkin lymphoma (FNHL), diffuse large B cell lymphoma (DLBCL), and Hodgkin lymphoma (HL). In studies of FNHL, Tregs have been largely defined as $CD4^{+}CD25^{+}$ $Foxp3^{+}$, shown to be functionally suppressive, and found to be highly concentrated in lymph node (LN) involved by lymphoma. FNHL-associated Tregs are therefore likely to actively inhibit the control of lymphoma by endogenous immunosurveillance (Yang et al. 2007, 2009). The enrichment of Treg within involved LN is likely due to expression of CCL22 by malignant B cells (Yang et al. 2006a). However, naïve peripheral $CD4^{+}$ T cells may

Table 1 Treg enumeration and function and clinical outcome correlation in hematological malignancies

Cancer type	Pts	Controls	Treg definition	Tissue	Immunology	Clinical observation	References
FNHL	24	5 (PB) 6 (Tonsil) 6 (LN)	$CD4^{+}CD25^{+}$ $FoxP3^{+}$ FC	Tumor biopsy	B cells express CCL22 Tregs suppress autologous anti-lymphoma CTL	NR	Yang et al. (2006a)
B cell NHL	28	ND	$CD4^{+}CD25^{+}$ $FoxP3^{+}$ IHC	Tumor biopsy	Tregs suppress CD8+ T cell function and number in LN	NR	Yang et al. (2006b)
FNHL	97	ND	$CD4^{+}CD25^{+}$ $FoxP3^{+}$IHC	Tumor biopsy	ND	Increased Tregs improved OS	Carreras et al. (2006)
FNHL	83	ND	FoxP3+ IHC	Tumor biopsy	ND	Increased Tregs improved OS	Tzankov et al. (2008)
DLBCL GC-like	81	ND	FoxP3+ IHC	Tumor biopsy	ND	Increased Tregs improved OS	
DLBCL Non-GC	98	ND	FoxP3+ IHC	Tumor biopsy	ND	Increased Tregs reduced OS	
HL	280	ND	FoxP3+ IHC	Tumor biopsy	ND	Increased Tregs improved OS and DFS	
HL	24	5	$CD4^{+}CD25^{+}$ FC	Tumor biopsy	IL-10 production, CTLA-4 expression and suppression of normal T cells	NR	Marshall et al. (2004)
HL	257	ND	$CD4^{+}CD25^{+}$ $FoxP3^{+}$IHC	Tumor biopsy		Decreased Tregs reduced OS	Alvaro et al. (2005)
CLL	60	10	$CD4^{+}CD25^{+}$ $FoxP3^{+}$ FC	Peripheral blood	ND	Tregs increased in CLL vs controls. Higher Tregs in more advanced disease. Tregs fell following thalidomide therapy	Giannopoulos et al. (2008)

MM	NS	NR	$CD4^+CD25^+$ FC	Peripheral blood	ND	Tregs higher in MM vs controls. Tregs lower at baseline in thalidomide responsive patients and increased on thalidomide	Yang et al. (2008)
MM	25	10	CD127dim $CD25^+$ $FoxP3^+$	Peripheral blood	ND	Tregs profoundly low in MM vs controls. Tregs increased on lenalidomide	Quach et al. 2008 (abstract 1696)
MM/MGUS	67/9	42	$CD4^+CD25^+$ FC	Peripheral blood	Treg expressed GITR, CTLA-4, IL-10 and TGF-β, and suppressed allogeneic MLR	Tregs elevated in MM and MGUS vs controls	Beyer et al. (2006)
AML			$CD4^+CD25^+$ $FoxP3^+$ FC	Peripheral blood	IL-10 and TGF-β production and suppression of normal T cells	Increased Tregs associated with reduced survival	Szczepanski et al. (2009)

Pts patients numbers in analysis, *FNHL* follicular non-Hodgkin lymphoma, *DLBCL* diffuse large B cell, *GC* germinal center cell, *HL* Hodgkin lymphoma, *CLL* chronic lymphocytic leukemia, *MM* multiple myeloma, *MGUS* monoclonal gammopathy of undetermined significance, *AML* acute myeloid leukemia, *NR* not reported, *ND* not done, *LN* lymph node, *FC* flow cytometry, *IHC* immunohistochemistry, *CTL* cytotoxic T lymphocyte, *GITR* glucocorticoid-induced TNF-R related protein, *MLR* mixed lymphocyte reaction, *OS* overall survival

Table 2 Treg enumeration and function and clinical outcome correlation in solid organ malignancy

Cancer type	Pts	Controls	Treg definition	Tissue	Immunology	Clinical observation	References
Epithelial malignancy	42	34	$CD4^+/CD25^+$ / $CD45RA^+$/ $CTLA\text{-}4^+$	Peripheral blood	TGF-β production and inhibitionof NK function	NR	Wolf et al. (2003)
Uterine cervix	14	4	CD4/CD25/$Nrp\text{-}1^+$	LN and peripheral blood	Nrp-1+ Tregs potently suppressive of T cell responses	Treg numbers in LN fall proportionally to tumor response	Battaglia et al. (2008)
Ovarian	104	–	$CD4^+CD25^+FoxP3^+$	Tumor biopsy and ascitic fluid	Tumor derived CCL22 enrich Tregs in tumor. Tregs suppress tumor specific T cells	High Treg numbers associated with poorer OS	Curiel et al. (2004)
Ovarian	306	–	$FoxP3^+$ IHC	Tumor biopsy	ND	High Treg numbers and high CD8: Treg ratio associated with improved survival in advanced metastatic disease	Leffers et al. (2009)
Ovarian	9	9	$CD4^+CD25^+$ FC	Tumor biopsy, ascitic fluid, peripheral blood	TGF-β production by Tregs	Increased Tregs in patients vs controls	Woo et al. (2001)
NSCLC	8			Tumor biopsy, Peripheral blood			
NSCLC	64	–	$CD3^+$ $FoxP3^+$ IHC	Tumor biopsy	ND	Low TIL: Treg ratio associated higher recurrence rate	Petersen et al. (2006)
Head and neck cancer	84	–	$CD4^+FoxP3^+$ IHC	Tumor biopsy	ND	Increased Tregs associated with improved 2 year survival (42% vs 89%)	Badoual et al. (2006)
HCC	84	53 (Non-malignant liver disease) 21 (healthy donors)	$CD4^+$ $CD25^+$ $CTLA4^+$ $GITR^+$ FC	Peripheral blood, LN, tumor biopsy	TIL Tregs and PB Tregs suppress T cell proliferation	Increased Tregs in PB of patients vs controls	Ormandy et al. (2005)

HCC	302	–	$FoxP3^+$ IHC	Tumor biopsy	CD3, CD4, CD8 granzyme B staining	Shows prognostic importance of CD8 to FoxP3 ratio	Gao et al. (2007)
Gastric cancer Esophageal cancer	20 10	16	$CD4^+CD25^+$	Peripheral blood and mucosal biopsies	IL-10 production and T cell inhibition	Increased Tregs in patients vs controls	Ichihara et al. (2003)
Gastric cancer	52	–	$CD4^+CD25^+FoxP3^+$ IHC	Tumor biopsy	ND	Increased Tregs associated with improved survival	Haas et al. (2009)
Gastro-intestinal malignancies	149	10	$CD4^+CD25^+$	Peripheral blood	IL4 and IL-10 production. Inhibition of cytokine production by T cells	High Treg numbers associated advanced disease and poorer OS in gastric cancer	Sasada et al. (2003)
Colorectal cancer	967	–	$CD4^+CD25^+FoxP3^+$ IHC	Tumor biopsy	ND	Higher Tregs associated with improved survival	Salama et al. (2009)
Pancreatic cancer Breast cancer	30 35	35	$CD4^+CD25^+$	Peripheral blood, LN, tumor biopsy	TGF-β and IL-10 production Tregs inhibit T cell cytokine production and proliferation	Increased Tregs in PB of patients vs controls	Liyanage et al. (2002)
Prostate	20	–	$CD4^+CD25^+$, $GITR^+$ FC, MA	Peripheral blood, tumor biopsy	CD4+ TILs skewed towards Tregs and Th17 cells. Tregs enriched in prostate vs PB	Increased Th17 cells in prostate associated with lower Gleason stage. No association between Tregs and Gleason stage	Sfanos et al. (2008)
Transitional cell cancer	93	38 (benign urinary) 37 (healthy donors)	$CD4^+CD25^+$ $CD127^{low}$	Peripheral blood	NR	Increased Tregs in patients vs controls Increased Tregs associated with higher stage disease and higher recurrence rate	Zhu et al. (2009)

(*continued*)

Table 2 (continued)

Cancer type	Pts	Controls	Treg definition	Tissue	Immunology	Clinical observation	References
						Tregs fell with tumor debulking	
Melanoma	12	–	$CD4^{+}CD25^{+}FoxP3^{+}$	Peripheral blood, LN	Tregs enriched in tumor LN compared to normal LN or PB Treg suppression of T cells Treg production of IL-10 and TGF-β	NR	Viguier et al. (2004)
Melanoma	30	–	$CD4^{+}CD25^{+}CD69^{-}$	Peripheral blood		Increased Tregs in PB of patients vs controls	Gray et al. (2003)

HCC hepatocellular carcinoma, *NSCLC* non-small cell lung cancer, *MA* micro-array, *NK* natural killer cell, *TIL* tumor infiltrating lymphocytes. See Table 1 for additional abbreviations also be driven by FNHL B cells to undergo Treg differentiation (Ai et al. 2009). Therefore, the Tregs associated with FNHL may be potentially induced at the sites of disease or enriched within the lymphoma under the influence of tumor-derived chemokines. Critically, FNHL B cells may skew the differentiation of CD4 T cells towards Tregs at the expense of Th17 cells (Yang et al. 2009) further promoting the immunosuppressive microenvironment within NHL LN affected.

Given the immunosuppressive capacity of Tregs, it seems paradoxical that increased Tregs have been repeatedly associated with an improved prognosis in FNHL (Carreras et al. 2006; Tzankov et al. 2008), the germinal center cell subtype of DLBCL (Tzankov et al. 2008), and HL (Alvaro et al. 2005; Tzankov et al. 2008) (Table 1). Three observations from these studies suggest that the subtype of lymphoma may determine both the enrichment of Tregs and the prognostic outcome. Firstly, a profoundly low (<5%) proportion of Tregs in FNHL is associated with a higher risk of refractivity to chemotherapy (Carreras et al. 2006). As B cell lymphoma evolves to increasing levels of malignancy (i.e., away from a follicular pattern and towards large cell disease), the ability for NHL cells to attract Treg infiltrates may also fall. This is supported by a second observation that Treg numbers fall precipitously when FNHL undergoes transformation to DLBCL (Carreras et al. 2006). Lastly, higher Treg numbers within lymphoma biopsies had negative prognostic impact in the setting of the poorer prognosis activated B-cell (ABC) subtype of DLBCL.

Treg biology in multiple myeloma (MM) remains the least clear of B cell malignancies (reviewed in Joshua et al. 2008). Much of the lack of clarity in MM likely stems from the use of potently immunosuppressive and lympholytic therapies, the wide range of disease stages assessed, and variations in the definition of Treg phenotype (Beyer et al. 2006; Yang et al. 2008) (Quach et al. 2008 Abstract 1696). In acute myeloid leukemia (AML), there is recent evidence that functionally suppressive Tregs accumulate in the peripheral blood of patients with AML (Szczepanski et al. 2009). AML associated Tregs may be due to the presentation of B7-H1 on DC-like leukemia cells (Ge et al. 2009). Furthermore, and in contradistinction to B cell lymphoma, increased Tregs in AML are associated with a poorer response to induction chemotherapy (Szczepanski et al. 2009). This clinical observation is in agreement with data from an AML mouse model that revealed that depletion of Tregs enhanced responses to adoptive CTL therapy in AML (Zhou et al. 2009a).

In solid organ malignancies, the prognostic impact of Treg number and function is less well described (Table 2). Early analyses have shown an increased frequency of peripheral blood TGF-β-producing $CD4^+CD25^+CD45RA^+CTLA\text{-}4^+$ T cells in peripheral blood compared to that of normal donors (Wolf et al. 2003). Subsets of Tregs have been shown to be elevated in the draining LN in patients with cervical cancer and were found to fall in proportion to the degree of tumor regression following therapy (Battaglia et al. 2008). Similarly, $CD4^+CD25^+Foxp3^+$ Tregs are over represented within ovarian cancer-associated lymphocytes in malignant ascites, likely due to the production of CCL22 (Curiel et al. 2004). In this study, Tregs were found to suppress tumor-specific T cell immunity and contribute to growth of human tumors in vivo resulting in reduced overall survival due to tumor progression (Curiel et al. 2004). Conversely, another study of ovarian cancer, analysis of Foxp3 expressing tumor infiltrating lymphocytes (TIL) showed that both increased Treg numbers and a high CD8 T cell:Treg ratio were independently associated with improved survival (Leffers et al. 2009). The reasons for these apparently conflicting findings may be partly explained by variation in tumor grade and stage at the time of Treg analysis; the definition of Tregs and the more recent use of Foxp3 as a specific (and sometimes sole) marker may overestimate the number of Tregs within the analyzed sample.

In colorectal cancer, suppression of the cytolytic capacity of peripheral blood CTL has also been demonstrated to be due to the production of TGF-β from Treg (Somasundaram et al. 2002). Peripheral blood and TIL Tregs are also increased in gastric and esophageal cancers. $CD4^{+}CD25^{+}$ cells in TIL and mucosal biopsies were highest in gastric cancer patients with advanced disease (Ichihara et al. 2003). Other studies in gastric carcinoma have shown that higher percentages of $CD4^{+}CD25^{+}$ T cells had a poorer prognosis. In addition, $CD4^{+}CD25^{+}$ T cells were present in greater proportions in the ascites from patients who had advanced-stage disease with peritoneal dissemination (Sasada et al. 2003). However, other studies have again given apparently conflicting prognostic data in gastric cancer of the stomach cardia, where increase in $Foxp3^{+}$ Tregs was associated with an improved clinical outcome (Haas et al. 2009). Patients with hepatocellular carcinoma (HCC) were found to have increased numbers Treg cells in their peripheral blood compared to that of both healthy donors and patients with non-malignant hepatic conditions. Tregs were also enriched in the ascitic fluid of patients with HCC in a manner analogous to that seen in ovarian cancer. (Ormandy et al. 2005).

Increased $CTLA\text{-}4^{+}CD45RO^{+}$ Tregs in PB, TILs, and regional lymph nodes have been shown in breast cancer and pancreatic cancer (Liyanage et al. 2002), and in LN positive metastatic melanoma, where Tregs were defined as $CD4^{+}CD25^{hi}Foxp3^{+}$ (Viguier et al. 2004). In both of these studies, Treg populations inhibited the proliferation and cytokine production of autologous $CD8^{+}$ T cells. Recently, Tregs in melanoma-infiltrating lymphocytes were found to express higher levels of ICOS compared to the Tregs in peripheral blood. $ICOS^{high}$ Treg mediated stronger $CD8^{+}$ T cell suppression compared to $ICOS^{low}$ Treg (Strauss et al. 2008).

In prostate cancer, high percentages of $CD4^{+}CD25^{+}$ $Foxp3^{+}$ and Th17 T cells have been shown in the majority (70%) of prostate TILs. Intriguingly, a Th17-profile in this study was associated with a lower pathologic Gleason score (Sfanos et al. 2008). Other tumor types associated with increased Tregs include non-small cell lung cancer (a predominance of TGF-β-producing, $CD4^{+}CD25^{+}$ T cells in TIL) (Woo et al. 2001) and urinary transitional cell carcinoma (TCC) (Zhu et al. 2009). In the Zhu et al. report, a strong correlation was found between the proportion of Tregs and the likelihood of tumor recurrence, number of lymph node metastasis, and pathological stage. Importantly, the proportion of Tregs fell following tumor resection suggesting that the resection of tumor bulk can induce a reduction of Tregs in peripheral blood.

6 Modification of Treg Biology as Cancer Immunotherapy

6.1 The Cellular Microenvironment

Tregs remain one of the major obstacles to successful cancer immunotherapy. Other leukocytes, including myeloid derived suppressor cells (MDSC), tumor associated macrophages (TAMs), type I/II NKT cells, mast cells, B cells, and subsets of DC have also been implicated in promoting tumor progression. In this section, we will first discuss how Tregs and other immunomodulatory cells are associated in tumor-mediated suppression before discussing clinical strategies to attenuate Treg function to improve current immunotherapeutic strategies.

During tumor development and progression, proinflammatory and immunosuppressive factors can be secreted from tumors or host cells into the tumor microenvironment that lead to immune evasion and promotion of tumor growth (de Visser and Coussens 2006; Mantovani et al. 2008). The major leukocyte population implicated in aiding tumor progression includes Tregs, MDSC (reviewed in Ostrand-Rosenberg and Sinha 2009), and TAMs (reviewed in Solinas et al. 2009). MDSC are a heterogeneous population of cells generally defined as Gr-1^{+}CD11b^{+}, and induced by proinflammatory cytokines such as IL-1β (Bunt et al. 2006; Song et al. 2005), IL-6 (Bunt et al. 2007), and the bioactive lipid PGE_2 (Sinha et al. 2007). Depending on the subpopulation of MDSC, Tregs can be induced through MDSC production of IL-10 and TGFβ (Huang et al. 2006), or arginase alone (Serafini et al. 2008).

TAMs originate from blood monocytes recruited to the tumor site (Mantovani et al. 1992) as a result of CCL2, M-CSF, and VEGF which are produced by neoplastic and stromal cells. Monocytes differentiate into TAMs upon exposure to CSFs, IL-4, IL-13, IL-10, and TGF-β. In turn, TAMs promote tumor survival by modifying neoplastic extracellular matrix (ECM) proteins, stimulating angiogenesis and inducing immunosuppression via the production of IL-10 and the secretion of chemokines (e.g., CCL17 and CCL22), which preferentially attract T cell subsets such as Tregs and Th2 (Balkwill 2004; Mantovani et al. 2004).

The relative hierarchy and importance of Tregs, MDSC, and TAMs in immune suppression and their temporal cross-regulation during the course of tumor progression still remain to be elucidated. It is likely that different cancer types or the location of the cancer dictates which immunomodulatory cells are preferentially recruited and/or induced to mediate immune suppression. In a study to evaluate the interplay between tumor and the different immunomodulatory cells during disease progression, Clark et el., generated a transgenic mouse model where expression of oncogenic $Kras^{G12D}$ was induced under the pancreas-specific promoters *Pdx-1* or *p48* (Clark et al. 2007). These mice spontaneously developed pancreatic ductal adenocarcinoma (PDA), which is markedly infiltrated by Tregs before the development of invasive disease (PanIN). Subsequently, macrophages (Gr-1^{-}CD11b^{+}) and then MDSC (Gr-1^{+}CD11b^{+}) infiltrate the tumor. Similar findings have been shown in the A20 B cell lymphoma tumor model, in which increased percentages of intratumoral and systemic Tregs are found, along with high intratumoral and systemic IL-10, and moderate levels of intratumoral TGF-β (Elpek et al. 2007). Additional studies reveal that A20 cells also express PD-L1 and secrete IL-10 and immunomodulatory IDO all of which contribute to the generation and function of iTregs (Baban et al. 2009). Importantly, this study also showed by depletion experiments that Tregs played a dominant role in early tumor progression in vivo. In contrast, a recent paper by Denardo et al., utilizing the MMTV-PyMT model of mammary carcinogenesis, demonstrated a tumor-promoting role for Th2-$CD4^+$IL-4 producing T cells, but not for Tregs, in sculpting the function of TAM to promote pulmonary metastasis of mammary adenocarcinomas (DeNardo et al. 2009). While some studies suggest that Tregs may often serve as the dominant immune escape mechanism early in tumor progression (Elpek et al. 2007), it should be noted that there are no mAbs that can specifically deplete all $Foxp3^+$ Tregs. Studies in which all $Foxp3^+$ Tregs can be depleted using Foxp3DTR mice (Kim et al. 2007; Lahl et al. 2007) will prove very useful for dissecting out the importance of Treg-mediated suppression in established tumors.

Generally, tumors progress when heavily infiltrated by inflammatory innate immune cells (i.e., macrophages, neutrophils, and mast cells) and they are rich in inflammatory cytokines, growth factors, and pro-angiogenic molecules (Badoual et al. 2009). It has been proposed that the presence of large numbers of local Tregs early on in inflammatory sites can delay or prevent inflammation-induced cancers (Haas et al. 2009). This is also supported by studies of $Apc^{Min/+}$ (multiple intestinal neoplasia (Min)) mice where the adoptive transfer of $CD4^+CD25^+$ lymphocytes induced tumor apoptosis, the regression of established adenomas, and down-regulation of COX-2 and proinflammatory cytokines within intestinal polyps (Erdman et al. 2005). The influx of mast cells (mastocytosis) was a necessary event for polyp outgrowth in $Apc^{\Delta 468}$ mice. A recent report by Gounaris et al. supported these relationships (Colombo and Piconese 2009; Gounaris et al. 2009). Interestingly, endogenous $Foxp3^+$ Tregs were found in elevated numbers in these polyp bearing $Apc^{\Delta 468}$ mice but intriguingly they had lost the ability to produce IL-10 with a proportion actually found to express the pro-inflammatory cytokine IL-17 preferentially produced by effector Th17 cells.

There are conflicting data on the role of IL-17 in carcinogenesis (Kryczek et al. 2009; Wang et al. 2009). Given that differentiation of Th17 cells requires TGF-β (plus IL-6 or IL-21), these cells may be developmentally linked to iTregs that also require TGF-β for differentiation. Tregs may differentiate into Th17 cells (reviewed in Lee et al. 2009; Zhou et al. 2009b), and $CD4^+Foxp3^+IL\text{-}17^+$ cells have recently been described in mice and humans (Voo et al. 2009; Xu et al. 2007). Furthermore, IL-17^+/$Foxp3^+$ Treg clones were recently shown to retain suppressive function and exhibited the plasticity to secrete IL-17 or suppress depending on the nature of the stimulus provided (Beriou et al. 2009). These findings suggest that exposure to pro-inflammatory cytokines can drive Tregs to secrete IL-17, and thereby promote an inflammatory microenvironment favoring tumor growth.

In addition to interacting with MDSC and TAMs, Tregs also interact and cross-regulate type-I-type II NKT cells. Type-I NKT cells are generally thought to be active in tumor immunosurveillance and enhance anti-tumor immunity, while type II NKT cells are thought to suppress these responses. Interestingly, in mouse tumor models where type II NKT cells have a major role in the suppression of tumor immunosurveillance, Tregs had a minimal role or no role in suppression. Intriguingly, the site of the tumor growth also appeared to determine whether type II NKT cells or Tregs were the major mediators of immune suppression (reviewed in Terabe and Berzofsky 2007). Further work to investigate the relationship between Tregs and NKT cells in a cancer setting will provide insight on the importance of these interactions.

6.2 *Strategies to Modulate Treg Number and Function*

Two opportunities exist to modify Treg biology in clinical studies to promote endogenous or induced anti-tumor immune responses. The first of these is to simply deplete Treg numbers, while the second is to modify Tregs function to limit their immunosuppressive capacity.

In light of the expression of CD25 by Tregs, this molecule has been an early target for both pre-clinical and clinical studies of Treg depletion. The administration of anti-CD25 mAbs in mouse models of cancer leads to $CD4^{+}CD25^{+}$ Treg depletion and a significant enhancement of anti-tumor activity, and the clinical utility of this approach has recently been described by Rech and Vonderheide (Rech and Vonderheide 2009). Tregs in mouse and human may also be targeted by CD25 fusion proteins such as LMB-2 which consists of a single-chain Fv fragment of a CD25-specific mAb linked to a 38 kDa fragment of Pseudomonas exotoxin A. Preclinical in vitro studies of human PBMCs successfully depleted $CD4^{+}CD25^{+}$ Tregs following incubation with LMB-2 (Attia et al. 2006). Administration of LMB-2 followed by peptide vaccination in patients with melanoma resulted in a profound fall of $Foxp3^{+}CD4^{+}CD25^{+}$ Tregs, although this did not result in clinical responses (Powell et al. 2007b). CD25-directed depletion of Tregs may also be achieved with Denileukin diftitox (DAB389IL-2/ ONTAK), which is comprised of a fusion protein of IL-2 and diphtheria toxin. This reagent profoundly depletes Tregs and enhances anti-tumor vaccines in mice (Litzinger et al. 2007). In clinical studies, Diftitox administration in advanced renal cell carcinoma before DC vaccination resulted in a reduction in peripheral Tregs and enhanced anti-tumor immune responses in vivo (Dannull et al. 2005). In a separate study in patients with melanoma, enhanced antigen-specific CD8 T-cell activity was seen following Diftitox-mediated Treg depletion (Mahnke et al. 2007). Despite these promising initial findings, a further study in melanoma with Diftitox failed to show either clinical benefit or alteration of peripheral Tregs number or function (Attia et al. 2005a).

The failure of Treg depletion therapies to result in significant promotion of anti-cancer immunity may in part be due to the rapid, and on occasions, refractory reaccumulation of suppressive $CD25^{+}$ $Foxp3^{+}$ Tregs (Dannull et al. 2005; Powell et al. 2007a). Alternatively, the lack of regression in established tumors following CD25 depletion raises the question of whether not enough Tregs were being eliminated to relieve suppression on anti-tumor immune cells or whether $CD25^+$ effector cells responsible for mediating anti-tumor response were concomitantly depleted. Potentially, this question can now be answered using mouse models where $Foxp3^+$ Tregs expressing the diphtheria toxin receptor can be completely eliminated following diphtheria toxin treatment.

A number of therapeutic agents have been used to deplete Treg numbers including conventional chemotherapeutic drugs although their exact mode of action remains largely unknown. The potential of the combined effects of non-specific lymphodepletion including depletion of Tregs to enhance anti-cancer immunotherapy has been most potently described when a combination of cyclophosphamide and fludarabine and total body irradiation was used prior to adoptive CTL immunotherapy for melanoma (Dudley et al. 2008; Rosenberg and Dudley 2009).

Of the available cytotoxic agents leading to Treg depletion, cyclophosphamide (Cy) is the best described, although the depletion of Tregs is not always reproducible (Audia et al. 2007). Cy is known to deplete $CD4^+CD25^+$ Tregs in vivo in mouse models (Ghiringhelli et al. 2004) and decreases the suppressive capacity of Tregs in vitro by reversibly decreasing the expression of GITR and FoxP3 (Lutsiak et al. 2005). When low-dose Cy was used in combination with GM-CSF secreting cellular vaccine (Gvax) in mice bearing endogenous prostate tumors (Pro-HA x TRAMP), a significant decrease in tumor burden was observed that correlated with decreased numbers of Tregs in the prostate and more activated DCs in the draining LN (Wada et al. 2009). Similarly, clinical trials have demonstrated that low-dose Cy used in a metronomic regimen showed increased anti-angiogenic and immunostimulatory properties and a decrease in Treg numbers in peripheral blood (Ghiringhelli et al. 2007; Lord et al. 2007), although without a clearly demonstrable relationship between clinical response and circulating Treg numbers. Other chemotherapy drugs with demonstrable actions on Treg function include fludarabine (Beyer et al. 2005; Hegde et al. 2008) and gemcitabine (Correale et al. 2005; Levitt et al. 2004). Additionally, Ozao-Choy et al. demonstrated that use of a tyrosine kinase inhibitor (sunitinib malate) also decreased Treg and MDSC numbers in the tumor microenvironment (Ozao-Choy et al. 2009).

6.3 Attenuating Treg Function

Given our improved understanding in Treg cell subsets and how they mediate their suppressive function, there are studies that advocate attenuating Treg function rather than simply depleting them (Colombo and Piconese 2007). Some of the strategies to attenuate Treg function include (1) blocking Treg suppression, (2) blocking Treg trafficking, and (3) blocking or subverting Treg differentiation (reviewed in Curiel 2008; Zou 2006).

Blocking or reversing Treg suppression through their cell surface markers has been a strategy investigated by many groups. Examples include antibodies to GITR (TNFRSF18), CTLA-4 (reviewed in Colombo and Piconese 2007), and more recently OX40 and TLR (Shevach 2009). However, as these surface markers are also expressed on non-Tregs, it has been difficult to conclude if the antibodies were just blocking Treg cell function or/and also stimulating non-Treg cells thereby rendering them resistant to suppression. Evidence for the latter was described in the GITR-GITRL setting and anti-OX40 mAbs (reviewed in Stephens et al. 2007 and Piconese et al. 2008). It must be considered however that OX40 agonists could drive Treg cell expansion under certain conditions (Ruby et al. 2009). Age of the tumor bearing host may also determine the outcome of these approaches as highlighted in a recent study by Ruby et al., where middle-aged and elderly tumor-bearing mice (12 and 20 months old, respectively) treated with anti-OX40 had decreased tumor-free survival because of a disproportionate decline of effector T cells compared with young mice (Ruby and Weinberg 2009).

Blockade of the suppressive molecule CTLA-4, which is expressed at high concentration on Tregs, may also attenuate Treg function. Gvax when used in combination with anti-CTLA-4 mAbs can mediate tumor rejection in a number of mouse tumor models, including the poorly immunogenic B16 melanoma (Peggs et al. 2009; Quezada et al. 2006, 2008). The latest study is the first to demonstrate the critical importance of synergy between the independent contributions of CTLA-4 blockade in cis and in trans to anti-tumor activity, illustrating that both Teff and Tregs are relevant targets for the therapeutic efficacy of anti-CTLA-4 mAbs (Peggs et al. 2009). This neutralizing mAb therapy has now reached clinical trials in many cancers with two humanized anti-CTLA-4 mAbs, MDX-010 (Ipilimumab) and CP-675 206 (Tremelimumab). In a phase I trial treating metastatic melanoma, 36% of patients showing grade III/IV autoimmune toxicity had tumor regression compared with 5% in patients without autoimmune symptoms (Attia et al. 2005b). In patients undergoing anti-CTLA-4 treatment for stage IV metastatic melanoma and renal cell carcinoma, no inhibition of the suppressive activity of $CD4^+$ $CD25^+$ T cells was observed, but an enhancement of effector cell function was seen (Maker et al. 2005). Tremelimumab has been successfully trialed in 39 patients with metastatic melanoma, of whom two patients had a complete response and two had a partial response, and there was an observed suppression of Treg activity (Ribas 2008).

Targeting of TLR2 on mice Tregs or TLR8 on human Tregs may also suppress Treg function (Liu et al. 2006a; Peng et al. 2005; Sutmuller et al. 2006a). However, a recent paper (Chen et al. 2009) has disputed the findings on TLR2 by using highly purified Treg cells from GFPFoxp3 trangenic mice and performing some of the studies in the previous papers. Their studies concluded that engagement of TLR2 did not reverse the suppressor function of Tregs but in fact reduced their threshold for activation and enhanced their survival.

The S1P receptor agonist FTY720 potently inhibits Treg proliferation in vitro and in vivo by impairing the IL-2 signaling pathway (Wolf et al. 2009). Their data suggested that inhibition of Tregs by S1P receptor agonists might represent an innovative adjuvant for cancer immunotherapy (e.g., in combination with DC vaccines) by limiting Treg expansion, while permitting generation of CTL.

It has recently been shown that different subsets of Tregs can control Th1, Th2, and Th17 responses by expressing the transcription factors Tbet, IRF4, and STAT3, respectively, that allow them to home on to the same inflammation sites at these effector cells (Chaudhry et al. 2009; Koch et al. 2009; Zheng et al. 2009). Potentially, the ability to disrupt the migratory specificity of Treg cells to a particular type of local inflammation, such as those induced by IL-12 and IFN-γ, may permit anti-tumor responses. In addition, given the plasticity of Tregs, some studies have suggested that exposure to some cytokines can result in Tregs downregulating Foxp3, losing their regulatory activity and under some conditions, becoming memory T cells capable of recognizing self-antigens and expressing effector cell activities such as IFN-γ production (Zhou and Littman 2009). More investigations will be required to understand the exact requirements needed to de-differentiate Tregs into effector cells.

Nonsteroidal anti-inflammatory drugs including aspirin have the ability to block the production of tumor-derived prostaglandin E2 (PGE2). This prostaglandin can induce Foxp3 expression and promote Treg inhibitory activity in vitro. The inhibition of PGE2 production therefore can be potentially used to limit Treg function in vivo. The specific use of COX-2 inhibitors, which reduce production of PGE2, significantly reduces Treg infiltration in mouse tumors. Furthermore, when PGE2 production was inhibited by Indomethacin in patients with colorectal cancer, Treg-mediated anti-tumor suppression was reversed (Yaqub et al. 2008). In addition, in patients with colon cancer randomized to treatment with either indomethacin/celebrex or a control drug prior to tumor resection, $CD8^+$ tumor-infiltrating T-cells were increased while decreased expression of Foxp3 and IL-10 was found in the COX2 inhibitor cohort (Lonnroth et al. 2008).

Perhaps, the most intriguing group of immunologically active drugs available for clinical use in recent years is that of the immunomodulatory drugs (IMiDs) thalidomide, lenalidomide, and pomalidomide (reviewed in Quach et al. 2009). In specific reference to the effect of these drugs on Tregs, much of the clinical data to date is in the setting of hematological malignancy. As such, the combined impact of specific disease and prior therapies on Treg number and function must be borne in mind when interpreting the effect of these drugs on Treg biology (see earlier discussion of Treg in myeloma). Nonetheless, IMiDs have shown potent modification of Treg numbers in a number of settings, including chronic lymphocytic leukemia (CLL) in which Tregs were substantially diminished by thalidomide therapy (Giannopoulos et al. 2008). A similar effect has also been shown in CLL with lenalidomide therapy. Moreover, lenalidomide therapy also drove the induction of Th17 cells, suggesting that this agent specifically modified $CD4^+$ T cell polarization (Idler et al. 2009). While the mechanism of action of these agents in humans is still being actively pursued, mouse studies indicate that both lenalidomide and pomalidomide inhibit the IL-2 mediated generation of $Foxp3^+CD25^+$ Tregs (Galustian et al. 2009).

7 Conclusions

Multiple lines of experimental and clinical data clearly identify regulatory T cells as an integral part of the host immune response to cancer. Treg associated with cancer are often, but not exclusively, associated with poor clinical outcomes and are therefore a major limitation to the development of effective anti-cancer immunotherapy. It is not clear what mechanisms are critical for Treg-mediated immunosuppression and the development of many conditional knockouts using FoxP3-cre mice will greatly aid this study in mouse models. Improved methods are required to surface mark iTregs from nTregs so that the role of each of these in tumor development and microenvironments can be better distinguished. Further studies are essential to determine the hierarchy between Tregs and other immunoregulatory tumor infiltrating leukocytes. Similarly, understanding the mechanisms by which Tregs contribute to the improved prognosis in many forms of lymphoma will provide further insight into Treg physiology more widely. Given the striking effects of fully depleting Tregs or modifying the behavior of Tregs in mouse tumor models, many opportunities exist to move effective depleting or immunomodulatory drug therapies into clinical studies either alone or as combination immunotherapies.

Acknowledgments MJS was supported by a National Health and Medical Research Council of Australia (NH&MRC) Research Program and Australia Fellowship. MWLT was supported by a NH&MRC Doherty Post-Doctoral Fellowship.

References

Abe M, Uchihashi K, Kazuto T, Osaka A, Yanagihara K, Tsukasaki K, Hasegawa H, Yamada Y, Kamihira S (2008) Foxp3 expression on normal and leukemic CD4+CD25+ T cells implicated in human T-cell leukemia virus type-1 is inconsistent with Treg cells. Eur J Haematol 81:209–217

Ai WZ, Hou JZ, Zeiser R, Czerwinski D, Negrin RS, Levy R (2009) Follicular lymphoma B cells induce the conversion of conventional CD4+ T cells to T-regulatory cells. Int J Cancer 124:239–244

Alvaro T, Lejeune M, Salvado MT, Bosch R, Garcia JF, Jaen J, Banham AH, Roncador G, Montalban C, Piris MA (2005) Outcome in Hodgkin's lymphoma can be predicted from the presence of accompanying cytotoxic and regulatory T cells. Clin Cancer Res 11:1467–1473

Attia P, Maker AV, Haworth LR, Rogers-Freezer L, Rosenberg SA (2005a) Inability of a fusion protein of IL-2 and diphtheria toxin (Denileukin Diftitox, DAB389IL-2, ONTAK) to eliminate regulatory T lymphocytes in patients with melanoma. J Immunother 28:582–592

Attia P, Phan GQ, Maker AV, Robinson MR, Quezado MM, Yang JC, Sherry RM, Topalian SL, Kammula US, Royal RE, Restifo NP, Haworth LR, Levy C, Mavroukakis SA, Nichol G, Yellin MJ, Rosenberg SA (2005b) Autoimmunity correlates with tumor regression in patients with metastatic melanoma treated with anti-cytotoxic T-lymphocyte antigen-4. J Clin Oncol 23:6043–6053

Attia P, Powell DJ Jr, Maker AV, Kreitman RJ, Pastan I, Rosenberg SA (2006) Selective elimination of human regulatory T lymphocytes in vitro with the recombinant immunotoxin LMB-2. J Immunother 29:208–214

Audia S, Nicolas A, Cathelin D, Larmonier N, Ferrand C, Foucher P, Fanton A, Bergoin E, Maynadie M, Arnould L, Bateman A, Lorcerie B, Solary E, Chauffert B, Bonnotte B (2007)

Increase of CD4+ CD25+ regulatory T cells in the peripheral blood of patients with metastatic carcinoma: a Phase I clinical trial using cyclophosphamide and immunotherapy to eliminate CD4+ CD25+ T lymphocytes. Clin Exp Immunol 150:523–530

Baban B, Chandler PR, Sharma MD, Pihkala J, Koni PA, Munn DH, Mellor AL (2009) IDO activates regulatory T cells and blocks their conversion into Th17-like T cells. J Immunol 183:2475–2483

Badoual C, Hans S, Rodriyuez J, Peyrard S, Klein C, Agueznay Nel H, Mosseri V, Laccaurrye O, Bruneval P, Fridman WH, Brasnu DF, Tartaur E (2006) Prognostic value of tumor-infulfrating CD4$^+$ T-cell populashons in head and neck cancers. Clin Cancer Res 12:465–472

Badoual C, Hans S, Fridman WH, Brasnu D, Erdman S, Tartour E (2009) Revisiting the prognostic value of regulatory T cells in patients with cancer. J Clin Oncol 27:e5–e6, author reply e7

Balkwill F (2004) Cancer and the chemokine network. Nat Rev Cancer 4:540–550

Baron U, Floess S, Wieczorek G, Baumann K, Grutzkau A, Dong J, Thiel A, Boeld TJ, Hoffmann P, Edinger M, Turbachova I, Hamann A, Olek S, Huehn J (2007) DNA demethylation in the human FOXP3 locus discriminates regulatory T cells from activated FOXP3(+) conventional T cells. Eur J Immunol 37:2378–2389

Battaglia A, Buzzonetti A, Monego G, Peri L, Ferrandina G, Fanfani F, Scambia G, Fattorossi A (2008) Neuropilin-1 expression identifies a subset of regulatory T cells in human lymph nodes that is modulated by preoperative chemoradiation therapy in cervical cancer. Immunology 123:129–138

Bennett CL, Christie J, Ramsdell F, Brunkow ME, Ferguson PJ, Whitesell L, Kelly TE, Saulsbury FT, Chance PF, Ochs HD (2001) The immune dysregulation, polyendocrinopathy, enteropathy, X-linked syndrome (IPEX) is caused by mutations of FOXP3. Nat Genet 27:20–21

Beriou G, Costantino CM, Ashley CW, Yang L, Kuchroo VK, Baecher-Allan C, Hafler DA (2009) IL-17-producing human peripheral regulatory T cells retain suppressive function. Blood 113:4240–4249

Beyer M, Schultze JL (2006) Regulatory T cells in cancer. Blood 108:804–811

Beyer M, Kochanek M, Darabi K, Popov A, Jensen M, Endl E, Knolle PA, Thomas RK, von Bergwelt-Baildon M, Debey S, Hallek M, Schultze JL (2005) Reduced frequencies and suppressive function of CD4+CD25hi regulatory T cells in patients with chronic lymphocytic leukemia after therapy with fludarabine. Blood 106:2018–2025

Beyer M, Kochanek M, Giese T, Endl E, Weihrauch MR, Knolle PA, Classen S, Schultze JL (2006) In vivo peripheral expansion of naive CD4+CD25high FoxP3+ regulatory T cells in patients with multiple myeloma. Blood 107:3940–3949

Bopp T, Becker C, Klein M, Klein-Hessling S, Palmetshofer A, Serfling E, Heib V, Becker M, Kubach J, Schmitt S, Stoll S, Schild H, Staege MS, Stassen M, Jonuleit H, Schmitt E (2007) Cyclic adenosine monophosphate is a key component of regulatory T cell-mediated suppression. J Exp Med 204:1303–1310

Bruder D, Probst-Kepper M, Westendorf AM, Geffers R, Beissert S, Loser K, von Boehmer H, Buer J, Hansen W (2004) Neuropilin-1: a surface marker of regulatory T cells. Eur J Immunol 34:623–630

Brunkow ME, Jeffery EW, Hjerrild KA, Paeper B, Clark LB, Yasayko SA, Wilkinson JE, Galas D, Ziegler SF, Ramsdell F (2001) Disruption of a new forkhead/winged-helix protein, scurfin, results in the fatal lymphoproliferative disorder of the scurfy mouse. Nat Genet 27:68–73

Bunt SK, Sinha P, Clements VK, Leips J, Ostrand-Rosenberg S (2006) Inflammation induces myeloid-derived suppressor cells that facilitate tumor progression. J Immunol 176:284–290

Bunt SK, Yang L, Sinha P, Clements VK, Leips J, Ostrand-Rosenberg S (2007) Reduced inflammation in the tumor microenvironment delays the accumulation of myeloid-derived suppressor cells and limits tumor progression. Cancer Res 67:10019–10026

Burmeister Y, Lischke T, Dahler AC, Mages HW, Lam KP, Coyle AJ, Kroczek RA, Hutloff A (2008) ICOS controls the pool size of effector-memory and regulatory T cells. J Immunol 180:774–782

Cao X, Cai SF, Fehniger TA, Song J, Collins LI, Piwnica-Worms DR, Ley TJ (2007) Granzyme B and perforin are important for regulatory T cell-mediated suppression of tumor clearance. Immunity 27:635–646

Carreras J, Lopez-Guillermo A, Fox BC, Colomo L, Martinez A, Roncador G, Montserrat E, Campo E, Banham AH (2006) High numbers of tumor-infiltrating FOXP3-positive regulatory T cells are associated with improved overall survival in follicular lymphoma. Blood 108:2957–2964

Carrier Y, Yuan J, Kuchroo VK, Weiner HL (2007) Th3 cells in peripheral tolerance. II. TGF-beta-transgenic Th3 cells rescue IL-2-deficient mice from autoimmunity. J Immunol 178:172–178

Chaudhry A, Rudra D, Treuting P, Samstein RM, Liang Y, Kas A, Rudensky AY (2009) CD4+ regulatory T cells control TH17 responses in a Stat3-dependent manner. Science 326:986–991

Chen Y, Kuchroo VK, Inobe J, Hafler DA, Weiner HL (1994) Regulatory T cell clones induced by oral tolerance: suppression of autoimmune encephalomyelitis. Science 265:1237–1240

Chen ML, Pittet MJ, Gorelik L, Flavell RA, Weissleder R, von Boehmer H, Khazaie K (2005) Regulatory T cells suppress tumor-specific CD8 T cell cytotoxicity through TGF-beta signals in vivo. Proc Natl Acad Sci USA 102:419–424

Chen X, Subleski JJ, Kopf H, Howard OM, Mannel DN, Oppenheim JJ (2008) Cutting edge: expression of TNFR2 defines a maximally suppressive subset of mouse CD4+CD25+FoxP3+ T regulatory cells: applicability to tumor-infiltrating T regulatory cells. J Immunol 180: 6467–6471

Chen Q, Davidson TS, Huter EN, Shevach EM (2009) Engagement of TLR2 does not reverse the suppressor function of mouse regulatory T cells, but promotes their survival. J Immunol 183:4458–4466

Clark CE, Hingorani SR, Mick R, Combs C, Tuveson DA, Vonderheide RH (2007) Dynamics of the immune reaction to pancreatic cancer from inception to invasion. Cancer Res 67: 9518–9527

Collison LW, Workman CJ, Kuo TT, Boyd K, Wang Y, Vignali KM, Cross R, Sehy D, Blumberg RS, Vignali DA (2007) The inhibitory cytokine IL-35 contributes to regulatory T-cell function. Nature 450:566–569

Colombo MP, Piconese S (2007) Regulatory-T-cell inhibition versus depletion: the right choice in cancer immunotherapy. Nat Rev Cancer 7:880–887

Colombo MP, Piconese S (2009) Polyps wrap mast cells and Treg within tumorigenic tentacles. Cancer Res 69:5619–5622

Correale P, Cusi MG, Tsang KY, Del Vecchio MT, Marsili S, Placa ML, Intrivici C, Aquino A, Micheli L, Nencini C, Ferrari F, Giorgi G, Bonmassar E, Francini G (2005) Chemo-immunotherapy of metastatic colorectal carcinoma with gemcitabine plus FOLFOX 4 followed by subcutaneous granulocyte macrophage colony-stimulating factor and interleukin-2 induces strong immunologic and antitumor activity in metastatic colon cancer patients. J Clin Oncol 23:8950–8958

Cosmi L, Liotta F, Lazzeri E, Francalanci M, Angeli R, Mazzinghi B, Santarlasci V, Manetti R, Vanini V, Romagnani P, Maggi E, Romagnani S, Annunziato F (2003) Human CD8+CD25+ thymocytes share phenotypic and functional features with CD4+CD25+ regulatory thymocytes. Blood 102:4107–4114

Crellin NK, Garcia RV, Hadisfar O, Allan SE, Steiner TS, Levings MK (2005) Human CD4+ T cells express TLR5 and its ligand flagellin enhances the suppressive capacity and expression of FOXP3 in CD4+CD25+ T regulatory cells. J Immunol 175:8051–8059

Curiel TJ (2008) Regulatory T cells and treatment of cancer. Curr Opin Immunol 20:241–246

Curiel TJ, Coukos G, Zou L, Alvarez X, Cheng P, Mottram P, Evdemon-Hogan M, Conejo-Garcia JR, Zhang L, Burow M, Zhu Y, Wei S, Kryczek I, Daniel B, Gordon A, Myers L, Lackner A, Disis ML, Knutson KL, Chen L, Zou W (2004) Specific recruitment of regulatory T cells in ovarian carcinoma fosters immune privilege and predicts reduced survival. Nat Med 10:942–949

Curotto de Lafaille MA, Lafaille JJ (2009) Natural and adaptive foxp3+ regulatory T cells: more of the same or a division of labor? Immunity 30:626–635

Dai J, Liu B, Li Z (2009) Regulatory T cells and Toll-like receptors: What is the missing link? International Immunopharmacology 9:528–533

Dannull J, Su Z, Rizzieri D, Yang BK, Coleman D, Yancey D, Zhang A, Dahm P, Chao N, Gilboa E, Vieweg J (2005) Enhancement of vaccine-mediated antitumor immunity in cancer patients after depletion of regulatory T cells. J Clin Invest 115:3623–3633

Darrasse-Jeze G, Bergot AS, Durgeau A, Billiard F, Salomon BL, Cohen JL, Bellier B, Podsypanina K, Klatzmann D (2009) Tumor emergence is sensed by self-specific CD44hi memory Tregs that create a dominant tolerogenic environment for tumors in mice. J Clin Invest 119:2648–2662

Davis JE, Smyth MJ, Trapani JA (2001) Granzyme A and B-deficient killer lymphocytes are defective in eliciting DNA fragmentation but retain potent in vivo anti-tumor capacity. Eur J Immunol 31:39–47

de Visser KE, Coussens LM (2006) The inflammatory tumor microenvironment and its impact on cancer development. Contrib Microbiol 13:118–137

Deaglio S, Dwyer KM, Gao W, Friedman D, Usheva A, Erat A, Chen JF, Enjyoji K, Linden J, Oukka M, Kuchroo VK, Strom TB, Robson SC (2007) Adenosine generation catalyzed by CD39 and CD73 expressed on regulatory T cells mediates immune suppression. J Exp Med 204:1257–1265

DeNardo DG, Barreto JB, Andreu P, Vasquez L, Tawfik D, Kolhatkar N, Coussens LM (2009) CD4(+) T cells regulate pulmonary metastasis of mammary carcinomas by enhancing protumor properties of macrophages. Cancer Cell 16:91–102

Dudley ME, Yang JC, Sherry R, Hughes MS, Royal R, Kammula U, Robbins PF, Huang J, Citrin DE, Leitman SF, Wunderlich J, Restifo NP, Thomasian A, Downey SG, Smith FO, Klapper J, Morton K, Laurencot C, White DE, Rosenberg SA (2008) Adoptive cell therapy for patients with metastatic melanoma: evaluation of intensive myeloablative chemoradiation preparative regimens. J Clin Oncol 26:5233–5239

Elpek KG, Lacelle C, Singh NP, Yolcu ES, Shirwan H (2007) CD4+CD25+ T regulatory cells dominate multiple immune evasion mechanisms in early but not late phases of tumor development in a B cell lymphoma model. J Immunol 178:6840–6848

Endharti AT, Rifa IM, Shi Z, Fukuoka Y, Nakahara Y, Kawamoto Y, Takeda K, Isobe K, Suzuki H (2005) Cutting edge: CD8+CD122+ regulatory T cells produce IL-10 to suppress IFN-gamma production and proliferation of CD8+ T cells. J Immunol 175:7093–7097

Erdman SE, Sohn JJ, Rao VP, Nambiar PR, Ge Z, Fox JG, Schauer DB (2005) CD4+CD25+ regulatory lymphocytes induce regression of intestinal tumors in ApcMin/+ mice. Cancer Res 65:3998–4004

Feuerer M, Hill JA, Mathis D, Benoist C (2009) Foxp3+ regulatory T cells: differentiation, specification, subphenotypes. Nat Immunol 10:689–695

Floess S, Freyer J, Siewert C, Baron U, Olek S, Polansky J, Schlawe K, Chang HD, Bopp T, Schmitt E, Klein-Hessling S, Serfling E, Hamann A, Huehn J (2007) Epigenetic control of the foxp3 locus in regulatory T cells. PLoS Biol 5:e38

Fontenot JD, Gavin MA, Rudensky AY (2003) Foxp3 programs the development and function of CD4+CD25+ regulatory T cells. Nat Immunol 4:330–336

Galustian C, Meyer B, Labarthe MC, Dredge K, Klaschka D, Henry J, Todryk S, Chen R, Muller G, Stirling D, Schafer P, Bartlett JB, Dalgleish AG (2009) The anti-cancer agents lenalidomide and pomalidomide inhibit the proliferation and function of T regulatory cells. Cancer Immunol Immunother 58:1033–1045

Gao Q, Qiu S, Fan J, Zhou J, Wang X, Xaio Y, Xu Y, Li Y, Tang Z (2007) Intratumoral balance of regulatory and cytotoxic T cells is associated with prognosis of hepatocellular carcinoma after resection. J Clin Oncol 25:2586–2593

Ge W, Ma X, Li X, Wang Y, Li C, Meng H, Liu X, Yu Z, You S, Qiu L (2009) B7-H1 up-regulation on dendritic-like leukemia cells suppresses T cell immune function through modulation of IL-10/IL-12 production and generation of Treg cells. Leuk Res 33:948–957

Ghiringhelli F, Larmonier N, Schmitt E, Parcellier A, Cathelin D, Garrido C, Chauffert B, Solary E, Bonnotte B, Martin F (2004) CD4+CD25+ regulatory T cells suppress tumor immunity but are sensitive to cyclophosphamide which allows immunotherapy of established tumors to be curative. Eur J Immunol 34:336–344

Ghiringhelli F, Menard C, Terme M, Flament C, Taieb J, Chaput N, Puig PE, Novault S, Escudier B, Vivier E, Lecesne A, Robert C, Blay JY, Bernard J, Caillat-Zucman S, Freitas A, Tursz T, Wagner-Ballon O, Capron C, Vainchencker W, Martin F, Zitvogel L (2005) CD4+CD25+ regulatory T cells inhibit natural killer cell functions in a transforming growth factor-beta-dependent manner. J Exp Med 202:1075–1085

Ghiringhelli F, Menard C, Puig PE, Ladoire S, Roux S, Martin F, Solary E, Le Cesne A, Zitvogel L, Chauffert B (2007) Metronomic cyclophosphamide regimen selectively depletes CD4+CD25+ regulatory T cells and restores T and NK effector functions in end stage cancer patients. Cancer Immunol Immunother 56:641–648

Giannopoulos K, Schmitt M, Wlasiuk P, Chen J, Bojarska-Junak A, Kowal M, Rolinski J, Dmoszynska A (2008) The high frequency of T regulatory cells in patients with B-cell chronic lymphocytic leukemia is diminished through treatment with thalidomide. Leukemia 22:222–224

Gobert M, Treilleux I, Bendriss-Vermare N, Bachelot T, Goddard-Leon S, Arfi V, Biota C, Doffin AC, Durand I, Olive D, Perez S, Pasqual N, Faure C, Ray-Coquard I, Puisieux A, Caux C, Blay JY, Menetrier-Caux C (2009) Regulatory T cells recruited through CCL22/CCR4 are selectively activated in lymphoid infiltrates surrounding primary breast tumors and lead to an adverse clinical outcome. Cancer Res 69:2000–2009

Gondek DC, Lu LF, Quezada SA, Sakaguchi S, Noelle RJ (2005) Cutting edge: contact-mediated suppression by CD4+CD25+ regulatory cells involves a granzyme B-dependent, perforin-independent mechanism. J Immunol 174:1783–1786

Gotsman I, Grabie N, Gupta R, Dacosta R, MacConmara M, Lederer J, Sukhova G, Witztum JL, Sharpe AH, Lichtman AH (2006) Impaired regulatory T-cell response and enhanced atherosclerosis in the absence of inducible costimulatory molecule. Circulation 114:2047–2055

Gounaris E, Blatner NR, Dennis K, Magnusson F, Gurish MF, Strom TB, Beckhove P, Gounari F, Khazaie K (2009) T-regulatory cells shift from a protective anti-inflammatory to a cancer-promoting proinflammatory phenotype in polyposis. Cancer Res 69:5490–5497

Gray CP, Arosio P, Hersey P (2003) Association of increased levels of heavy chain ferritin with increased $CD4^+$ $CD25^+$ regulatory T-cell levels in patients with melanema. Clin Cancer Res 9:2551–2559

Groux H, O'Garra A, Bigler M, Rouleau M, Antonenko S, de Vries JE, Roncarolo MG (1997) A CD4+T-cell subset inhibits antigen-specific T-cell responses and prevents colitis. Nature 389:737–742

Haas M, Dimmler A, Hohenberger W, Grabenbauer GG, Niedobitek G, Distel LV (2009) Stromal regulatory T-cells are associated with a favourable prognosis in gastric cancer of the cardia. BMC Gastroenterol 9:65

Hartigan-O'Connor DJ, Poon C, Sinclair E, McCune JM (2007) Human CD4+ regulatory T cells express lower levels of the IL-7 receptor alpha chain (CD127), allowing consistent identification and sorting of live cells. J Immunol Methods 319:41–52

Hegde U, Chhabra A, Chattopadhyay S, Das R, Ray S, Chakraborty NG (2008) Presence of low dose of fludarabine in cultures blocks regulatory T cell expansion and maintains tumor-specific cytotoxic T lymphocyte activity generated with peripheral blood lymphocytes. Pathobiology 75:200–208

Hori S, Nomura T, Sakaguchi S (2003) Control of regulatory T cell development by the transcription factor Foxp3. Science 299:1057–1061

Huang B, Pan PY, Li Q, Sato AI, Levy DE, Bromberg J, Divino CM, Chen SH (2006) Gr-1 +CD115+ immature myeloid suppressor cells mediate the development of tumor-induced T regulatory cells and T-cell anergy in tumor-bearing host. Cancer Res 66:1123–1131

Huehn J, Hamann A (2005) Homing to suppress: address codes for Treg migration. Trends Immunol 26:632–636

Huehn J, Siegmund K, Lehmann JC, Siewert C, Haubold U, Feuerer M, Debes GF, Lauber J, Frey O, Przybylski GK, Niesner U, de la Rosa M, Schmidt CA, Brauer R, Buer J, Scheffold A, Hamann A (2004) Developmental stage, phenotype, and migration distinguish naive- and effector/memory-like CD4+ regulatory T cells. J Exp Med 199:303–313

Huehn J, Polansky JK, Hamann A (2009) Epigenetic control of FOXP3 expression: the key to a stable regulatory T-cell lineage? Nat Rev Immunol 9:83–89

Ichihara F, Kono K, Takahashi A, Kawaida H, Sugai H, Fujii H (2003) Increased populations of regulatory T cells in peripheral blood and tumor-infiltrating lymphocytes in patients with gastric and esophageal cancers. Clin Cancer Res 9:4404–4408

Idler I, Giannopoulos K, Zenz T, Bhattacharya N, Nothing M, Dohner H, Stilgenbauer S, Mertens D (2009) Lenalidomide treatment of chronic lymphocytic leukaemia patients reduces regulatory T cells and induces Th17 T helper cells. Br J Haematol. Nov 30, Epub ahead of print

Jarnicki AG, Lysaght J, Todryk S, Mills KH (2006) Suppression of antitumor immunity by IL-10 and TGF-beta-producing T cells infiltrating the growing tumor: influence of tumor environment on the induction of CD4+ and CD8+ regulatory T cells. J Immunol 177:896–904

Jonuleit H, Schmitt E, Stassen M, Tuettenberg A, Knop J, Enk AH (2001) Identification and functional characterization of human CD4(+)CD25(+) T cells with regulatory properties isolated from peripheral blood. J Exp Med 193:1285–1294

Joosten SA, van Meijgaarden KE, Savage ND, de Boer T, Triebel F, van der Wal A, de Heer E, Klein MR, Geluk A, Ottenhoff TH (2007) Identification of a human CD8+ regulatory T cell subset that mediates suppression through the chemokine CC chemokine ligand 4. Proc Natl Acad Sci USA 104:8029–8034

Josefowicz SZ, Rudensky A (2009) Control of regulatory T cell lineage commitment and maintenance. Immunity 30:616–625

Joshua DE, Brown RD, Ho PJ, Gibson J (2008) Regulatory T cells and multiple myeloma. Clin Lymphoma Myeloma 8:283–286

Kabelitz D (2007) Expression and function of Toll-like receptors in T lymphocytes. Curr Opin Immunol 19:39–45

Karube K, Ohshima K, Tsuchiya T, Yamaguchi T, Kawano R, Suzumiya J, Utsunomiya A, Harada M, Kikuchi M (2004) Expression of FoxP3, a key molecule in CD4CD25 regulatory T cells, in adult T-cell leukaemia/lymphoma cells. Br J Haematol 126:81–84

Kim HP, Leonard WJ (2007) CREB/ATF-dependent T cell receptor-induced FoxP3 gene expression: a role for DNA methylation. J Exp Med 204:1543–1551

Kim JM, Rasmussen JP, Rudensky AY (2007) Regulatory T cells prevent catastrophic autoimmunity throughout the lifespan of mice. Nat Immunol 8:191–197

Kiniwa Y, Miyahara Y, Wang HY, Peng W, Peng G, Wheeler TM, Thompson TC, Old LJ, Wang RF (2007) CD8+ Foxp3+ regulatory T cells mediate immunosuppression in prostate cancer. Clin Cancer Res 13:6947–6958

Kobie JJ, Shah PR, Yang L, Rebhahn JA, Fowell DJ, Mosmann TR (2006) T regulatory and primed uncommitted CD4 T cells express CD73, which suppresses effector CD4 T cells by converting 5′-adenosine monophosphate to adenosine. J Immunol 177:6780–6786

Koch MA, Tucker-Heard G, Perdue NR, Killebrew JR, Urdahl KB, Campbell DJ (2009) The transcription factor T-bet controls regulatory T cell homeostasis and function during type 1 inflammation. Nat Immunol 10:595–602

Krejsgaard T, Gjerdrum LM, Ralfkiaer E, Lauenborg B, Eriksen KW, Mathiesen AM, Bovin LF, Gniadecki R, Geisler C, Ryder LP, Zhang Q, Wasik MA, Odum N, Woetmann A (2008) Malignant Tregs express low molecular splice forms of FOXP3 in Sezary syndrome. Leukemia 22:2230–2239

Kryczek I, Wei S, Szeliga W, Vatan L, Zou W (2009) Endogenous IL-17 contributes to reduced tumor growth and metastasis. Blood 114:357–359

Lahl K, Loddenkemper C, Drouin C, Freyer J, Arnason J, Eberl G, Hamann A, Wagner H, Huehn J, Sparwasser T (2007) Selective depletion of Foxp3+ regulatory T cells induces a scurfy-like disease. J Exp Med 204:57–63

Larmonier N, Marron M, Zeng Y, Cantrell J, Romanoski A, Sepassi M, Thompson S, Chen X, Andreansky S, Katsanis E (2007) Tumor-derived CD4(+)CD25(+) regulatory T cell suppression of dendritic cell function involves TGF-beta and IL-10. Cancer Immunol Immunother 56:48–59

Lee YK, Mukasa R, Hatton RD, Weaver CT (2009) Developmental plasticity of Th17 and Treg cells. Curr Opin Immunol 21:274–280

Leffers N, Gooden MJ, de Jong RA, Hoogeboom BN, ten Hoor KA, Hollema H, Boezen HM, van der Zee AG, Daemen T, Nijman HW (2009) Prognostic significance of tumor-infiltrating T-lymphocytes in primary and metastatic lesions of advanced stage ovarian cancer. Cancer Immunol Immunother 58:449–459

Levitt ML, Kassem B, Gooding WE, Miketic LM, Landreneau RJ, Ferson PF, Keenan R, Yousem SA, Lindberg CA, Trenn MR, Ponas RS, Tarasoff P, Sabatine JM, Friberg D, Whiteside TL (2004) Phase I study of gemcitabine given weekly as a short infusion for non-small cell lung cancer: results and possible immune system-related mechanisms. Lung Cancer 43:335–344

Liang B, Workman C, Lee J, Chew C, Dale BM, Colonna L, Flores M, Li N, Schweighoffer E, Greenberg S, Tybulewicz V, Vignali D, Clynes R (2008) Regulatory T cells inhibit dendritic cells by lymphocyte activation gene-3 engagement of MHC class II. J Immunol 180: 5916–5926

Lin YC, Chang LY, Huang CT, Peng HM, Dutta A, Chen TC, Yeh CT, Lin CY (2009) Effector/memory but not naive regulatory T cells are responsible for the loss of concomitant tumor immunity. J Immunol 182:6095–6104

Litzinger MT, Fernando R, Curiel TJ, Grosenbach DW, Schlom J, Palena C (2007) IL-2 immunotoxin denileukin diftitox reduces regulatory T cells and enhances vaccine-mediated T-cell immunity. Blood 110:3192–3201

Liu H, Komai-Koma M, Xu D, Liew FY (2006a) Toll-like receptor 2 signaling modulates the functions of CD4+ CD25+ regulatory T cells. Proc Natl Acad Sci USA 103:7048–7053

Liu W, Putnam AL, Xu-Yu Z, Szot GL, Lee MR, Zhu S, Gottlieb PA, Kapranov P, Gingeras TR, de St F, Groth B, Clayberger C, Soper DM, Ziegler SF, Bluestone JA (2006b) CD127 expression inversely correlates with FoxP3 and suppressive function of human CD4+ T reg cells. J Exp Med 203:1701–1711

Liyanage UK, Moore TT, Joo H-G, Tanaka Y, Herrmann V, Doherty G, Drebin JA, Strasberg SM, Eberlein TJ, Goedegebuure PS, Linehan DC (2002) Prevalence of Regulatory T Cells Is Increased in Peripheral Blood and Tumor Microenvironment of Patients with Pancreas or Breast Adenocarcinoma. J Immunol 169:2756–2761

Lonnroth C, Andersson M, Arvidsson A, Nordgren S, Brevinge H, Lagerstedt K, Lundholm K (2008) Preoperative treatment with a non-steroidal anti-inflammatory drug (NSAID) increases tumor tissue infiltration of seemingly activated immune cells in colorectal cancer. Cancer Immun 8:5

Lord R, Nair S, Schache A, Spicer J, Somaihah N, Khoo V, Pandha H (2007) Low dose metronomic oral cyclophosphamide for hormone resistant prostate cancer: a phase II study. J Urol 177:2136–2140, discussion 2140

Loser K, Apelt J, Voskort M, Mohaupt M, Balkow S, Schwarz T, Grabbe S, Beissert S (2007) IL-10 controls ultraviolet-induced carcinogenesis in mice. J Immunol 179:365–371

Lutsiak ME, Semnani RT, De Pascalis R, Kashmiri SV, Schlom J, Sabzevari H (2005) Inhibition of CD4(+)25+ T regulatory cell function implicated in enhanced immune response by low-dose cyclophosphamide. Blood 105:2862–2868

Mahnke K, Schonfeld K, Fondel S, Ring S, Karakhanova S, Wiedemeyer K, Bedke T, Johnson TS, Storn V, Schallenberg S, Enk AH (2007) Depletion of CD4+CD25+ human regulatory T cells in vivo: kinetics of Treg depletion and alterations in immune functions in vivo and in vitro. Int J Cancer 120:2723–2733

Mailloux AW, Young MR (2009) NK-dependent increases in CCL22 secretion selectively recruits regulatory T cells to the tumor microenvironment. J Immunol 182:2753–2765

Maker AV, Attia P, Rosenberg SA (2005) Analysis of the cellular mechanism of antitumor responses and autoimmunity in patients treated with CTLA-4 blockade. J Immunol 175:7746–7754

Mantovani A, Bottazzi B, Colotta F, Sozzani S, Ruco L (1992) The origin and function of tumor-associated macrophages. Immunol Today 13:265–270

Mantovani A, Sica A, Sozzani S, Allavena P, Vecchi A, Locati M (2004) The chemokine system in diverse forms of macrophage activation and polarization. Trends Immunol 25:677–686
Mantovani A, Allavena P, Sica A, Balkwill F (2008) Cancer-related inflammation. Nature 454:436–444
Marshall NA, Christie LE, Munro LR, Culligan DJ, Johnston PW, Basher RN, Vickers MA (2004) Immunosuppressive regulatory T-cells are abundant in the reactive lymphocytes of Hodgkin lymphoma. Blood 103:1755–1762
Marzano AV, Vezzoli P, Fanoni D, Venegoni L, Berti E (2009) Primary cutaneous T-cell lymphoma expressing FOXP3: a case report supporting the existence of malignancies of regulatory T cells. J Am Acad Dermatol 61:348–355
Maynard CL, Harrington LE, Janowski KM, Oliver JR, Zindl CL, Rudensky AY, Weaver CT (2007) Regulatory T cells expressing interleukin 10 develop from Foxp3+ and Foxp3- precursor cells in the absence of interleukin 10. Nat Immunol 8:931–941
Miyara M, Yoshioka Y, Kitoh A, Shima T, Wing K, Niwa A, Parizot C, Taflin C, Heike T, Valeyre D, Mathian A, Nakahata T, Yamaguchi T, Nomura T, Ono M, Amoura Z, Gorochov G, Sakaguchi S (2009) Functional delineation and differentiation dynamics of human CD4+ T cells expressing the FoxP3 transcription factor. Immunity 30:899–911
Mizukami Y, Kono K, Kawaguchi Y, Akaike H, Kamimura K, Sugai H, Fujii H (2008) CCL17 and CCL22 chemokines within tumor microenvironment are related to accumulation of Foxp3+ regulatory T cells in gastric cancer. Int J Cancer 122:2286–2293
Nagar M, Vernitsky H, Cohen Y, Dominissini D, Berkun Y, Rechavi G, Amariglio N, Goldstein I (2008) Epigenetic inheritance of DNA methylation limits activation-induced expression of FOXP3 in conventional human CD25-CD4+ T cells. Int Immunol 20:1041–1055
Olkhanud PB, Baatar D, Bodogai M, Hakim F, Gress R, Anderson RL, Deng J, Xu M, Briest S, Biragyn A (2009) Breast cancer lung metastasis requires expression of chemokine receptor CCR4 and regulatory T cells. Cancer Res 69:5996–6004
Ormandy LA, Hillemann T, Wedemeyer H, Manns MP, Greten TF, Korangy F (2005) Increased populations of regulatory T cells in peripheral blood of patients with hepatocellular carcinoma. Cancer Res 65:2457–2464
Ostrand-Rosenberg S, Sinha P (2009) Myeloid-Derived Suppressor Cells: Linking Inflammation and Cancer. J Immunol 182:4499–4506
Ozao-Choy J, Ma G, Kao J, Wang GX, Meseck M, Sung M, Schwartz M, Divino CM, Pan PY, Chen SH (2009) The novel role of tyrosine kinase inhibitor in the reversal of immune suppression and modulation of tumor microenvironment for immune-based cancer therapies. Cancer Res 69:2514–2522
Peggs KS, Quezada SA, Chambers CA, Korman AJ, Allison JP (2009) Blockade of CTLA-4 on both effector and regulatory T cell compartments contributes to the antitumor activity of anti-CTLA-4 antibodies. J Exp Med 206:1717–1725
Peng G, Guo Z, Kiniwa Y, Voo KS, Peng W, Fu T, Wang DY, Li Y, Wang HY, Wang RF (2005) Toll-like receptor 8-mediated reversal of CD4+ regulatory T cell function. Science 309:1380–1384
Peterson RP, Campa MJ, Sperlazza J, Conon D, Joshi MB, Harpole PH Jr, Patz EF Jr (2006) Tumer intiltrating Foxp3+ regulatory T-cells are associated with reaccurrence in pathology stage INSCLC patients. Cancer 107:2866–2872
Petrausch U, Jensen SM, Twitty C, Poehlein CH, Haley DP, Walker EB, Fox BA (2009) Disruption of TGF-beta signaling prevents the generation of tumor-sensitized regulatory T cells and facilitates therapeutic antitumor immunity. J Immunol 183:3682–3689
Piconese S, Valzasina B, Colombo MP (2008) OX40 triggering blocks suppression by regulatory T cells and facilitates tumor rejection. J Exp Med 205:825–839
Piersma SJ, Welters MJ, van der Burg SH (2008) Tumor-specific regulatory T cells in cancer patients. Hum Immunol 69:241–249
Polansky JK, Kretschmer K, Freyer J, Floess S, Garbe A, Baron U, Olek S, Hamann A, von Boehmer H, Huehn J (2008) DNA methylation controls Foxp3 gene expression. Eur J Immunol 38:1654–1663

Powell DJ Jr, de Vries CR, Allen T, Ahmadzadeh M, Rosenberg SA (2007a) Inability to mediate prolonged reduction of regulatory T Cells after transfer of autologous CD25-depleted PBMC and interleukin-2 after lymphodepleting chemotherapy. J Immunother 30:438–447

Powell DJ Jr, Felipe-Silva A, Merino MJ, Ahmadzadeh M, Allen T, Levy C, White DE, Mavroukakis S, Kreitman RJ, Rosenberg SA, Pastan I (2007b) Administration of a CD25-directed immunotoxin, LMB-2, to patients with metastatic melanoma induces a selective partial reduction in regulatory T cells in vivo. J Immunol 179:4919–4928

Quach H, Ritchie D, Neeson P, Harrison S, Tai T, Taviton K, Lynch K, Prince HMP (2008) Regulatory T-cell (Treg) are depressed in patients with relapsed/refractory multiple mydoma (MM) and increases towards normal range in responding patients treated with lenalidomide (LEN). Blood (ASH, Annual meeting abstracts), Nov 2008; 112:1696

Quach H, Ritchie D, Stewart AK, Neeson P, Harrison S, Smyth MJ, Prince HM (2010) Mechanism of action of immunomodulatory drugs (IMiDS) in multiple myeloma. Leukemia 24:22–32

Quezada SA, Peggs KS, Curran MA, Allison JP (2006) CTLA4 blockade and GM-CSF combination immunotherapy alters the intratumor balance of effector and regulatory T cells. The Journal of Clinical Investigation 116:1935–1945

Quezada SA, Peggs KS, Simpson TR, Shen Y, Littman DR, Allison JP (2008) Limited tumor infiltration by activated T effector cells restricts the therapeutic activity of regulatory T cell depletion against established melanoma. J Exp Med 205:2125–2138

Rajashree P, Das SD (2008) Infection with prevalent clinical strains of Mycobacterium tuberculosis leads to differential maturation of monocyte derived dendritic cells. Immunol Lett 117:174–180

Ralainirina N, Poli A, Michel T, Poos L, Andres E, Hentges F, Zimmer J (2007) Control of NK cell functions by CD4+CD25+ regulatory T cells. J Leukoc Biol 81:144–153

Rech AJ, Vonderheide RH (2009) Clinical use of anti-CD25 antibody daclizumab to enhance immune responses to tumor antigen vaccination by targeting regulatory T cells. Ann N Y Acad Sci 1174:99–106

Ribas A (2008) Overcoming Immunologic Tolerance to Melanoma: Targeting CTLA-4 with Tremelimumab (CP-675, 206). Oncologist 13:10–15

Roncador G, Brown PJ, Maestre L, Hue S, Martinez-Torrecuadrada JL, Ling KL, Pratap S, Toms C, Fox BC, Cerundolo V, Powrie F, Banham AH (2005) Analysis of FOXP3 protein expression in human CD4+CD25+ regulatory T cells at the single-cell level. Eur J Immunol 35:1681–1691

Rosenberg SA, Dudley ME (2009) Adoptive cell therapy for the treatment of patients with metastatic melanoma. Curr Opin Immunol 21:233–240

Rubtsov YP, Rasmussen JP, Chi EY, Fontenot J, Castelli L, Ye X, Treuting P, Siewe L, Roers A, Henderson WR Jr, Muller W, Rudensky AY (2008) Regulatory T cell-derived interleukin-10 limits inflammation at environmental interfaces. Immunity 28:546–558

Ruby CE, Weinberg AD (2009) OX40-enhanced tumor rejection and effector T cell differentiation decreases with age. J Immunol 182:1481–1489

Ruby CE, Yates MA, Hirschhorn-Cymerman D, Chlebeck P, Wolchok JD, Houghton AN, Offner H, Weinberg AD (2009) Cutting Edge: OX40 agonists can drive regulatory T cell expansion if the cytokine milieu is right. J Immunol 183:4853–4857

Sakaguchi S, Sakaguchi N, Asano M, Itoh M, Toda M (1995) Immunologic self-tolerance maintained by activated T cells expressing IL-2 receptor alpha-chains (CD25). Breakdown of a single mechanism of self-tolerance causes various autoimmune diseases. J Immunol 155:1151–1164

Sakaguchi S, Yamaguchi T, Nomura T, Ono M (2008) Regulatory T cells and immune tolerance. Cell 133:775–787

Salama P, Phillips M, Grieu F, Morris M, Zeps N, Joseph D, Platell C, Iacopetta B (2009) Tumor infiltrating FoxP3+ T regulatory cells show strong prognostic significance in colorectal cancer. J Clin Oncol 27:186–192

Sarris M, Andersen KG, Randow F, Mayr L, Betz AG (2008) Neuropilin-1 expression on regulatory T cells enhances their interactions with dendritic cells during antigen recognition. Immunity 28:402–413

Sasada T, Kimura M, Yoshida Y, Kanai M, Takabayashi A (2003) CD4+CD25+ regulatory T cells in patients with gastrointestinal malignancies: possible involvement of regulatory T cells in disease progression. Cancer 98:1089–1099

Seddiki N, Santner-Nanan B, Martinson J, Zaunders J, Sasson S, Landay A, Solomon M, Selby W, Alexander SI, Nanan R, Kelleher A, de St F, Groth B (2006a) Expression of interleukin (IL)-2 and IL-7 receptors discriminates between human regulatory and activated T cells. J Exp Med 203:1693–1700

Seddiki N, Santner-Nanan B, Tangye SG, Alexander SI, Solomon M, Lee S, Nanan R, de Saint F, Groth B (2006b) Persistence of naive CD45RA+ regulatory T cells in adult life. Blood 107:2830–2838

Serafini P, Mgebroff S, Noonan K, Borrello I (2008) Myeloid-derived suppressor cells promote cross-tolerance in B-cell lymphoma by expanding regulatory T cells. Cancer Res 68: 5439–5449

Sfanos KS, Bruno TC, Maris CH, Xu L, Thoburn CJ, DeMarzo AM, Meeker AK, Isaacs WB, Drake CG (2008) Phenotypic analysis of prostate-infiltrating lymphocytes reveals TH17 and Treg skewing. Clin Cancer Res 14:3254–3261

Shevach EM (2006) From vanilla to 28 flavors: multiple varieties of T regulatory cells. Immunity 25:195–201

Shevach EM (2009) Mechanisms of foxp3+ T regulatory cell-mediated suppression. Immunity 30:636–645

Shevach EM, Tran DQ, Davidson TS, Andersson J (2008) The critical contribution of TGF-beta to the induction of Foxp3 expression and regulatory T cell function. Eur J Immunol 38:915–917

Siegmund K, Feuerer M, Siewert C, Ghani S, Haubold U, Dankof A, Krenn V, Schon MP, Scheffold A, Lowe JB, Hamann A, Syrbe U, Huehn J (2005) Migration matters: regulatory T-cell compartmentalization determines suppressive activity in vivo. Blood 106:3097–3104

Siewert C, Menning A, Dudda J, Siegmund K, Lauer U, Floess S, Campbell DJ, Hamann A, Huehn J (2007) Induction of organ-selective CD4+ regulatory T cell homing. Eur J Immunol 37:978–989

Sinha P, Clements VK, Fulton AM, Ostrand-Rosenberg S (2007) Prostaglandin E2 promotes tumor progression by inducing myeloid-derived suppressor cells. Cancer Res 67:4507–4513

Smyth MJ, Street SE, Trapani JA (2003) Cutting edge: granzymes A and B are not essential for perforin-mediated tumor rejection. J Immunol 171:515–518

Smyth MJ, Teng MW, Swann J, Kyparissoudis K, Godfrey DI, Hayakawa Y (2006) CD4+CD25+ T regulatory cells suppress NK cell-mediated immunotherapy of cancer. J Immunol 176: 1582–1587

So T, Lee SW, Croft M (2008) Immune regulation and control of regulatory T cells by OX40 and 4-1BB. Cytokine Growth Factor Rev 19:253–262

Solinas G, Germano G, Mantovani A, Allavena P (2009) Tumor-associated macrophages (TAM) as major players of the cancer-related inflammation. J Leukoc Biol 86:1065–1073

Somasundaram R, Jacob L, Swoboda R, Caputo L, Song H, Basak S, Monos D, Peritt D, Marincola F, Cai D, Birebent B, Bloome E, Kim J, Berencsi K, Mastrangelo M, Herlyn D (2002) Inhibition of cytolytic T lymphocyte proliferation by autologous CD4+/CD25+ regulatory T cells in a colorectal carcinoma patient is mediated by transforming growth factor-beta. Cancer Res 62:5267–5272

Song X, Krelin Y, Dvorkin T, Bjorkdahl O, Segal S, Dinarello CA, Voronov E, Apte RN (2005) CD11b+/Gr-1+ immature myeloid cells mediate suppression of T cells in mice bearing tumors of IL-1beta-secreting cells. J Immunol 175:8200–8208

Stephens GL, Andersson J, Shevach EM (2007) Distinct subsets of FoxP3+ regulatory T cells participate in the control of immune responses. J Immunol 178:6901–6911

Strauss L, Bergmann C, Szczepanski MJ, Lang S, Kirkwood JM, Whiteside TL (2008) Expression of ICOS on human melanoma-infiltrating CD4+CD25highFoxp3+ T regulatory cells: implications and impact on tumor-mediated immune suppression. J Immunol 180:2967–2980

Sutmuller RP, den Brok MH, Kramer M, Bennink EJ, Toonen LW, Kullberg BJ, Joosten LA, Akira S, Netea MG, Adema GJ (2006a) Toll-like receptor 2 controls expansion and function of regulatory T cells. J Clin Invest 116:485–494

Sutmuller RP, Morgan ME, Netea MG, Grauer O, Adema GJ (2006b) Toll-like receptors on regulatory T cells: expanding immune regulation. Trends Immunol 27:387–393

Szczepanski MJ, Szajnik M, Czystowska M, Mandapathil M, Strauss L, Welsh A, Foon KA, Whiteside TL, Boyiadzis M (2009) Increased Frequency and Suppression by Regulatory T Cells in Patients with Acute Myelogenous Leukemia. Clinical Cancer Research 15:3325–3332

Takegawa S, Jin Z, Nakayama T, Oyama T, Hieshima K, Nagakubo D, Shirakawa AK, Tsuzuki T, Nakamura S, Yoshie O (2008) Expression of CCL17 and CCL22 by latent membrane protein 1-positive tumor cells in age-related Epstein-Barr virus-associated B-cell lymphoproliferative disorder. Cancer Sci 99:296–302

Tan MC, Goedegebuure PS, Belt BA, Flaherty B, Sankpal N, Gillanders WE, Eberlein TJ, Hsieh CS, Linehan DC (2009) Disruption of CCR5-dependent homing of regulatory T cells inhibits tumor growth in a murine model of pancreatic cancer. J Immunol 182:1746–1755

Tang Q, Bluestone JA (2008) The Foxp3+ regulatory T cell: a jack of all trades, master of regulation. Nat Immunol 9:239–244

Terabe M, Berzofsky JA (2007) NKT cells in immunoregulation of tumor immunity: a new immunoregulatory axis. Trends Immunol 28:491–496

Tzankov A, Meier C, Hirschmann P, Went P, Pileri SA, Dirnhofer S (2008) Correlation of high numbers of intratumoral FOXP3+ regulatory T cells with improved survival in germinal center-like diffuse large B-cell lymphoma, follicular lymphoma and classical Hodgkin's lymphoma. Haematologica 93:193–200

Vignali DA, Collison LW, Workman CJ (2008) How regulatory T cells work. Nat Rev Immunol 8:523–532

Viguier M, Lemaitre F, Verola O, Cho MS, Gorochov G, Dubertret L, Bachelez H, Kourilsky P, Ferradini L (2004) Foxp3 expressing CD4+CD25(high) regulatory T cells are overrepresented in human metastatic melanoma lymph nodes and inhibit the function of infiltrating T cells. J Immunol 173:1444–1453

Voo KS, Wang YH, Santori FR, Boggiano C, Arima K, Bover L, Hanabuchi S, Khalili J, Marinova E, Zheng B, Littman DR, Liu YJ (2009) Identification of IL-17-producing FOXP3+ regulatory T cells in humans. Proc Natl Acad Sci USA 106:4793–4798

Vu MD, Xiao X, Gao W, Degauque N, Chen M, Kroemer A, Killeen N, Ishii N, Chang Li X (2007) OX40 costimulation turns off Foxp3+ Tregs. Blood 110:2501–2510

Wada S, Yoshimura K, Hipkiss EL, Harris TJ, Yen HR, Goldberg MV, Grosso JF, Getnet D, Demarzo AM, Netto GJ, Anders R, Pardoll DM, Drake CG (2009) Cyclophosphamide augments antitumor immunity: studies in an autochthonous prostate cancer model. Cancer Res 69:4309–4318

Wan YY, Flavell RA (2007) Regulatory T-cell functions are subverted and converted owing to attenuated Foxp3 expression. Nature 445:766–770

Wang HY, Wang RF (2007) Regulatory T cells and cancer. Curr Opin Immunol 19:217–223

Wang L, Yi T, Kortylewski M, Pardoll DM, Zeng D, Yu H (2009) IL-17 can promote tumor growth through an IL-6-Stat3 signaling pathway. J Exp Med 206:1457–1464

Weaver CT, Hatton RD (2009) Interplay between the TH17 and TReg cell lineages: a (co-) evolutionary perspective. Nat Rev Immunol 9:883–889

Wei S, Kryczek I, Zou L, Daniel B, Cheng P, Mottram P, Curiel T, Lange A, Zou W (2005) Plasmacytoid dendritic cells induce CD8+ regulatory T cells in human ovarian carcinoma. Cancer Res 65:5020–5026

Wildin RS, Ramsdell F, Peake J, Faravelli F, Casanova JL, Buist N, Levy-Lahad E, Mazzella M, Goulet O, Perroni L, Bricarelli FD, Byrne G, McEuen M, Proll S, Appleby M, Brunkow ME

(2001) X-linked neonatal diabetes mellitus, enteropathy and endocrinopathy syndrome is the human equivalent of mouse scurfy. Nat Genet 27:18–20

Williams LM, Rudensky AY (2007) Maintenance of the Foxp3-dependent developmental program in mature regulatory T cells requires continued expression of Foxp3. Nat Immunol 8:277–284

Wing K, Onishi Y, Prieto-Martin P, Yamaguchi T, Miyara M, Fehervari Z, Nomura T, Sakaguchi S (2008) CTLA-4 control over Foxp3+ regulatory T cell function. Science 322:271–275

Wolf AM, Wolf D, Steurer M, Gastl G, Gunsilius E, Grubeck-Loebenstein B (2003) Increase of regulatory T cells in the peripheral blood of cancer patients. Clin Cancer Res 9:606–612

Wolf AM, Eller K, Zeiser R, Durr C, Gerlach UV, Sixt M, Markut L, Gastl G, Rosenkranz AR, Wolf D (2009) The sphingosine 1-phosphate receptor agonist FTY720 potently inhibits regulatory T cell proliferation in vitro and in vivo. J Immunol 183:3751–3760

Woo EY, Chu CS, Goletz TJ, Schlienger K, Yeh H, Coukos G, Rubin SC, Kaiser LR, June CH (2001) Regulatory CD4(+)CD25(+) T cells in tumors from patients with early-stage non-small cell lung cancer and late-stage ovarian cancer. Cancer Res 61:4766–4772

Wrzesinski SH, Wan YY, Flavell RA (2007) Transforming growth factor-beta and the immune response: implications for anticancer therapy. Clin Cancer Res 13:5262–5270

Xu L, Kitani A, Fuss I, Strober W (2007) Cutting edge: regulatory T cells induce CD4+CD25-Foxp3- T cells or are self-induced to become Th17 cells in the absence of exogenous TGF-beta. J Immunol 178:6725–6729

Yagi H, Nomura T, Nakamura K, Yamazaki S, Kitawaki T, Hori S, Maeda M, Onodera M, Uchiyama T, Fujii S, Sakaguchi S (2004) Crucial role of FOXP3 in the development and function of human CD25+CD4+ regulatory T cells. Int Immunol 16:1643–1656

Yamaguchi T, Hirota K, Nagahama K, Ohkawa K, Takahashi T, Nomura T, Sakaguchi S (2007) Control of immune responses by antigen-specific regulatory T cells expressing the folate receptor. Immunity 27:145–159

Yang ZZ, Novak AJ, Stenson MJ, Witzig TE, Ansell SM (2006) Intratumoral CD4+CD25+ regulatory T-cell-mediated suppression of infiltrating CD4+ T cells in B-cell non-Hodgkin lymphoma. Blood 107:3639–3646

Yang ZZ, Novak AJ, Ziesmer SC, Witzig TE, Ansell SM (2007) CD70+ non-Hodgkin lymphoma B cells induce Foxp3 expression and regulatory function in intratumoral CD4+CD25 T cells. Blood 110:2537–2544

Yang Y, Zhang WG, He AL, Yang HY, Wang JL, Tian W (2008) Effects of thalidomide on CD4 (+)CD25(+) T regulatory cells in patients with multiple myeloma. Zhongguo Shi Yan Xue Ye Xue Za Zhi 16:538–542

Yang ZZ, Novak AJ, Ziesmer SC, Witzig TE, Ansell SM (2009) Malignant B cells skew the balance of regulatory T cells and TH17 cells in B-cell non-Hodgkin's lymphoma. Cancer Res 69:5522–5530

Yaqub S, Henjum K, Mahic M, Jahnsen FL, Aandahl EM, Bjornbeth BA, Tasken K (2008) Regulatory T cells in colorectal cancer patients suppress anti-tumor immune activity in a COX-2 dependent manner. Cancer Immunol Immunother 57:813–821

Zhao DM, Thornton AM, DiPaolo RJ, Shevach EM (2006) Activated CD4+CD25+ T cells selectively kill B lymphocytes. Blood 107:3925–3932

Zheng Y, Chaudhry A, Kas A, deRoos P, Kim JM, Chu TT, Corcoran L, Treuting P, Klein U, Rudensky AY (2009) Regulatory T-cell suppressor program co-opts transcription factor IRF4 to control T(H)2 responses. Nature 458:351–356

Zhou L, Littman DR (2009) Transcriptional regulatory networks in Th17 cell differentiation. Curr Opin Immunol 21:146–152

Zhou Q, Bucher C, Munger ME, Highfill SL, Tolar J, Munn DH, Levine BL, Riddle M, June CH, Vallera DA, Weigel BJ, Blazar BR (2009a) Depletion of endogenous tumor-associated regulatory T cells improves the efficacy of adoptive cytotoxic T-cell immunotherapy in murine acute myeloid leukemia. Blood 114:3793–3802

Zhou X, Bailey-Bucktrout S, Jeker LT, Bluestone JA (2009b) Plasticity of CD4(+) FoxP3(+) T cells. Curr Opin Immunol 21:281–285

Zhu X, Ma LL, Ye T (2009) Expression of CD4(+)CD25(high)CD127(low/-) regulatory T cells in transitional cell carcinoma patients and its significance. J Clin Lab Anal 23:197–201

Zou W (2006) Regulatory T cells, tumour immunity and immunotherapy. Nat Rev Immunol 6:295–307

Concepts and Ways to Amplify the Antitumor Immune Response

Bent Rubin and Jean Edouard Gairin

Contents

1 Introduction 98
2 Pharmacology of Tumor Cell–Immune Cell Interactions 100
3 Tumor Cell Development and Its Danger Signals 101
3.1 Neoplastic Cells 102
3.2 Chronic Inflammation 103
3.3 Stroma 105
4 Expression and Presentation of Tumor Antigens 105
5 Mouse Models of Cancer 107
5.1 The LCMV Model to Study the Regulation of MHCI Expression 107
5.2 The L12R4 Vaccination Model 109
5.3 The SR/CR Mouse Model 110
6 Cellular and Molecular Regulation of Tumor Immunity 113
7 Discussion 117
References 122

Abstract In this chapter, a detailed description of how the innate and adaptive immune responses interact with malignant cells is presented. In addition, we discuss how developing tumors establish themselves, and how they benefit on one hand and organize their defense against the immune system on the other hand. New data from three tumor model systems in mice are discussed; in particular, the intricate interactions between the immune cells and the tumor cells are highlighted. With the present data and knowledge, we conclude that a first prerequisite for the

B. Rubin
Institut de Sciences et Technologies du Médicament de Toulouse, UMR 2587 CNRS-Pierre Fabre, 3, rue des Satellites, 31400 Toulouse, France

J.E. Gairin (✉)
Institut de Sciences et Technologies du Médicament de Toulouse, UMR 2587 CNRS-Pierre Fabre, 3, rue des Satellites, 31400 Toulouse, France
Faculté de Pharmacie, Université Paul Sabatier, 31400 Toulouse, France
e-mail: jean-edouard.gairin@istmt.cnrs.fr

G. Dranoff (ed.), *Cancer Immunology and Immunotherapy*,
Current Topics in Microbiology and Immunology 344, DOI 10.1007/82_2010_89

combat against tumors is the activation of the innate immune system via external danger signals or damage signals and internal danger signals. The second prerequisite for efficient tumor cell eradication is combined therapeutic approaches of physical, chemical, pharmacological, and immunological origin. Finally, we propose new ways for further investigation of the relationship linking tumor cells and our defense system. It appears mandatory to understand how the malignant cells render the adaptive immune cells tolerant instead of turning them into aggressive effectors and memory cells. Perhaps, the most important thing, for immunologists and clinicians, to understand is that tumor cells must not be viewed just as antigens but much more.

1 Introduction

Communication between the immune system and tumor cells takes place via both cell–cell contact-dependent receptor–ligand interactions and released cytokines/chemokines. T lymphocytes of the adaptive immune system learn in the thymus to distinguish various self or altered self-structures from non-self-structures presented as peptides bound to major histocompatibility complex (MHC) class I or class II antigens (pMHC) (Krogsgaard and Davis 2005; Call and Wucherpfennig 2007). pMHC molecules represent the antigenic universe to αβ-T lymphocytes, both the self and the non-self-repertoire. γδ-T lymphocytes recognize small phosphorylated molecules or non-classical MHCI antigens in a non-MHC restricted manner (Allison et al. 2001; Gao et al. 2003; Adams et al. 2008), and B lymphocytes recognize tertiary or quaternary structures of antigens using immunoglobulins (Ig) (Jerne 1984, Davies and Cohen 1996). A third type of recognition is used by cells of the innate immune system: natural killer (NK) and natural killer T (NKT) cells recognize lack of expression of self (missing self), i.e., absence or low cell-surface levels of MHCI and/or MHCII molecules (Kärre et al. 1986; Godfrey et al. 2004). Furthermore, antigen-presenting cells (APC) such as dendritic cells (DC), macrophages, and granulocytes can recognize non-self-structures via toll-like receptors (TLR) or C-type lectin receptors (CLRs) (Janeway 1989; Figdor et al. 2002). Activation of T cells, NKT, or NK cells happens via the interaction of activating receptors (KAR) associated with signaling molecules expressing immuno-tyrosine-activation-motif (ITAM) signal-motifs in their cytoplasmic region. T lymphocytes and NKT cells express T-cell receptor (TCR)/CD3 complexes, and T, NKT, or NK cells express KARs such as NKG2D associated with DAP10 signal-transduction molecules and Ly49D associated with DAP12 molecules (Call and Wucherpfennig 2007; Vivier and Anfossi 2004). It appears that the high number (~10) of ITAMs associated with TCR molecules is necessary to avoid autoimmunity (Holst et al. 2008). Inhibition of cell activation by inhibitory receptors (KIRs) such as NKG2A/CD94 is related to the expression by KIRs of ITIM inhibitory motifs in their cytoplasmic tails (Call and Wucherpfennig 2007; Kane et al. 2001).

Helper T (Th) cells trigger differentiation of precursor cells into $CD8^+$ cytotoxic T lymphocytes (CTL) or antibody-producing B cells. The so-called Th1 cells induce preferentially the production of IL-2 and IFNγ and the differentiation of CTL, whereas Th2 cells induce mostly the production of IL-4, IL-5, and IL-13 and the differentiation of B cells into antibody-producing plasma cells (Kalinski and Moser 2005). When administered to elicit specific immune responses and memory but not tolerance, the antigens have to be presented in the form of cells, particles, or aggregates, or emulsified in adjuvants such as Freund's adjuvants or aluminum salt precipitates (McKee et al. 2007). A unifying concept of these phenomena was proposed by late Charlie Janeway (Janeway 1989). The innate immune system, NKT cells, NK cells, DC, macrophages, and granulocytes are activated by pathogen-associated molecular patterns (PAMPs) by means of TLR (Janeway 1989; Medzhitov 2001) or CLRs (Figdor et al. 2002). The DC differentiates from immature, phagocytosing cells to mature, non-phagocytosing cells with increased levels of co-stimulatory molecules such as MHCII, CD40, CD80, and CD86 and enhanced antigen-presenting activity (Janeway 1989; Carnaud et al. 1999; Fernandez et al. 1999). Cells from the innate immune system release inflammatory cytokines that induce the priming of $CD4^+$ Th subpopulations (Th1, Th2, and Th17). Immediately after stimulation, NKT cells release preformed IFNγ and IL-4 which direct Th1 and Th2 cell differentiation, respectively. IFNγ triggers DC to produce IL-12, which induces preferential Th1-priming and NK cell production of IFNγ and cytotoxicity (Carnaud et al. 1999; Fernandez et al. 1999). A subset of DCs, $CD8^+CD205^+$ dendritic cells, produces endogenous TGFβ and is specialized to induce $Foxp3^+$ T_{reg} cells, whereas another subset, $CD8^-CD205^-$ and $DCIR\text{-}2^+$ (DC inhibitory receptor-2), participates in Th2 responses (Yamazaki et al. 2008).

Although stimulation of the innate immune system may greatly help the initiation of adaptive cellular and humoral immune responses, over-activation of the innate immune system represents a risk due to a possible "fatal cytokine storm" (Smyth and Godfrey 2000; Kim et al. 2007). However, the cytokine storm is prevented by $CD4^+$ Th or $CD8^+$ CTL, which down-regulate the activity of the innate immune cells by a cell–cell contact, MHC-dependent mechanism (Kim et al. 2007). It seems clear that memory T cells are derived from effector T cells by avoiding antigen-induced cell death (Harrington et al. 2008). In contrast, the subdivision of $CD4^+$ T cells into Th1, Th2, Th9, Th17, and T_{reg} cells is more malleable and demonstrates more functional plasticity than previously thought. Inexperienced, naïve T cells appear to receive different types of "secondary education" when they encounter antigen at various regional sites including tumor microenvironments (Tato and Cua 2008). Besides possessing different effector functions, DC and T cells should be able to migrate to and within tissues. Adhesion via L-selectin induces rolling, activation, and transmigration via chemokine receptors such as CCR7. The interaction between CCR7 and its ligands, CCL19 and CCL21, may balance immunity and tolerance (Homey et al. 2002; Förster et al. 2008).

T lymphocytes do not react with self-structures that are expressed in normal physiological conditions, i.e., the organism is tolerant to self-structures. However, thymus negative selection (central tolerance) is not infallible, and self-reactive

T cells with low-avidity TCR do emigrate from the thymus. Such self-reactive T cells are regulated by $CD4^{+}CD25^{+}$ T regulatory (T_{reg}) cells (peripheral tolerance) (Vignali et al. 2008). Thus, since many antitumor immune responses are "autoimmune" reactions, these are often weak in both quantity and quality (Pardoll 2002). It is important to distinguish between the following three levels of low responsiveness to malignant cells: (1) tumor-specific T cells with high-avidity TCR have been eliminated in the thymus; (2) tumor cells or their products may induce tolerance (in the sense of unresponsiveness), i.e., tumor-specific T cells are present but are rendered anergic; (3) immune effectors recognize tumor cells but are prohibited from performing their natural function due to tumor-associated inhibitory molecules and/or cells. The latter two phenomena are linked to the fact that resting DC or macrophages in the tumor induces and maintains peripheral tolerance and functional anergy in $CD8^{+}$ T cells, NKT cells, and NK cells through PD-1 and CTLA-4-related mechanisms (Probst et al. 2005; Chang et al. 2008).

In this review, we discuss the possible ways in which the interactions between immune cells and tumor cells can be increased and consequently mediate tumor cell destruction. Both genetic and mechanical (chemical or physical) interventions can render established tumors more vulnerable to the immune cells. These mechanisms as well as active defenses by the tumor cells releasing cytokines/chemokines/hormones inhibitory to the function of the immune cells are taken into consideration (Entin et al. 2003; Ganss et al. 2004).

2 Pharmacology of Tumor Cell–Immune Cell Interactions

The discussion on molecules that can augment the interactions between immune cells and tumor cells is based on three different possible mechanisms: molecules that can interfere with (1) specific, clonal interactions; (2) specific, non-clonal interactions; or (3) non-specific, global reactions. The big disadvantage of the latter two possibilities is that such treatments may also attain functions other than the specific immune cell–tumor cell interaction. Interactions between KARs, co-receptors, or immunoglobulins (Ig) and tumor cells are mediated by receptors reacting with their membrane-bound ligands on the tumor cells (Bendelac et al. 2001). The interaction between the TCRs and tumor cells is more complex for several reasons:

- First, TCR recognizes composite ligands (pMHC) with such a low avidity that a simultaneous interaction of co-receptors (e.g., CD4, CD8, CD28, and CD154) and/or adhesion receptors (e.g., CD2, LFA-1) is necessary to trigger T cell activation. These two co-signals augment the messages sent through the different intracellular signal transmission pathways. Consequently, not only the TCR–pMHC interaction (the clonal signal 1) is a target for potentiating drugs but also the interactions between the co-receptors or adhesion receptors (the non-clonal signal 2) on T cells and their ligands on APC are possible, non-specific drug targets.

- Second, there are two levels of interactions between TCR and tumor antigens: (1) initial activation recognition and (2) effector cell recognition. In responses against tumor cells, these two processes are separated by the fact that $CD4^+$ Th cells need MHCII to be triggered and the $CD8^+$ effector CTL are MHCI restricted (Krogsgaard and Davis 2005; Kärre et al. 1986, Janeway 1989). As tumor cells are frequently $MHCII^-$, the Th cell activation process has to take place via a cross-presentation procedure, where APC takes up tumor cell antigen as immature DC in the local tumor, process it, and present it on the outer cell surface of mature DC in association with MHCII molecules in the draining lymph nodes (Corthay et al. 2005). Activated $CD4^+$ Th1 cells produce IL-2, which appears necessary and sufficient for CTL differentiation (Denizot and Rubin 1985). Furthermore, $CD8^+$ CTL activation is also dependent on the presence of mature DCs to initiate their differentiation program (van Stipdonk et al. 2003).
- Third, once the $CD8^+$ effector cells are activated and have matured, they can interact with tumor cell ligands directly, provided that the tumor cells do present tumor cell-specific peptides associated with MHCI molecules on their cell surface.

In the following sections, we will discuss the characteristics of tumor cell development, the nature of the tumor antigens, and the way such antigens are presented to the immune system. The common denominator of these sections will be the definition of what the immune system "see" on tumor cells. After this, we will discuss the innate and adaptive immune systems in three different tumor model systems in mice. The purpose is to understand how the interaction between tumor cells and immune cells can be efficiently manipulated for prevention or therapeutic purpose. In these discussions, it is important to keep in mind that (1) a possible drawback of induction of antitumor immune responses is the potential risk of concomitant autoimmune reactions (Ludewig et al. 2000), and (2) tumor cells are not "just" antigens, but cells that are self-sufficient in growth signals are insensitive to growth-inhibitory signals, evade programmed cell death (apoptosis), have limitless replicative potential, have sustained angiogenesis, have tissue invasive and metastatic properties (Hanahan and Wienberg 2000), and have apparent resistance to the immune system once organized as an established tumor (Curiel 2007).

3 Tumor Cell Development and Its Danger Signals

Cancer develops from "sub-threshold neoplastic states" caused by viral, physical, or chemical carcinogens, or UV or X-ray radiations that involve DNA change or damage. Tumor progression is a selection for cells that survive and accumulate. The selection results in a stepwise loss of growth control mechanisms and up-regulation of growth mechanisms. Regulatory mechanisms such as checkpoint control and apoptosis are absent or ineffective in tumor cells. Thus, developing tumor cells are self-cells with abnormalities caused by structural changes in or altered levels of expression of household proteins. These abnormalities may be due to irreversible genomic instability in the tumor cells or due to reversible selection exerted on regulatory elements for genes encoding cell growth factors (Mueller and Fusenig 2004; Singh et al. 1992; Coussens and Werb 2002; Dunn et al. 2004). The most common genetic changes found in neoplasia are the somatic mutations in the p53 gene. The p53 tumor-suppressor protein is a sequence-specific DNA-binding protein that functions as a DNA repair factor. DNA damage activates p53, which in turn induces expression of proteins that halt the cell-division cycle to allow for DNA repair. Activation of p53 can also initiate programs of cell death (apoptosis) or permanent growth arrest (senescence) if the DNA damage is persistent and severe. Restoration of p53 expression leads to tumor regression (Xue et al. 2007). A p53 response may also contribute to innate immunity by enhancing IFN-α activity independently of its function as a proapoptotic and tumor-suppressor gene (Munoz-Fontela et al. 2008).

3.1 Neoplastic Cells

Neoplastic cells may express membrane-bound molecules, which they did not express before (or only in low quantities), or mutated membrane molecules. As a selective response to immune destruction, tumor cells may use several escape strategies, many of which involve down-regulation of MHCI molecules or other molecules implicated in the antigen-presentation pathway (Ganss et al. 2004; Mueller and Fusenig 2004; Singh et al. 1992; Coussens and Werb 2002; Dunn et al. 2004; Schüler and Blankenstein 2003; Seliger et al. 2001). Such tumor cells do not express tumor-specific peptides on the outer membrane, and consequently they cannot be recognized by CTLs. Tumor cells may also directly inhibit the recognition or the function of immune cells by releasing immune inhibitory molecules, e.g., IL-10 or TGFβ. However, cells other than CTL attack tumor cells: NK cells, polymorphonuclear leukocytes (PMN), and macrophages/DC do not recognize tumor cells via peptide/MHCI ligands. These cells seem to be involved in the recently described, natural immunity against tumor cells (Cui et al. 2003). Moreover, mice deficient in the innate immune system show higher incidence of tumor cell induction and outgrowth compared to wild-type mice (Ljunggren and Kärre 1985; Gorelik et al. 1988; Kawano et al. 1986). Thus, cells from the innate immune system may play a role both in the destruction of the tumor cells and in the regulation of MHCI expression on cells with which they interact (Rubin et al. 2008). However, an important question in the discussion is whether the so-called selective response of tumor cells to immune destruction is (1) *a global inductible response of all tumor cells*, i.e., the immune system induces the tumor cells to change character in such a way that the tumor cells become less sensitive to the immune effectors, or (2) *a selective response of surviving tumor cells*, i.e., the immune effectors kill sensitive tumor cells but not mutated tumor cells or tumor cells that have changed (down-regulated) certain characters, which render them invulnerable to the immune attack (Rubin et al. 2008).

To activate the immune system, neoplastic cells must, in addition to the expression of tumor-associated antigens (TAA), induce cellular stress signals, danger signals, or damage-associated signals that alert the innate immune system (Janeway 1989; Gardai et al. 2006). Cell death, damage-associated molecular-pattern molecules (DAMPs), and endogenous danger signals are all associated with expression of heat-shock proteins (HSP), chromatin-associated protein high-mobility group box 1 (HMGB1), and others. This is followed by the expression of "eat me" signals and suppression of "don't eat me" signals (i.e., CD31 and CD47) on the "troubled" cells, which are then taken-up by immature DCs. The consequence of the DC-"troubled" cells interaction will greatly differ, depending on the necrotic versus apoptotic status of the "troubled" cells. If the "troubled" cells are necrotic, then they release inflammatory molecules that induce the immature DCs to mature and elicit cross-priming of the immune system. Necrotic cell death releases HMGB1 and proteins derived from the tissue injury, such as hyaluronan fragments and non-protein purinergic molecules such as ATP and uric acid, and induces inflammation due to IL-1β, IFNγ, and TNFα (Sha et al. 2008). DAMPs activate cells of the innate immune system by triggering TLR or other alarm-signal receptors (Bianchi 2007; Rubartelli and Lotze 2007). In contrast, if the immature DCs take up "troubled" cells undergoing apoptotic cell death, they turn into tolerogenic DCs due in part to the activity of caspases 3 and 7 that render HMGB1 inactive. This causes absence of induction of inflammation and no differentiation of immature DCs to mature DCs (Kazama et al. 2008). In addition to DAMPs and endogenous danger signals, tumor cells may release effector molecules that stimulate the immune cells to collaborate in tumor growth in the sub-threshold neoplastic states (Prehn and Prehn 2008; de Visser et al. 2006). The complement system, in particular C5a and properdin, seems to play an important role in this process by amplifying the production of reactive oxygen and nitrogen species by myeloid-derived suppressor cells (MDSC) (Markiewski et al. 2008; Kemper et al. 2008). In fact, growing neoplastic cells may be considered by the tissue as a physical wound, and the tissue response to such "intrusion" is wound healing. This means attraction of stromal, endothelial, and epithelial cells, release of chemokines and cytokines as well as molecules of the blood-clotting system (Fig. 1).

Thus, both normal repair systems, different danger signals, and the immune system may take part in the initiation process from a transformed neoplastic cell to an established, solid tumor.

3.2 Chronic Inflammation

Chronic inflammation increases the risk of the development of transformed cells and aggravates the development of established malignancies. Some of the properties of inflammation that contribute to these processes are understood, such as the promotion of angiogenesis, the induction of tumor-promoting cytokines, the up-regulation of anti-apoptotic genes, and uncontrolled feed-forward signaling in

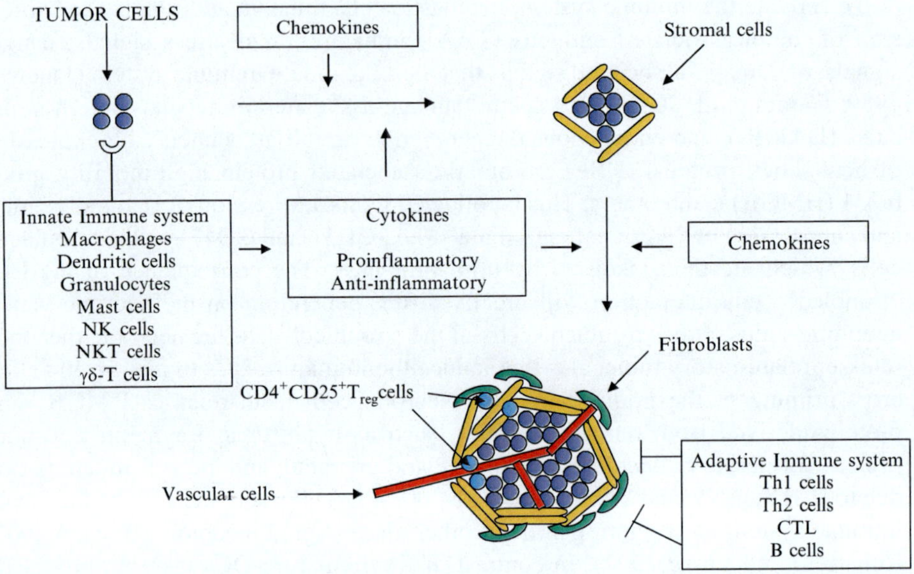

Fig. 1 Interactions between growing tumor cells and the immune system. Tumor cells (*violet circles*) develop due to changes in DNA (damage or mutation) or to virus infection. Cells from the innate immune system recognize small growing tumors as a wound, and a wound healing process is initiated. This may accelerate tumor development due to production of growth factors, chemokines, and cytokines. Stromal cells (*yellow*) are attracted, and they create a type of maternal–fetus relationship protecting the developing tumor cells from the adaptive immune system. Among stromal cells are hematopoietic cells mediating suppressor function such as macrophages and T_{reg} cells (*light blue*). When the tumor attains a certain size, nutrients and oxygen cannot reach the more interior parts of the tumor. Consequently, VEGF is produced by the tumor cells and/or stromal cells, and vascularization is established and secures continuous growth of the tumor (*red*). The vascular cells express low amounts of integrins necessary for immune cells to enter the tumor. For further details, see text. Any reagent which can either block the interactions marked with arrows or cancel the blockage of access to and function of the adaptive immune system may increase the chance to fight tumor growth. Due to the complexity of the tumor–immune system interactions, combined chemo-, radio-, and immunotherapy would be the most serious

tumor cells through cell surface receptors such as the receptor for advanced glycosylation end-products (RAGE). Many of these mechanisms are due to perturbations in the tumor microenvironment that co-opt innate immunity to favor tumor initiation and progression (Prehn and Prehn 2008; de Visser et al. 2006). Inflammation also promotes tumor progression by blocking adaptive immunity through the induction of MDSC (Zou 2006), which prevent the activation of $CD4^+$ and $CD8^+$ T cells. The inflammatory stimuli are either the proinflammatory cytokines IL-1β and IL-6 or PGE_2. Mice with heightened levels of IL-1β or IL-6 in the tumor microenvironment accumulate MDSC with enhanced suppressive activity. S100 proteins are calcium-binding proteins released by MDSC. These intracellular molecules are released into extracellular compartments in response to cell damage, infection, or inflammation, and they function as proinflammatory danger signals.

The proteins are chemotactic for leukocytes, thereby amplifying the local proinflammatory microenvironment, and they interact with plasma membrane receptors on endothelial cells, macrophages and DC-like heparan sulfate, TLR4, or carboxyl *N*-glycans. MDSC from tumor-bearing mice have receptors for S100 proteins, and they synthesize S100 proteins providing an autocrine pathway of MDSC accumulation (Sinha et al. 2008). Inhibition of cyclooxygenase 2 (COX-2) leads to marked lymphocytic infiltration of the tumor and reduced tumor growth. Treatment of mice with anti-PGE_2 mAb replicates the growth reduction seen in tumor-bearing mice treated with COX-2 inhibitors. It is concluded that abrogation of COX-2 expression promotes antitumor reactivity by restoring the balance of IL-10 and IL-12 in vivo (Stolina et al. 2000).

3.3 *Stroma*

All solid tumors are composed of malignant cells that are embedded in stroma consisting of a variety of non-malignant cells and extracellular matrix. Stromal cells include bone marrow-derived cells, such as macrophages, granulocytes, and lymphocytes, and non-bone marrow-derived cells, such as endothelium and other cells of vasculature and fibroblasts. Stroma is essential for the tumor growth as it provides nutrition, growth factors, and cytokines (Mueller and Fusenig 2004). Thus, a solid tumor is not just an accumulation of tumor cells, but forms an *organ* in which transformed cells are surrounded and nurtured by the stroma cells (Fig. 1). The effectiveness of antitumor strategies declines significantly with tumor size. Stromal cells are known to produce factors that promote tumorigenesis and may also contribute to immune evasion for instance by preventing DC maturation (Ganss et al. 2004).

Thus, there is a fine balance between immune recognition and elimination of tumor cells on one hand, and growth and organization of solid tumors on the other hand. The more organized the tumor cells are, the more insensitive the tumor cells become to both innate and adaptive immune cells.

4 Expression and Presentation of Tumor Antigens

TAA represent the consequences of the genetic and epigenetic alterations in cancer cells. TAA may be released glycoproteins or glycolipids, i.e., glycosphingolipids (Sriram et al. 2002; Wu et al. 2003), or they may be membrane-bound glycolipids, proteins, or glycoproteins. The latter two may be classified into five groups: (1) tumor-specific shared antigens, (2) antigens encoded by mutated genes, (3) differentiation antigens, (4) over-expressed or ubiquitously expressed proteins, and (5) virus-derived antigens (Sugiyama 2008). As discussed above, tumor cells dying by necrotic or apoptotic mechanisms induce immunogenic or tolerogenic dendritic cells, respectively (Sauter et al. 2000; Steinman et al. 2000). Soluble or membrane-bound

TAA may be presented to the immune system by uptake and degradation/processing by APC. Processed TAA may be associated with MHCI, MHCII, or non-classical MHCI such as CD1 molecules and thus, in principle, activate T cells or NKT cells. If the TAA are normal self-structures, they may be expressed in increased amounts as a consequence of carcinogenesis; e.g., Rae1 and H60 MHCI-like molecules are expressed in tumor cells, and less or not at all in normal cells (Sauter et al. 2000). The MHCI-like molecules may also be induced by cellular stress such as oncogene transformation, infection, heat shock, or DNA damage. The up-regulation of MHCI-like molecules alerts the immune system for the presence of damaged and potentially dangerous cells via NKG2D and other receptors (Diefenbach et al. 2001). Furthermore, glycolipid-loaded DC induce tumor cell immunity by NKT–DC interactions dependent on CD40-CD40L reactions (Corthay et al. 2005), and such interactions induce tumor-specific memory (Fujii 2008). A novel way to induce antitumor immunity is to vaccinate with GD2 ganglioside mimotopes, which induces $CD8^+$ T cells with reactivity to cell adhesion molecules on the tumor cells, i.e., activated leukocyte adhesion molecule ALCAM/CD166 (Wierzbicki et al. 2008). In contrast, if the TAA are mutated household proteins, they represent a new "foreign" structure and the foreignness may be presented to the T cells by any of the various MHC molecules. Thus, haptenated self-proteins or cells induce immune responses of normal type and magnitude (Rubin and Wigzell 1973; Preckel et al. 1997). Migrating phagocytes routinely ingest moribund neighboring cells, infecting microbes and particulate debris. If the fragments are derived from non-self-structures, the phagocytes (in particular, DC) add indicators of the alien status of the ingest on the cell surface. Protein antigens delivered, e.g., via *Escherichia coli*, which would be expected to activate TLR4, were fully processed into peptide-loaded MHCII complexes and expressed at the DC surface. In contrast, proteins delivered by phagocytosis of apoptotic cells, which lack TLR ligands, were not presented by MHCII molecules on the DC surface (Blander and Medzhitov 2006). Mincle is a transmembrane CLR, which is expressed on macrophages, and is augmented by stimulation with bacterial LPS or various fungi. Mincle recognizes a soluble factor, spliceosome-associated protein 130 (SAP130), released by necrotic cells (Yamasaki et al. 2008). The tumor necrosis factor superfamily member, LIGHT, seems to bind to a herpesvirus entry receptor expressed on T cells (causing T-cell priming) and to the lymphotoxin-β receptor expressed on stroma cells (causing induction of T-cell attractive chemokines). LIGHT may be considered as a "double-edged sword" for the immune system that can be turned from a barrier against the immune cells to a participant in immune responses against cancer (Yu et al. 2004).

Post-translational modifications that occur during cellular transformation, infection, or inflammation may result in the display of MHC-associated neoantigens. Evidence suggests that peptides containing post-translational modifications such as deamination, cysteinylation, glycosylation, or phosphorylation contribute to the pool of MHCI-bound peptides presented on the cell surface, and they represent potential targets for T-cell recognition. Therefore, transformed neoplastic cells may have an altered self-repertoire (Rubin and Sönderstrup 2004; Mohammed et al.

2008). The main message is that TAA associated with TLR or CLR induce DC maturation with presentation of tumor-specific peptides to $CD4^+$ Th1 cells that initiate the $CD8^+$ CTL response.

The level of MHC expression on live cells is a sensor for T, NK, or NKT cell recognition and activation (Kärre et al. 1986; Cerwenka and Lanier 2001). A key question is "What level of MHCI expression is advantageous for tumor cells in their interactions with the immune system?" High levels of MHCI expression may suppress CTL responses due to the action of inhibitory receptors (Vivier and Anfossi, 2004), intermediate levels of MHCI expression would favor CTL killing, and low levels of MHCI expression favor NK and NKT cell cytotoxicity (Krogsgaard and Davis 2005; Cerwenka and Lanier 2001). At the start of neoplastic cell development, it would be an advantage for the tumor cells to maintain high levels of MHCI expression, as the frequency of tumor-specific CTL is very low and the number of NKT and NK cells is high: $MHCI^{low}$ tumor cells produced fewer tumor colonies compared to MHC^{high} tumor cells when injected into naïve mice, indicating that innate effector cells are involved in this phenomenon (Ljunggren and Kärre 1985; Gorelik et al. 1988; Kawano et al. 1986). However, these considerations may change as a function of the immunogenicity of the TAA. In summary, to activate an adaptive tumor-specific immune response and memory, the innate immune system has to recognize the "danger" of the presence of neoplastic cells.

In the next chapter, we discuss the results from tumor model systems in mice, where important mechanisms in the "pas de deux" between immune cells and tumor cells have been highlighted.

5 Mouse Models of Cancer

Several tumor models use, as tumor-specific antigens, peptides from proteins against which specific TCRαβ transgenic mice have been made (Ganss et al. 2004; Schüler and Blankenstein 2003; Prévost-Blondel et al. 1998; Mocikat et al. 2003). These models systems have demonstrated that tumor cells may be killed directly by specific $CD8^+$ CTL and/or indirectly by released IFNγ. However, most systems showed that despite an overwhelming excess of tumor-specific T cells in the transgenic mice, the tumor cells still grow and kill the hosts (Ganss et al. 2004; Prévost-Blondel et al. 1998). Are these tumor-specific T cells activated, or do they ignore the tumor cells, and in either case, why?

5.1 The LCMV Model to Study the Regulation of MHCI Expression

LCMV peptide gp33-41 expressing B16.F10 (B16gp) melanoma cells expressed low levels of MHCI at the cell surface, and this low level of MHCI expression could be augmented by treatment with IFNγ (Seliger et al. 2001; Böhm et al. 1998).

As host for these B16gp cells were used TCR-transgenic mice bearing a TCRαβ with specificity against the gp33-41 LCMV peptide, called P14 mice, were used as hosts for these B16gp cell. Using this model, we investigated whether in vitro incubation of B16gp cells with normal spleen cells (NSC) could augment MHCI expression and thereby renders the B16gp cells vulnerable to CTL killing by P14 transgenic CTL. The rational was that NSC may either kill most $MHCI^{low}$ B16gp cells and consequently *select* cells with medium–high MHCI expression, or release IFNγ upon recognition of the low levels of MHCI and subsequently induce MHCI expression on $MHCI^{low-medium}$ B16 cells that escaped NK killing. Our experiments showed that (1) NSC induce high MHCI expression on $B16gp^{low}$ cells in a cell–cell contact and IFNγ-dependent manner, and (2) as expected, such $MHCI^{high}$ B16gp cells were very sensitive to CTL killing. The observed phenomenon was executed by a collaboration of $CD4^+$, CD1-independent NKT cells, $CD4^+$, $CD11c^+$ DC, $NK1.1^+$, and $NK1.1^+$, $DX5^-$NK cells. The phenomenon is not observed with $MHCI^{high}$ tumor cells (Rubin et al. 2008). Our conclusion is that cells from the innate immune system regulate MHCI expression on $MHCI^{low}$ tumor cells. The combination of the described NKT, DC, and NK cells is present in highest numbers in spleen and lymph nodes, and in low levels in the peritoneum, thymus, or bone marrow. These data have recently been confirmed in vivo using GFP-labeled B16 cells (Riond et al. 2009). Therefore, P14-transgenic mice (raised in SPF conditions) should be able to reject injected B16gp cells by a combined increase in MHCI expression induced by NSC and P14-CTL-mediated killing. However, the fact is that the tumor cells grow apparently undisturbed (Prévost-Blondel et al. 1998; Roehm et al. 2002). Possible reasons for the failure of P14-transgenic mice to reject the B16gp tumor cells could be that the tumor cells quickly protect themselves with stromal cells and/or that they release inhibitory cytokines that down-regulate the immune response. Another possibility is that the high amounts of B16gp-specific P14-CTL are not activated, or activated too late. B16gp cells are $MHCII^-$, which means that they cannot activate $CD4^+$ Th1 cells directly. Immature DCs recruited to the tumor site have to phagocytose the tumor cells or tumor cell debris, process possible TAA on B16gp cells, and express TAA peptides associated with MHCII on mature DCs. Only then, $CD4^+$ Th1 cells are activated and ready to trigger the P14-CTLs. This process may take too long, and in the meantime the tumor cells have organized themselves as a solid tumor, and neither the innate NKT–DC–NK cells nor the activated $CD8^+$ P14-CTLs have access to the tumor cells within the solid tumor. The apparent failure of the P14-mice to combat and eradicate the B16gp cells is likely the non-activated innate immune system. If the P14 TCRαβ transgenic mice are first immunized with live LCMV, then they become resistant to tumor growth (Prévost-Blondel et al. 1998; Roehm et al. 2002). This indicates that components of the innate immune system may have to be activated (probably via Toll-like receptors interacting with DNA or RNA from dying virus) to trigger the $CD4^+$ Th1 cells and tumor-specific CTL. As discussed below, this idea is supported by our findings that tumor-specific responses are much higher in conventional mice compared to SPF mice due to an inefficiently activated innate immune system in SPF mice (Rubin 2009). Moreover, injection of TLR ligands in SPF mice increases significantly the tumor-specific responses (Rubin 2009; Garbi et al. 2004). It should be investigated which of the innate immune cells in the LCMV-immunized mice are the inducer and/or effector cells of tumor cell resistance. This could be done by in vivo cell transfer of, e.g., LCMV-immune cells fractionated into macrophages, DC, NK, NKT, granulocytes, or others. Identification of this subpopulation of innate immune cells may lead to protocols or the development of drugs that can directly activate such cells without immunization with either virus or inactivated/attenuated tumor cells. Yet another possibility is that a direct interaction between the P14 CTLs and B16gp cells leads to tolerance or anergy of the tumor-specific $CD8^+$ T cells due to lack of co-stimulation.

Then, we investigated whether MHCI down-regulation was an induced or a selective phenomenon. We used the L12R4 lymphoma cells (see below) as targets and P14 CTLs as effectors. Cell culture of gp33 peptide-loaded L12R4 cells in the presence of P14-CTL resulted in the killing of about 95% of the L12R4 cells. The surviving cells expressed lower levels of MHCI compared to wild-type cells. Then, the surviving cells were re-incubated with gp33 peptide and subjected to P14-CTL. Again more than 95% of the cells were killed, and 1–2 weeks later the surviving cells had further decreased their level of MHCI expression. Further rounds of selection culture were performed until we obtained a L12R4 variant cell line with almost no MHCI expression. Without further immuno-selection, this $MHCI^{low}$ phenotype lasted for about 2–3 weeks, after which the L12R4 variant cells gradually regained the $MHCI^{high}$ phenotype. Cloning of the MHC^{low} L12R4 cells after the last P14-CTL selection resulted in only $MHCI^{high}$ L12R4 clones. Mammalian cells go through cell-cycle-dependent variations in surface membrane protein expression; momentarily $MHCI^{low}$ L12R4 cells may survive the action of P14-CTLs. Supernatants from cultures of gp33-loaded L12R4 cells and P14-CTLs contained no substances that could down-regulate or maintain already down-regulated MHCI expression on L12R4 $MHCI^{low}$ variant. Thus, MHCI down-regulation is most probably a selective process; however, it is not excluded that CTLs may "impose on" the tumor cells to stay $MHCI^{low}$ for a certain period of time by a cell–cell contact-dependent mechanism. In conclusion, both the innate and the adaptive immune systems play an important role in the regulation of MHCI expression on tumor cells.

5.2 *The L12R4 Vaccination Model*

Vaccination of syngeneic mice (i.p.) with mitomycin C-treated L12R4 ($L12R4^M$) lymphoma cells induces a tumor-specific immune response with life-long specific memory: the mice are resistant to further inoculation with live tumor cells even in high quantities (Rubin 2009; Gonthier et al. 2004). In this model, $CD4^+$ Th1 cells are activated by L12R4-processed material associated with MHCII molecules on mature DCs (Corthay et al. 2005), and the activated Th1 cells help the activation and differentiation of $CD8^+$ L12R4-specific CTL and memory cells (Denizot and

Rubin 1985). These CTLs are specific for variable region epitope(s) on the TCR expressed by the L12R4 cells (Vα10/Vβ12), or for unknown household protein epitope(s). Thus, this is an example of a tumor-specific "antigen" which is normally present in the antigenic repertoire of self; however, a special Vα/Vβ combination with multiple CDR3 variations may be present in such low concentrations that the negative selection in the thymus neglects such epitopes and lets the TCR repertoire against such epitopes to migrate to the periphery. Here, they can serve as precursors of anti-T-lymphoma effector T cells. There are at least two interesting and non-solved problems in this model: (1) immunization with the L12R4 cells in Freund's complete adjuvant (FCA) induces a non-protective Th2-immune response, which actually inhibits subsequent induction of Th1 responses in the same animals. Thus, the route of vaccination and the physical state of the vaccinating tumor material (the L12R4 cells in FCA are mostly dead necrotic cells, whereas L12R4^{M} cells may survive up to 3 days) play an important role in orienting the subsequent type of immune response; (2) immunization of mice with already established tumors does not protect the mice. Thus, everything takes place as if the growing tumor was ignored by a highly activated immune system. The stromal cells may protect the tumor cells from invading immune cells. The immune cells sense something "dangerous," but interaction with the stromal cells (which do not display danger signals) convinces them that they were mistaken. The L12R4 cells grow as an ascites tumor (single cell suspension, not protected by stromal cells), yet only vaccination before challenge with live tumor cells saves the mice. Furthermore, adoptive transfer of L12R4-specific CD8^{+} CTL can protect the mice from live tumor cells, however, only if the immune T cells are given before or with the tumor cells, and not afterward (Böhm et al. 1998; Rubin 2009). Thus, pre-established L12R4 tumors possess sufficiently powerful arms against the immune system to avoid the immune attack. Further experimentation is necessary to elucidate these problems.

An important observation is that if the vaccination with L12R4^{M} cells is carried out in SPF mice, the success of inducing a protective immune response and tumor-specific memory is very low. The tumor-specific responses are much higher in conventional mice compared to SPF mice due to an inefficiently activated innate immune system in SPF mice (Rubin 2009). Injection of TLR ligands in SPF mice may increase significantly the tumor-specific responses (Rubin 2009; Garbi et al. 2004), and transfer of SPF mice to a natural environment induces conditions required for successful vaccination (Fig. 2).

Thus, as in the B16gp/P14 mouse model, pre-activation of the innate immune system appears indispensable for induction of efficient tumor-specific immunity. Furthermore, the data indicate that only Th1 immune responses are protective against tumor cells.

5.3 *The SR/CR Mouse Model*

The SR/CR mice are resistant to multiple transplantable tumor cell lines. They were developed from a BALB/c mouse that resisted the inoculation of virulent ascites

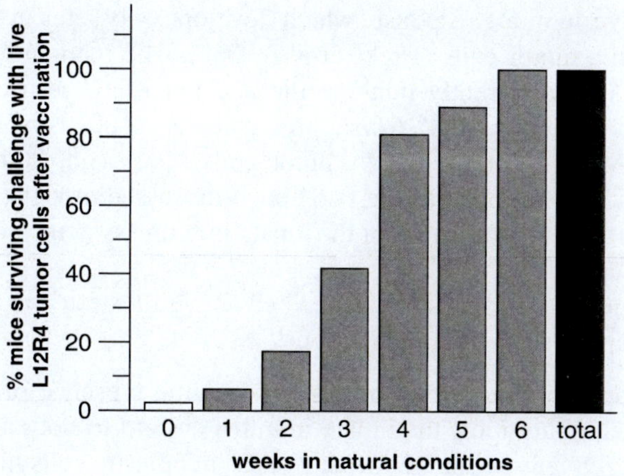

Fig. 2 Effect of exposure to natural environment on the success of vaccination. C57Bl/6 mice (126) born and raised on SPF conditions were divided into 7 groups of 18 mice. An additional group of 18 C57Bl/6 mice born and raised in conventional (natural) conditions was used as control (total, meaning all the time in conventional conditions). Of the seven groups, one was kept under SPF conditions, and the six others were transferred to a farm house, where they lived in a natural environment with natural food (vegetables, grains, and source water). After 1, 2, 3, 4, 5, or 6 weeks, they were immunized 3× with mitomycin C-treated L12R4 lymphoma cells. The mice kept under SPF or conventional conditions all their life were vaccinated at the same time as the SPF mice having been in a natural environment for 6 weeks. After 3 weeks of rest, the mice were challenged with 10^5 live L12R4 cells and protective immunity was observed. Each column indicates the percentage of vaccinated mice that survived challenge with live L12R4 cells (vaccination-protected mice)

tumor cells. In the SR/CR mice, the killing of tumor cells requires three distinct phases. First, the migration of the leukocytes to the site of tumor cells after sensing their presence. Second, the recognition by leukocytes of the unique properties of the tumor cell surface and make tight contact with it. Third, the delivery of the effector mechanisms to target cells. The difference between SR/CR mice and wild-type mice seems to lie in one of the first two phases. Upon challenge with tumor cells, wild-type mice lack leukocyte infiltration and rosette formation. Apparently, a stable, heritable, and unknown mutation in SR/CR mice renders the leukocytes capable of sensing unique diffusible and surface signals from tumor cells, and of responding to the activation signals by migration and physical contact. Once the first two phases are accomplished, unleashing the pre-existing effector mechanisms for killing seems to ensue by default. The major effectors appear to be macrophages, which kill tumor cells via apoptosis induced by reactive oxygen species and serine proteases. The mutated gene(s) in SR/CR mice may determine whether leukocytes interpret the "signals" from the tumor cells as neglect or inhibition (wild-type mice) or as activation of migration and of tumor cell recognition (SR/CR leukocytes) (Cui et al. 2003; Hicks et al. 2006a,b). The mutated innate immune cells can even recognize and kill the tumor cells autonomously without interference from an adaptive immune response, which develops only later in the mice that are able to reject the tumor cells (Hicks et al. 2006a). The recognition mechanism is unknown, but it is apparently non-specific and not MHC restricted, i.e., SR/CR mice reject the original $MHCI^{low}$ fibrosarcoma cells, S180, as well as other MHC-incompatible MHC^{low} or $MHCI^{high}$ tumor cells (Cui et al. 2003). Therefore, it seems that this tumor model, as the two above-discussed models, strongly emphasizes the importance of activation of the innate immune system and its participation in tumor eradication.

The three mouse model systems described above illustrate the major challenges in tumor cell–immune system interactions.

- First, the innate immune system has to sense the presence of neoplastic cells: under normal conditions, the innate immune system in both a natural environment and a SPF environment does not sense neoplastic cells immediately. Only when the tumor cells and surrounding tissue send out danger signals, the innate immune cells react, and innate immune cells partially activated in response to a natural environment react much more efficiently than innate immune cells from SPF mice (Rubin 2009; Gonthier et al. 2004). The sensing of tumor cells is particularly strong in SR/CR mice, where the mutation(s) has rendered the innate immune cells extremely sensitive to the presence of neoplastic cells (Cui et al. 2003; Gonthier et al. 2004; Hicks et al. 2006a). Thus, it seems that this tumor cell model, as the two above-discussed models, strongly emphasizes the importance of the innate immune system. Furthermore, the SR/CR model demonstrates that the innate immune system may combat tumor cells very efficiently and autonomously by a mechanism which is strictly regulated in normal mice.
- Second, with the assistance from the innate immune system, the TAA-specific $CD4^+$ Th1 cells have to be present in a state (Corthay et al. 2005) where they can be activated. As TAA may be self-structures, the relevant $CD4^+$ Th1 cells may be absent, anergized, or kept silent by $CD4^+CD25^+$ T_{reg} cells (see below). Furthermore, the activation of the $CD4^+$ Th1 cells may be dependent on cross-presentation by mature DCs (Corthay et al. 2005). In addition, the activation must take place in such a way that only Th1 cells are activated (presence of IFNγ and IL-12 among others), since Th2 responses are non-protective and inhibitory for the development of protective Th1 responses (Rubin 2009). Unfortunately, it is not clear which mechanisms are at play in the Th2-cell differentiation pathway (MacDonald and Maizels 2008). Therefore, it is very important to clearly establish, in a tumor model, how DCs process TAA and avoid the induction of both TAA-specific tolerance and Th2-cell differentiation.
- Third, it is indispensable to know how a given tumor defends itself against the immune system. The tissue response to developing neoplastic cells is like a wound-type response, i.e., repair (Coussens and Werb 2002). Thus, neoplastic cells become protected relatively quickly by stromal cells that do not present TAA peptides on their MHC molecules and do not release danger signals. In addition, tumor cells may release a series of inhibitory molecules, which decrease the efficiency of the immune system: VEGF (which induces tumor

vascularization and inhibits DC maturation), IL-6 and M-CSF (which push DC into macrophage differentiation), prostaglandin E2, IL-10, TGFβ, and gangliosides (which all suppress DC maturation and function). The abundance of these molecules causes presence of low concentrations of important immune stimulatory cytokines in the tumor environment: GM-CSF, IL-4 (DC activation and differentiation), IL-12, and IFNγ (Th1 cell activation and development) (Zou 2005; Rabinovich et al. 2007). Such an inhibitory, protective milieu may well be the main reason for the inefficiency of tumor cell vaccination in individuals with already established tumors (Ganss et al. 2004; Prévost-Blondel et al. 1998; Rubin 2009; Gonthier et al. 2004).

6 Cellular and Molecular Regulation of Tumor Immunity

As discussed previously, $CD4^+$ T cells are necessary for induction of TAA-specific $CD8^+$ CTL (Corthay et al. 2005; Denizot and Rubin 1985; van Stipdonk et al. 2003). When the $CD4^+$ T cells are alerted and migrate to the tumor, they have the immediate risk of being tolerized by the tumor cells that often do not express either MHCII or co-receptor ligand molecules and by DCs that are in an immature state. Not only may the $CD4^+$ T cells be tolerized, but they may differentiate into TAA-specific T_{reg} cells (Chen et al. 2003), or they may simply ignore the tumor cells and stay naïve T cells. The problem in the clinical situation is that the presence or absence of tumors is a matter of detection, i.e., we are always confronted with a therapeutic situation (Van Elsas et al. 2001).

T-cell activation requires two signals, one provided by TCR–pMHC interactions and another mediated by co-receptors such as CD28 or ICOS (see Sect. 1). CD28 interacts with CD80 (B7.1) and CD86 (B7.2), whereas ICOS has B7h as a ligand. Absence of CD28 and ICOS co-stimulation causes induction of anergy or functional tolerance in both $CD4^+$ and $CD8^+$ T cells, seemingly due to low IL-2 production. Expression of two crucial components in T-cell activation, PLCγ1 and PKC0, is very low in anergized T cells, and signal pathways through MAP kinases, NK-kB, and NFAT are impaired. Furthermore, expression of Th1 and Th2 as well as CTL lineage commitment regulators (T-bet, GATA-3 and Eomes, respectively) is greatly reduced. However, it seems that naïve T cells receiving only TCR–pMHC stimulation are not anergized. The necessary activators of anergy on APC may come from negative co-stimulatory molecules such as CTLA-4, PD-1, B7-H3, and B7-H4. The master regulator appears to be IL-2 that when produced in high concentrations induces immunity (positive co-stimulation via CD28 and ICOS) but when produced in low concentrations induces tolerance (negative CTLA-4, PD-1, B7-H3/H4 co-stimulation). Thus, concerning possible anergized tumor-specific T cells, it would be advantageous to augment positive co-stimulation and block negative co-stimulation (Nurieva et al. 2006).

So, how can the host immune system be regulated in such a way that it mounts stronger and, more importantly, protective tumor-specific immune responses?

Many new therapeutic axes are available such as novel adjuvants, DC-based immunotherapy, and adoptive T-cell immunotherapy. In case of tumor cells with mutated self-proteins or with expression of viral proteins, the T-cell repertoire would be of normal size and avidity. However, if the tumor cells express deregulated quantities of self-proteins or differentiation proteins, the T-cell repertoire is rather low and self-reactive T cells have TCR with low avidity. These cells can be activated and induced into memory T cells with a significantly higher response potential than naïve T cells (Morgan et al. 1998; Cordaro et al. 2002). Possible ways to activate low-avidity T cells are (1) the use of high vaccinating antigen concentration [eventually using tumor TAA peptides inserted into the variable region of immunoglobulins (Lee et al. 2008)], (2) the use of altered peptides (Slansky et al. 2000), and (3) the inhibition of the action of inhibitory molecules (e.g., CTLA-4) or cells (such as $CD4^{+}CD25^{+}$ T_{reg} cells) (Van Elsas et al. 2001). Often tumor antigenic peptides do bind reasonably well to the MHC molecules; the weak point is the interaction between the TCR and pMHC. One approach is to keep the MHC anchor residues and change the TCR-binding residues. This may increase immunogenicity up to 100 times and presents a promising way to augment tumor-specific immune responses (Slansky et al. 2000). However, the difficulty is that when diagnosing cancer in a given patient, you first have to identify the TAA, then the dominant immunogenic peptide, and then alter this peptide to increase effectiveness. This treatment is long and expensive, but tumor-specific and with possible induction of T-cell memory. It is important to note that peptide-vaccination regimes should favor induction of Th1 responses, which are solely responsible for significant tumor-specific $CD8^{+}$ CTL responses (Pardoll 2002; van Stipdonk et al. 2003; Schüler and Blankenstein 2003; Mocikat et al. 2003; Gonthier et al. 2004). The production of IL-12 by DCs, of IFNγ by macrophages, DC, NK, and NKT cells, and absence of the production of IL-4 by Th-2 have to be controlled (Lee et al. 2008).

Immune consequences of chemotherapy and/or X-ray radiation of solid tumors are (1) increased immunogenicity through cross-presentation (Ganss et al. 2004; Bhardwaj 2007), (2) increased TAA concentration and stromal cell load (Zhang et al. 2007), (3) enhanced MHCI expression, (4) increased expression of ligands for NK cells, and (5) enhanced NK cell activity (Reits et al. 2006). Adoptive transfer of tumor-specific CTL may lead to complete tumor rejection (Bhardwaj 2007; Zhang et al. 2007; Reits et al. 2006). Thus, a combined therapy of physico-chemical destruction and of adoptive CTL transfer may convert the situation in tumor cell–immune cell interactions from: "not enough of a good thing" and "too much of a bad thing" (Curiel 2007) to the advantage of the patient.

The thymus accomplishes two essential tasks concerning maintenance of immunological tolerance: (1) negative selection (clonal deletion) of potentially hazardous self-reactive T cells, and (2) production of $CD4^{+}CD25^{+}$ T_{reg} cells, which act in the periphery to control self-reactive T cells that have escaped negative selection in the thymus. It appears that expression of AIRE on medullary thymic epithelial cells and of FOXP3 by maturing T_{reg} cells play an important role in both thymic negative selection and generation of T_{reg} cells. Compared with the thymic selection of conventional T cells, the selection of T_{reg} cells requires agonistic interactions of higher avidity between T cell receptors in developing thymocytes and self-peptide/MHC on thymic stromal cells (Sakaguchi et al. 2006; Hsieh et al. 2006; Nomura and Sakagushi 2007; Aschenbrenner et al. 2007). Furthermore, it appears that conventional effector T cells and T_{reg} cells have very similar repertoires, even though the T_{reg} cells do only constitute about 5–10% of $CD4^+$ T cells. Despite the higher TCR avidity of T_{reg} cells, they do no apparent harm to the host, because triggering of their TCR does not induce proinflammatory cytokines (Sakaguchi et al. 2006). $CD4^+CD25^+$ T_{reg} cells may not be strictly lineage-specific; it has been shown that $CD4^+CD25^-$ naïve or effector T cells can convert into $CD4^+CD25^+$ T_{reg} cells upon stimulation with TGFβ (Chen et al. 2003), and Th2 cells may convert into Th17 or Th9 cells (Tato and Cua 2008). This may have important bearing on therapies involving T_{reg} cell elimination by treatment with anti-CTLA4 or anti-CD25 mAb.

T_{reg} cells are antigen-specific in their differentiation and activation, but they may exert their function in an antigen-independent manner whether through soluble or cell–cell contact-dependent mechanisms. They deregulate effector cell function by at least four different mechanisms: (1) suppression by inhibitory cytokines, (2) suppression by cytolysis, (3) suppression by metabolic disruption, or (4) suppression by targeting DC. T_{reg} cells suppress profoundly APC, T cells, and NK cells probably by the inhibitory cytokines IL-10, IL-35, and TGFβ. In contrast to normal effector T cells, T_{reg} cells express the high-avidity IL-2 receptor, IL-2Rα (CD25)/IL-2Rβ (CD122)/IL-2Rγ (CD132). Consequently, they may suppress effector T-cell function by IL-2 competition or consumption (Vignali et al. 2008; Curiel 2007; Zou 2005, 2006; Mills 2008; Pasare and Medzhitov 2003). T_{reg} cells migrate to and colonize the tumor mass by unknown mechanisms; however, it seems as if MDSCs expressing B7-H1 or B7-H4 are involved in this process via interactions with CTLA4 on the T_{reg} cells. The production of IL-10 by T_{reg} cells modulates selectively the expression of B7 family members so as to tilt the balance toward immune suppressive B7-H1 and B7-H4 up-regulation and co-receptor ligand B7.1 (CD80) or B7.2 (CD86) down-regulation. Presence of T_{reg} cells and $B7\text{-}H4^+$ macrophages is frequent in the tumor environment. The interaction of CTLA4 on T_{reg} cells and CD80 or CD86 on APC induces the latter to produce indoleamine-2,3-dioxygenase (IDO) or arginase-1, which degrades the essential amino acids, tryptophan and arginine, respectively, that are indispensable for T-cell activation and function (Curiel 2007; Zou 2005, 2006). Activation of TLR9 by DNA or of other TLRs by bacterial products may inhibit T_{reg} cell activity by IL-6 dependent or independent mechanisms. This ascertains that immune responses can – and should – take the advantage over suppression (Mills 2008; Pasare and Medzhitov 2003).

Tumor cells generate chemokines that attract T_{reg} cells to the tumor microenvironment, an effect inhibited by IL-6 (Pasare and Medzhitov 2003; Moutsopoulos et al. 2008). If $CD4^+CD25^+$ T_{reg} cells are not removed before establishment of a solid tumor, these T_{reg} cells infiltrate the tumor and participate in the change of tumor vasculature to become less permeable to activated T cells. Both ICAM and VCAM adhesion molecules are not up-regulated on tumor vasculature; anti-CD25 mAb treatment does decrease circulating T_{reg} cells and augment effector T-cell generation but it does not decrease T_{reg} in the tumor (Quezada et al. 2008). The function of tumor-specific $CD4^{+}CD25^{+}$ T_{reg} cells can be inhibited/attenuated by several mechanisms: (1) inhibition of the production by tumor cells of cyclooxygenase-2 (Moutsopoulos et al. 2008), CD70, Galectin-1, TGFβ, and IDO (Gajewsky et al. 2006); (2) non-specific depletion by treatment with anti-CD25 mAb, with IL-2-diphteria toxin, with cyclophosphamide, by vaccination against FOXP3 or CpG treatment; (3) treatment with TAA-peptide to which T_{reg} cell TCR binds with much higher avidity compared to tumor-specific effector CTL, raising the effector cell threshold by means of treatment with anti-CTLA4 antibodies (Chambers et al. 2001); and (4) blocking of T_{reg} cell trafficking, effector function, or differentiation (Curiel 2007). Expression and function of CTLA-4 can be regulated using anti-CTLA4 antibody therapy (Quezada et al. 2008). Imatinib mesylate inhibits $CD4^{+}CD25^{+}$ T_{reg} cell activity and enhances active immunotherapy by a cell–cell contact-dependent mechanism (Larmonier et al. 2008).

Tumor-associated macrophages are recruited to tumors and promote tumor growth by enhancing inflammation and angiogenesis. Therapies, which neutralize pathways of chronic production of proinflammatory cytokines, may limit tumor growth (Bhardwaj 2007). TGFβ is first produced by developing tumor cells, and then by infiltrating TILs, NK cells, macrophages (in particular, MDSC), epithelial cells, and stromal cells, all recruited by the tumor-produced TGFβ. TGFβ pervades the milieu and profoundly influences the behavior of both tumor cells, stromal cells, and immune cells. Tumor progression is promoted synergistically by epiregulin, matrix metalloproteinases, and COX-2. TGFβ together with IL-6 and IL-21 induces Th17 cell differentiation, which has been linked to tumorigenesis. IL-17 is implicated in recruitment of phagocytes and with increased angiogenesis (via CXCR2). Th17 cells produce IL-21, IL-22, and TNFα, all proinflammatory cytokines that may foment a tumor-supportive niche. TGFβ has multiple actions: i) it promotes Treg function, ii) it induces diminished DC maturation (with decreased expression of MHCII and co-receptor ligands) and migration, iii) it increases DC sensitivity to apoptosis, iv) it induces VEGF and vascularization, and v) it suppresses $CD4^{+}$, $CD8^{+}$ T cell, and NK cell recognition, expansion, and function (Moutsopoulos et al. 2008). Transgenic mice, in which $CD4^{+}$ and $CD8^{+}$ T cells cannot signal through TGFβ, can mount a potent tumor-specific CTL response that results in tumor eradication. However, $TGF\beta R^{-/-}$ T cells can only protect if given at the same time or up to 3 days after the tumor cells. $TGF\beta R^{-/-}$ mice that have rejected tumors do not develop tissue-specific immune destruction. It appears that only tumor-specific T-cell responses are enhanced in the absence of TGFβ signaling (Gorelik and Flavell 2001).

T cells are dependent on a minimal number of TCR/CD3 complexes on the cell surface for optimal effector function. Therefore, one efficient way to diminish T-cell effector function (induction of tolerance or anergy) is to down-regulate TCR/CD3 surface membrane expression. TCR/CD3 cell surface expression is mainly controlled by CD3ζ (Geisler et al. 1992). Consequently, an efficient way to attenuate T-cell effector function is to decrease CD3ζ biosynthesis, intracellular transport, and surface membrane expression. An impressive number of tumors and chronic inflammatory diseases cause induction of nitric oxide (NO), reactive oxygen species (ROS), arginase-1 (Rodriguez et al. 2002), or TNFα (see above), all of which provoke CD3ζ down-regulation (Kiessling 1997; Baniyash 2004). These activities are produced by tolerogenic DC, suppressive macrophages, or MDSC. Furthermore, the tumor microenvironment produces inhibitory factors such as hyaluronan fragments, which down-regulate CD3ε (Kuang et al. 2008). As suppression by these activities is reversible, it is possible to avoid this form of immunosuppression by reagents which neutralize these activities.

In summary, an ultimate goal in the enhancement of antitumor cell immune responses is to master the effects of T_{reg} cells, Th17 cells, MDSC, and their inhibitory molecules (Kryczek et al. 2007). A promising way is to render effector T cells resistant to regulation by regulatory cells (Schneider et al. 2008; Toscano et al. 2007). Both cytokines like TNFα, IL-4, IL-6, IL-7, IL-12, IL-15, and IL-21 impair T_{reg} function (Schneider et al. 2008; Toscano et al. 2007), and the level of glycosylation on the surface of Th1, Th2, or Th17 (Toscano et al. 2007) influences the sensitivity of effector T cells to T_{reg} cells.

7 Discussion

In the preceding chapters, we have described how developing and established tumors interact with the microenvironment and the immune system. In addition, we have given a description of the different aspects of the immune system. In this final discussion, we summarize what the immune system can do to combat the tumors, and, conversely, what the tumors can do to avoid the immune system (Table 1). Through this discussion, the idea is to focus on possible ways to amplify the antitumor immune response to render it efficient. As we have seen, the neoplastic cells develop as a consequence of natural or imposed changes in the genome of host cells. The presence of "changed" cells is interpreted by the host environment as a wound that should be healed to re-establish order. However, the neoplastic cells by themselves may have gained uncontrolled cell growth, and/or they may be helped in the growth by stromal cells including immune cells and molecules. In this situation, the tumor cells establish as a solid tumor at the same time, as the immune system is triggered by the danger or damage signals sent out from the tumor. Sometimes the immune system takes the advantage in this race, and sometimes it is the tumor cells that take over. In the human situation, most often we are dealing with established tumors and an inefficient immune system. Thus, the question is how can we attenuate/eradicate the tumor cells and amplify the destructive effect of the immune system. Solid tumors can in principle be removed by surgery, and eventual residual tumor cells can be eradicated by chemotherapy and/or irradiation. Pharmacological drugs with high efficiency against rapidly growing cells are available, and pharmacological companies are developing increasingly efficient anti-proliferation drugs (Muller and Scherle 2006; Zitvogel et al. 2008). For immunotherapy, the three main problems are: (1) the specific activation of

Table 1 Parameters in the immune system – tumor cell fight

1. What the immune system can do against tumors?
(a) Innate immune cells such as NK and NKT cells survey cells with anomalous expression of MHCI molecules
(b) Innate immune cells such as macrophages or DCs sense "troubled" host cells. Innate immune cells from SR/CR mice are particularly sensitive in this respect. Apoptotic cell death leads to induction of tolerogenic DCs. Necrotic cell death leads to induction of immunogenic DCs, which induces cross-priming of Th1 cells
(c) Innate immune cells help the establishment of neoplastic cells into solid tumors
(d) Vaccination increases the frequency and efficiency of tumor-specific effector cells and induces specific memory
(e) Immune cells should avoid or fight against suppressive molecules or cells induced by tumor cells
(f) Immune cells should have increased capacity to migrate and penetrate into tumors, i.e., increased expression of receptors for chemokines and adhesion molecules
(g) Augment the production of GM-CSF that converts immature DCs to mature DCs
(h) Increase production of IL-12 to enhance Th1 responses
(i) Tumor-specific effector T cells acquire resistance to T_{reg} cells (IL-21)
(j) Avoid differentiation of $CD8^+CD205^+$ DCs, which are specialized to induce $Foxp3^+$ T_{reg} cells
(k) Avoid Th17 cell differentiation by TGFβ, IL-6 and IL-21, or block IL-17 release (induce phagocyte recruitment to tumor site and angiogenesis)

2. What the tumors can do to avoid the immune system?
(a) Get protected by stromal cells and nurtured by vascularization
(b) Make as little "noise" as possible by avoiding production of inflammation and danger signals
(c) Produce inhibitory substances against innate immune cells, adaptive immune cells, against cell interactions or cell migration (chemo-attractants such as CXCL12 and cytokines such as IL-10 and TGFβ)
(d) Use selective procedures as lack of tumor-associated antigens, of MHCI expression or of molecules in the antigen-presentation pathway
(e) Convert tumor-specific Th1 cells into either Th2 cells or $CD4^+CD25^+$ T_{reg} cells
(f) Induce death of activated T cells by, e.g., Fas (CD95) – FasL, or PD-1/PD-2 – ligand interactions
(g) Become resistant to apoptosis induction (expression of FLIP and Survivin)
(h) Trigger differentiation of either TAM, MDSC, or $CD8^+CD205^+$ DCs, which can induce T_{reg} cells
(i) Induce tumor-specific tolerance
(j) Recruit inhibitory macrophages, MDSC and $CD4^+CD25^+$ T_{reg} cells, or Th17 cells to tumor niche
(k) Avoid expression of integrin and chemokine receptors on tumor cells, stromal cells, and vascular cells

3. What can the researchers do amplify the immune cells and attenuate the tumor cells?
(a) Monoclonal antibodies against inhibitory cytokines/chemokines/hormones/growth factors in the tumor microenvironment should be carried to and released in the solid tumor
(b) Tumor-specific monoclonal antibody-coupled liposomes (or other carriers) with encapsulated tumor drugs should be targeted to and phagocytized by the tumor cells (Serre et al. 1998)
(c) Production of stable (not easily degradable) peptides which enhance interactions between TCR and pMHCI, or block unsuitable interactions of integrins, adhesion receptors, cytokine receptors, and chemokine receptors with their ligands
(d) Production of inhibitors against suppressor cells such as MDSC or natural or activated T_{reg} cells
(e) Production of reagents that block the activity of TGFβ, IL-10, IL-35, and VEGF and can be delivered locally (Homey et al. 2002)

(f) Inhibit antigen-induced, activated T-cell death (Chang et al. 2008; Lu and Finn 2008; Nurieva et al. 2006)
(g) Avoid induction of T-cell tolerance (unresponsiveness) by down-regulation of T_{reg} cell activity and up-regulation of low-avidity T-cell reactivity (Cordaro et al. 2002; Morgan et al. 1998; Slansky et al. 2000)
(h) Induction of T_{reg} cell resistance in tumor-specific effector T cells (Schneider et al. 2008; Toscano et al. 2007)
(i) Blocking Treg cell trafficking (anti-CCL22 mAb) (Zou 2006)
(j) Restoration of normal p53 gene function and p53 protein stability (Xue et al. 2007)
(k) Avoid treatment with glucocorticoids during chemotherapy, and avoid removal of tumor-draining lymph nodes (Zitvogel et al. 2008)
(l) Therapeutic induction of lymphopenia (Zitvogel et al. 2008)
(m) Combined treatment with IL-12 and doxorubicin (anthracycline) therapy (Zitvogel et al. 2008)
(n) Activate Vγ9Vδ2 T cells that augment antitumor immunotherapy (Caccamo et al. 2008; Vantourout et al. 2008)
(o) Activate the innate immune system via TLR and/or CLR
(p) Immunize against ganglioside mimotopes (Wierzbicki et al. 2008)
(q) Altered tumor peptide therapy (Slansky et al. 2000)
(r) Control the chemokine balance in the tumor environment (Kiessling 1997)
(s) Small molecule inhibitors of IDO, ARG, iNOS, COX2, TGFβR1, JAK/STAT, VEGFR1, CCR4, CXCR4, and CCR2 (Homey et al. 2002; Muller and Scherle 2006)
(t) Reactivate CD3ζ expression (Baniyash 2004; Geisler et al. 1992; Kiessling 1997; Rodriguez et al. 2002)

T cells in a situation where mechanisms of tumor-specific T-cell tolerance are already present, (2) whether the tumor-specific T cells have the capacity to migrate to and penetrate into the tumor (Rudd et al. 2008), and (3) the sensitivity of effector T cells to tumor cell-produced inhibition (Muller and Scherle 2006). These processes are regulated by $CD4^+CD25^+$ T_{reg} cells, Th17 cells, and MDSC. Therefore, a first step in attempting to increase tumor-specific immunity is by trying to diminish the effect of these cells. A relatively straightforward method would be to eliminate/inactivate T_{reg} cells by treatment with mAb against CD25, CTLA-4, GITR, or Foxp3 (Curiel 2007; Zou 2006; Van Elsas et al. 2001; Chambers et al. 2001). One promising way is to activate natural immunity, which mediates a continuously activated innate immune system (Rubin 2009). Thus, activation of TLR on APC by ligands such as CpG (TLR9), LPS (TLR4), or double-stranded DNA (TLR3) induces increased TCR triggering (by slowing pMHCI decay rates on the APC) (Rudd et al. 2008) and T_{reg} cell activity inhibition (Zou 2006; Mills 2008). The property of T_{reg} cell TCRs in general to have a higher avidity than that of TAA-specific effector T cells may be used to induce TAA-specific tolerance of the T_{reg} cells with appropriate doses of altered peptide (Hsieh et al. 2006; Mills 2008).

In the injured tissue, macrophages are supplemented from the circulation, and the activities of the inflammatory cells are biased toward phagocytosis, extracellular proteolysis, and production of factors that promote growth and repair (Hume 2008). Endothelial cells express two endothelin receptors, ETRA and ETBR. In the presence of endothelin, the adhesion of lymphocytes to endothelial cells is reduced. This effect can be reversed by the ETBR inhibitor peptide, BQ-788, which upregulates expression of ICAM-1. ETBR ligation induces nitric oxide production that plays a role in leukocyte recruitment to tissues, but also in production of VEGF. Treatment of mice with BQ-788 could inhibit tumor growth and was associated with increased lymphocyte infiltration into tumors (Buckanivich et al. 2008). Activated DCs express the chemokine receptor, CCR7, which facilitates their migration to lymph nodes and initiates DC maturation (Homey et al. 2002; Förster et al. 2008). DCs can be "alarmed" by products (alarmins) of injured or dying host cells. G protein-coupled receptors mediate a wide variety of sensory functions by interacting with ligands as distinct as photons, hormones, neurotransmitters, or proteins (peptides). One such receptor, GPR91, functions as a receptor for succinate, which in addition to its metabolic function in cellular respiration (Krebs cycle) may alert the innate system of immunological danger. Immature DCs express high levels of GPR91, which bind to succinate released locally or in the circulation and induces DC maturation. In this process, the DCs lose GPR91 expression (Rubic et al. 2008). These processes augment T-cell migration to and penetration into the tumors.

One of the mechanisms to evade effective immunosurveillance is induction of T-cell death by tumor cells. Chronic stimulation of T cells by tumors leads to activation-induced cell death (AICD). Abortive stimulation of T cells by tolerogenic DC loaded with tumor antigens or caused by cytokine withdrawal leads to autonomous death of tumor-specific T cells (ACAD). Possible mechanisms are the expression by tumor cells of Fas or B7-H1/H4, which interact with FasL or PD-1 or PD-2 on activated T cells. Hyaluronan (a damage signal) participates in the maturation of DCs and thereby activation of naïve T cells. This causes expansion of specific T cells. Thus, activated T cells express CD44 which binds hyaluronan and mediates cell death (Ruffell and Johnson 2008) via a non-Fas (CD95)-dependent but Bim-dependent mechanism (Green 2008). Therapeutic approaches that prevent T-cell death in the tumor microenvironment and tumor-draining lymph nodes, therefore, should be used. However, AICD and ACAD are also natural regulatory pathways that control and stop normal immune responses, when these are no more needed (Lu and Finn 2008).

Most patients do not experience tumor regressions in response to active immunization. For tumor rejection to occur, activated effector T cells must migrate into the tumor sites and gain contact with antigen-expressing tumor cells. In addition, they must maintain their effector functions for a sufficient time to eradicate the population of tumor cells. Th1 cells and $CD8^+$ CTL express CCR2 [which binds monocyte chemotactic proteins (MCPs) MCP-1, MCP-2, and MCP-3], CCR5 [macrophage inflammatory protein 1α (MIP-1α) and MIP-1β], and CXCR3 (which binds IP-10, Mig, and I-TAC). In contrast, Th2 cells express CCR3, CCR4, CCR8, and CXCR4 arguing that a partially distinct set of chemokines is responsible for establishing this T-cell differentiation state. T_{reg} cells are attracted by a separate set of chemokines, i.e., thymus and activation-regulated chemokine (TARC) and macrophage-derived chemoattractant (MDC) via CCR4. These observations suggest that expression of the appropriate array of chemokines within a tumor microenvironment that are chemotactic for IFNγ-producing Th1 cells, with minimal expression of the T_{reg} cell-recruiting TARC and MDC, might be important for establishing the most effective microenvironment for executing the effector phase of the antitumor immune response (Zou 2005; Wang et al. 2004).

The fact that tumors acquire such a complex program of immune evasion mechanisms is striking. At first glance, it may not seem logical that tumor cells should so readily orchestrate an immunosuppressive microenvironment. However, from the evolutionary perspective, there is a clear developmental context in which such a tolerogenic environment must be generated in normal physiology, which is at the maternal/fetal interface. The mechanisms by which the placenta prevents immune-mediated rejection of the semi-allogeneic fetus are strikingly similar to those present in tumors (Petroff 2005).

From the discussion emerge some therapeutic opportunities (see also Table 1):

1. The greatest information can be gained by gene expression profiling on tumor samples that capture the spectrum of cells in the tumor microenvironment (Wang et al. 2004).
2. Intratumoral introduction of chemokines through the use of viral vectors would serve as a proof of concept. Transduction of tumor cells to express specific chemokines has shown benefit in some experimental murine models (Zitvogel et al. 2008; Yingling et al. 2004).
3. Anergy of antitumor T cells is amenable to reversal or prevention in vivo. One strategy may be to use homeostatic proliferation (Nair et al. 2003).
4. Another strategy would be to restore the expression of co-stimulatory ligands and to decrease the expression of inhibitory ligands within the tumor microenvironment.
5. Depletion of T_{reg} cells or interfering with their regulatory function (Schneider et al. 2008; Toscano et al. 2007).
6. Interfere with intratumoral migration of T_{reg} by blocking TARC or MDC and/or inhibiting the engagement of CCR4 (Homey et al. 2002; Förster et al. 2008; Buckanivich et al. 2008).
7. Try to counter metabolic dysregulation at tumor sites (Stolina et al. 2000; Gajewsky et al. 2006).
8. Inhibit STAT3 function. STAT3 inhibitors have been shown to augment the attraction of effector T cells to the tumor site, in addition to their effect as negative regulators of vascularization (inhibition of VEGF production). Down-regulation of VEGF further avoids interference with DC generation and maturation (Wang et al. 2004).
9. Tumor cells are relatively resistant to apoptosis in contrast to stromal cells. Therefore, one should use the lower threshold of stromal cell killing compared to tumor cells.
10. Combined immunotherapy against tumor antigens and VEGF or VEGFR-2 causes tumor cell rejection even when given after tumor cell implantation (Nair et al. 2003).

In summary, we have discussed that even when tumor antigen-specific T cells are appropriately activated and home to tumor tissues, they must maintain their effector function and overcome local mechanisms of immune suppression in the tumor microenvironment for tumor eradication to be achieved. There are multiple possible combinations of different types of therapies, and only our imagination may be at default. However, the main message is that all environmental factors which can activate the innate immune system and maintain its activity are beneficial in our combat against cancer. In addition, effector T cells have to be rendered insensitive to tumor environment-related inhibition.

Acknowledgement We wish to thank the CNRS, Pierre Fabre Laboratories, the french Association for Research on Cancer ARC and the European Union for grants and financial supports.

References

Adams EJ, Strop P, Shin S, Chien YH, Garcia KC (2008) An autonomous CDR3δ is sufficient for recognition of the nonclassical MHCI molecules T10 and T22 by γδ T cells. Nat Immunol 9:777–784

Allison TJ, Winter CC, Fournié JJ, Bonneville M, Garboczi DN (2001) Structure of a human γδ T-cell antigen receptor. Nature 411:820–824

Aschenbrenner K, D'Cruz LM, Vollmann EH, Hinterberger M, Emmerich J, Swee LM, Rolink A, Klein L (2007) Selection of $FOXP3^+$ regulatory T cells specific for self antigen expressed and presented by $AIRE^+$ medullary thymic epithelial cells. Nat Immunol 8:351–358

Baniyash M (2004) TCRζ-chain downregulation: curtailing an excessive inflammatory immune response. Nat Rev Immunol 4:675–687

Bendelac A, Bonneville M, Kearney JF (2001) Autoreactivity by design: innate B and T lymphocytes. Nat Rev Immunol 1:177–186

Bhardwaj N (2007) Harnessing the immune system to treat cancer. J Clin Invest 117:1130–1136

Bianchi ME (2007) DAMPs, PAMPs and alarmins: all we need to know about danger. J Leuk Biol 81:1–5

Blander JM, Medzhitov R (2006) Toll-dependent selection of microbial antigens for presentation by dendritic cells. Nature 440:808–812

Böhm W, Thoma S, Leithäuser F, Möller P, Schirrmbeck R, Reimann J (1998) T cell-mediated, IFNγ-facilitated rejection of murine B16 melanomas. J Immunol 161:897–908

Buckanivich RJ, Facciabene A, Kim S, Benencia F, Sasaroli D, Balint K, Katsaros D, O'Brien-Jenkins A, Gimotty PA, Coukos G (2008) Endothelin B receptor mediates the endothelial barrier to T-cell homing to tumors and disables immune therapy. Nat Med 14:28–36

Caccamo N, Meravgilia S, Scarpa F, Mendola CL, Santini D, Bonanno CT, Missiano G, Dieli F, Salerno A (2008) Aminobisphosphonate-activated γδ T cells in immunotherapy of cancer: doubts no more. Expert Opin Biol Ther 8:875–883

Call ME, Wucherpfennig KW (2007) Common themes in the assembly and architecture of activating immune receptors. Nat Rev Immunol 7:841–850

Carnaud C, Lee D, Donnars O, Park SH, Beavis A, Koezuka Y, Bendelac A (1999) Cross-talk between cells of the innate immune system: NKT cells rapidly activate NK cells. J Immunol 163:4647–4650

Cerwenka A, Lanier LL (2001) Natural killer cells, viruses and cancer. Nat Rev Immunol 1:41–49

Chambers CA, Kuhns MS, Egen JG, Allison JP (2001) CTLA4-mediated inhibition in regulation of T-cell responses: mechanisms and manipulation in tumor immunotherapy. Ann Rev Immunol 19:565–594

Chang WS, Kim JY, Kim YJ, Kim YS, Lee JM, Azuma M, Yagita H, Kang CY (2008) Programmed death-1/programmed death ligand interaction regulates the induction and maintenance of NKT cell anergy. J Immunol 181:6707–6710

Chen W, Jin W, Hardegen N, Lei K, Li L, Marinos N, McGrady G, Wahl SM (2003) Conversion of peripheral $CD4^{+}CD25^{-}$ naive T cells to $CD4^{+}CD25^{+}$ regulatory T cells by TGFβ induction of transcription factor Foxp3. J Exp Med 198:1875–1886

Cordaro TA, de Visser KE, Tirion FH, Schumacher TNM, Kruisbeek AM (2002) Can the low-avidity self-specific T cell repertoire be exploited for tumor rejection? J Immunol 168:651–660

Corthay A, Skovstedt DK, Lundin KU, Rösjö E, Omholt H, Hofgaard PO, Haraldsen G, Bogen B (2005) Primary anti-tumor immune response mediated by $CD4^{+}$ T cells. Immunity 22:371–383

Coussens LM, Werb Z (2002) Inflammation and cancer. Nature 420:860–867

Cui Z, Willingham MC, Hicks AM, Alexander-Miller MA, Howard TD, Hawkins GA, Miller MS, Weir HM, Du W, Delong CJ (2003) Spontaneous regression of advanced cancer: Identification of a unique genetically determined, age-dependent trait in mice. Proc Natl Acad Sci USA 100:6682–6687

Curiel TJ (2007) T_{reg} cells and rethinking cancer immunotherapy. J Clin Invest 117:1167–1174

Davies DR, Cohen GH (1996) Interactions of protein antigens with antibodies. Proc Natl Acad Sci USA 93:7–12

de Visser KE, Eichten A, Coussens LM (2006) Paradoxical roles of the immune system during cancer development. Nat Rev Cancer 6:24–37

Denizot F, Rubin B (1985) Murine and human T-cell factors that induce the differentiation of normal mouse lymphocytes into cytotoxic cells copurify with interleukin-2. Scand J Immunol 22:401–413

Diefenbach A, Jensen ER, Jamieson AM, Raulet DH (2001) Rae1 and H60 ligands of the NKG2D receptor stimulate tumour immunity. Nature 413:165–171

Dunn GP, Old LJ, Schreiber RD (2004) The three aces of cancer immunoediting. Ann Rev Immunol 22:329–360

Entin I, Plotnikov A, Korenstein R, Keisari Y (2003) Tumor growth retardation, cure, and induction of anti-tumor immunity in B16 melanoma-bearing mice by mow electric field-enhanced chemotherapy. Clin Cancer Res 9:3190–3197

Fernandez NC, Lozier A, Flament C, Ricciardi-Castagnoli P, Bellet D, Suter M, Perricaudet M, Tursz T, Maraskovsky E, Zitvogel L (1999) Dendritic cells directly trigger NK cell functions: cross-talk relevant in innate anti-tumor immune responses in vivo. Nat Med 5:405–411

Figdor CG, van Kooyk Y, Adema GJ (2002) C-type lectin receptors on dendritic cells and langerhans cells. Nat Rev Immunol 2:77–84

Förster R, Davalos-Misslitz AC, Rot A (2008) CCR7 and its ligands: balancing immunity and tolerance. Nat Rev Immunol 8:362–371

Fujii SI (2008) Exploiting dendritic cells and natural killer T cells in immunotherapy against malignancies. Trends Immunol 29:242–249

Gajewsky TF, Meng Y, Blank C, Brown I, Kacha A, Kline J, Harlin H (2006) Immune resistance orchestrated by the tumor microenvironment. Immunol Rev 213:131–145

Ganss R, Arnold B, Hämmerling GJ (2004) Overcoming tumor-intrinsic resistance to immune effector function. Eur J Immunol 34:2635–2641

Gao Y, Yang W, Pan M, Scully E, Girardi M, Augenlicht LH, Craft J, Yin Z (2003) γδ T cells provide an early source of interferon γ in tumor immunity. J Exp Med 198:433–442

Garbi N, Arnold B, Gordon S, Hämmerling GJ, Ganss R (2004) CpG motifs as proinflammatory factors render autochthonous tumors permissive for infiltration and destruction. J Immunol 172:5861–5869

Gardai SJ, Bratton DL, Ogden CA, Henson PM (2006) Recognition ligands on apoptotic cells: a perspective. J Leuk Biol 79:896–903

Geisler C, Rubin B, Bauguil-Caspar S, Champagne E, Vangsted A, Hou X, Gajhede M (1992) Structural mutations of C-domains in members of the immunoglobulin superfamily:

consequences for the interaction between the T cell antigen receptor and the CD3-ζ homodimer. J Immunol 148:3469–3477

Godfrey DI, MacDonald HR, Kronenberg M, Smyth MJ, Van Kaer L (2004) NKT cells: what's in a name? Nat Rev Immunol 4:231–237

Gonthier M, Llobera R, Arnaud J, Rubin B (2004) Self-reactive T cell receptor-reactive $CD8^+$ T cells inhibit T cell lymphoma growth in vivo. J Immunol 173:7062–7069

Gorelik L, Flavell RA (2001) Immune-mediated eradication of tumors through the blockade of transforming growth factor-β signaling in T cells. Nat Med 7:1118–1122

Gorelik E, Gunji Y, Herberman RB (1988) H-2 antigen expression and sensitivity of BL6 melanoma cells to natural killer cell cytotoxicity. J Immunol 140:2096–2102

Green DR (2008) Fas Bim Boom! Immunity 28:141–143

Hanahan D, Wienberg RA (2000) The hallmarks of cancer. Cell 100:57–70

Harrington LE, Janowski KM, Oliver JR, Zajac AJ, Weaver CT (2008) Memory CD4 T cells emerge from effector T-cell progenitors. Nature 452:356–361

Hicks AM, Riedlinger G, Willingham MC, Alexander-Miller MA, von Kap-Herr C, Pettenati MJ, Sanders AM, Weir HM, Du W, Kim J, Simpson AJG, Old LJ, Cui Z (2006a) Transferable anticancer innate immunity in spontaneous regression/complete resistance mice. Proc Natl Acad Sci USA 103:7753–7758

Hicks AM, Willingham MC, Du W, Pang CS, Old LJ, Cui Z (2006b) Effector mechanisms of the anti-cancer immune response of macrophages in SR/CR mice. Cancer Immun 6:11–20

Holst J, Wang H, Eder KD, Workman CJ, Boyd KL, Baquet Z, Singh H, Forbes K, Chruscinski A, Smeyne R, van Oers NSC, Utz PJ, Vignali DAA (2008) Scalable signaling mediated by T cell antigen receptor-CD3 ITAMs ensures effective negative selection and prevents autoimmunity. Nat Immunol 9:658–666

Homey B, Müller A, Zlotnik A (2002) Chemokines: agents for the immunotherapy of cancer. Nat Rev Immunol 2:175–184

Hsieh CS, Zheng Y, Liang Y, Fontenot JD, Rudensky AY (2006) An intersection between the self-reactive regulatory and nonregulatory T-cell receptor repertoires. Nat Immunol 7:401–410

Hume DA (2008) Macrophages as APC and the dendritic cell myth. J Immunol 181:5829–5835

Janeway CA Jr (1989) Approaching the asymptote? Evolution and revolution in immunology. Cold Spring Harb Symp Quant Biol 54:1–13

Jerne NK (1984) Idiotypic networks and other preconceived ideas. Immunol Rev 79:5–24

Kalinski P, Moser M (2005) Consensual immunity: success-driven development of Th1 and Th2 responses. Nat Rev Immunol 5:251–260

Kane KP, Silver ET, Hazes B (2001) Specificity and function of activating Ly-49 receptors. Immunol Rev 181:104–114

Kärre K, Ljunggren HG, Piontel G, Kiessling R (1986) Selective rejection of H-2-deficient lymphoma variants suggests alternative immune defence strategy. Nature 319:675–678

Kawano YI, Tanigushi K, Toshitani A, Nomoto K (1986) Synergistic defense system by cooperative natural effectors against metastasis of B16 melanoma cells in H-2 associated control: different behavior of $H\text{-}2^+$ and $H\text{-}2^-$ cells in metastatic processes. J Immunol 136:4729–4734

Kazama H, Ricci JE, Herndon JM, Hoppe G, Green DR, Ferguson TA (2008) Induction of immunological tolerance by apoptotic cells requires caspase-dependent oxidation of high-mobility group box-1 protein. Immunity 29:21–32

Kemper C, Mitchell LM, Zhang L, Hourcade DE (2008) The complement protein properdin binds apoptotic T cells and promotes complement activation and phagocytosis. Proc Natl Acad Sci USA 105:9023–9028

Kiessling R (1997) Signals from lymphocytes in colon cancer. Gut 40:153–158

Kim KD, Zhao J, Auh S, Yang X, Du P, Tang H, Fu YX (2007) Adaptive immune cells temper initial innate responses. Nat Med 13:1248–1252

Krogsgaard M, Davis MM (2005) How T cells "see" antigen. Nat Immunol 6:239–247

Kryczek I, Wei S, Zou L, Altuwaijri S, Szeliga W, Kolls J, Chang A, Zou W (2007) Th17 and regulatory T cell dynamics and the regulation by IL-2 in the tumor microenvironment. J Immunol 178:6730–6733

Kuang DM, Zhao Q, Xu J, Yun JP, Wu C, Zheng L (2008) Tumor-educated tolerogenic dendritic cells induce CD3ε down-regulation and apoptosis of T cells through oxygen-dependent pathways. J Immunol 181:3089–3098

Larmonier N, Janikashvili N, LaCasse CJ, Larmonier CB, Cantrell J, Situ E, Lundeen T, Bonnotte B, Katsanis E (2008) Imatinib mesylate inhibits $CD4^{+}CD25^{+}$ regulatory T-cell activity and enhances active immunotherapy against BCR-ABL- tumors. J Immunol 181:6955–6965

Lee HH, Hoeman CM, Hardaway JC, Guloglu FB, Ellis JS, Jain R, Divekar R, Tartar DM, Haymaker CL, Zaghouani H (2008) Delayed maturation of an IL-12 producing dendritic cell subset explains the early Th2 bias in neonatal immunity. J Exp Med 205:2269–2280

Ljunggren HG, Kärre K (1985) Host resistance directed selectively against H-2-deficient lymphoma variants. Analysis of the mechanism. J Exp Med 162:1745–1759

Lu B, Finn OJ (2008) T-cell death and cancer immune tolerance. Cell Death Differ 15:70–79

Ludewig B, Ochsenbein AE, Odermatt B, Paulin D, Hengartner H, Zinkernagel RM (2000) Immunotherapy with dendritic cells directed against tumor antigens shared with normal host cells results in severe autoimmune disease. J Exp Med 191:795–803

MacDonald AS, Maizels RM (2008) Alarming dendritic cells for Th2 induction. J Exp Med 205:13–17

Markiewski MM, DeAngelis RA, Benencia F, Ricklin-Lichtsteiner SK, Koutoulaki A, Gerard C, Coukos G, Lambris JD (2008) Modulation of the antitumor immune response by complement. Nat Immunol 9:1225–1235

McKee AS, Munks MW, Marrack P (2007) How do adjuvants work? Important considerations for new generation adjuvants. Immunity 27:687–690

Medzhitov R (2001) Toll-like receptors and innate immunity. Nat Rev Immunol 1:135–145

Mills KHG (2008) TLR9 turns the tide on T_{reg} cells. Immunity 29:518–520

Mocikat R, Braumüller H, Gumy A, Egeter O, Ziegler H, Reusch U, Bubeck A, Louis J, Mailhammer R, Riethmuller G, Koszinowski U, Rocken M (2003) Natural killer cells activated by MHC class I^{low} targets prime dendritic cells to induce protective CD8 T cell responses. Immunity 19:561–569

Mohammed F, Cobbold M, Zarling AL, Salim M, Barrett-Wilt GA, Shabanowitz J, Hunt DF, Engelhard VH, Willcox BE (2008) Phosphorylation-dependent interaction between antigenic peptides and MHCI: a molecular basis for the presentation of transformed self. Nat Immunol 9:1236–1243

Morgan DJ, Kreuwel HTC, Fleck S, Levitsky HL, Pardoll DM, Sherman LA (1998) Activation of low avidity CTL specific for a self epitope results in tumor rejection but not autoimmunity. J Immunol 160:643–651

Moutsopoulos NM, Wen J, Wahl SM (2008) TGFβ and tumors – an ill-fated alliance. Curr Opin Immunol 20:234–240

Mueller MM, Fusenig NE (2004) Friends or foes – Bipolar effects of the tumor stroma in cancer. Nat Rev Cancer 4:839–849

Muller AJ, Scherle PA (2006) Targeting the mechanisms of tumoral immune tolerance with small-molecule inhibitors. Nat Rev Cancer 6:613–625

Munoz-Fontela C, Macip S, Martinez-Sobrido L, Brown L, Ashour J, Garcia-Sastre A, Lee SW, Aaronson SA (2008) Transcriptional role of p53 in interferon-mediated antiviral immunity. J Exp Med 205:1929–1938

Nair S, Boczkowski D, Moeller B, Dewhirst M, Vieweg J, Gilboa E (2003) Synergy between tumor immunotherapy and antiangiogenic therapy. Blood 102:964–971

Nomura T, Sakagushi S (2007) FOXP3 and AIRE in thymus-generated Treg cells: a link in self-tolerance. Nat Immunol 8:333–334

Nurieva R, Thomas S, Nguyen T, Martin-Orozco N, Wang Y, Kaja MK, Yu XZ, Dong C (2006) T-cell tolerance or function is determined by combinatorial costimulatory signals. EMBO J 25:2623–2633
Pardoll DM (2002) Spinning molecular immunology into successful immunotherapy. Nat Rev Immunol 2:227–238
Pasare C, Medzhitov R (2003) Toll pathway-dependent blockade of $CD4^{+}CD25^{+}$ T cell-mediated suppression by dendritic cells. Science 299:1033–1036
Petroff MG (2005) Immune interactions at the maternal-fetal interface. J Reprod Immunol 68:1–13
Preckel T, Grimm R, Martin S, Weltzien HU (1997) Altered hapten ligands antagonize trinitrophenyl-specific cytotoxic T cells and block internalization of hapten-specific receptors. J Exp Med 185:1803–1813
Prehn RT, Prehn LM (2008) The flip side of immune surveillance: immune dependency. Immunol Rev 222:341–356
Prévost-Blondel A, Zimmermann C, Stemmer C, Kulmburg P, Rosenthal FM, Pircher H (1998) Tumor-infiltrating lymphocytes exhibiting high ex vivo cytolytic activity fail to prevent murine melanoma tumor growth in vivo. J Immunol 161:2187–2194
Probst HC, McCoy K, Okazaki T, Honjo T, van den Broek M (2005) Resting dendritic cells induce peripheral $CD8^{+}$ T cell tolerance through PD-1 and CTLA-4. Nat Immunol 6:280–286
Quezada SA, Peggs KS, Simpson TR, Shen Y, Littman DR, Allison JP (2008) Limited tumor infiltration by activated T effector cells restricts the therapeutic activity of regulatory T cell depletion against established melanoma. J Exp Med 205:2125–2138
Rabinovich GA, Gabrilovich D, Sotomayor EM (2007) Immunosuppressive strategies that are mediated by tumor cells. Ann Rev Immunol 25:267–296
Reits EA, Hodge JW, Herberts CA, Groothuis TA, Chakraborty M, Wansley EK, Camphausen K, Luiten RM, de Ru AH, Neijssen J, Griekspoor A, Mesman E, Verreck FA, Spits H, Schlom J, van Veelen P, Neefjes JJ (2006) Radiation modulates the peptide repertoire, enhances MHCI expression, and induces successful antitumor immunotherapy. J Exp Med 203:1259–1271
Riond J, Rodriguez S, Nicolau ML, al Saati T, Gairin JE (2009) In vivo major histocompatibility complex class I (MHCI) expression on $MHCI^{low}$ tumor cells is regulated by $\gamma\delta$ T and NK cells during the early steps of tumor growth. Cancer Immun 9:10
Rodriguez PC, Zea AH, Culotta KS, Zabaletta J, Ochoa JB, Ochoa AC (2002) Regulation of T-cell receptor CD3zeta chain expression by L-arginine. J Biol Chem 277:21123–21128
Roehm U, Roth E, Brommer K, Dumrese T, Rosenthal FM, Pircher H (2002) Lack of effector cell function and altered tetramer binding of tumor-infiltrating lymphocytes. J Immunol 169:5522–5530
Rubartelli A, Lotze MT (2007) Inside, outside, upside down: damage-associated molecular-pattern molecules (DAMPs) and redox. Trends Immunol 28:429–436
Rubic T, Lametschwandtner G, Jost S, Hinteregger S, Kund J, Carballido-Perrig N, Schwärzler C, Junt T, Vosbol H, Meingassner JG, Mao X, Werner G, Rot A, Carballido JM (2008) Triggering the succinate receptor GPR91 on dendritic cells enhances immunity. Nat Immunol 9:1261–1269
Rubin B (2009) Natural immunity has significant impact on the immune response against cancer. Scand J Immunol 69:275–290
Rubin B, Sönderstrup G (2004) Citrullination of self-proteins and autoimmunity. Scand J Immunol 60:112–120
Rubin B, Wigzell H (1973) On the nature of hapten-reactive lymphocytes. Nature 242:467–469
Rubin B, Riond J, Courtiade L, Roullet N and Gairin JE (2008) The innate immune system recognizes and regulates MHCI expression on $MHCI^{low}$ tumor cells. Cancer Immun 8:14–25
Rudd BD, Brien JD, Davenport MP, Nikolich-Zugich J (2008) TLR ligands increase TCR triggering by slowing pMHCI decay rates. J Immunol 181:5199–5203
Ruffell B, Johnson P (2008) Hyaluronan induces cell death in activated T cells through CD44. J Immunol 181:7044–7054

Sakaguchi S, Ono M, Setoguchi R, Yagi H, Hon S, Fehervari Z, Shimizu J, Takahashi T, Nomura T (2006) Foxp3$^+$ CD25$^+$CD4$^+$ natural regulatory T cells in dominant self-tolerance and autoimmune disease. Immunol Rev 212:8–27

Sauter B, Albert ML, Francisco L, Larsson M, Somersan S, Bhardwaj N (2000) Consequences of cell death: Exposure to necrotic tumor cells, but not primary tissue cells or apoptotic cells, induces the maturation of immunostimulatory dendritic cells. J Exp Med 191:423–433

Schneider A, Rieck M, Sanda S, Pihoker C, Greenbaum C, Buckner JH (2008) The effector T cells of Diabetic subjects are resistant to regulation via CD4$^+$CD25$^+$ regulatory T cells. J Immunol 181:7350–7355

Schüler T, Blankenstein T (2003) CD8$^+$ effector T cells reject tumors by direct antigen recognition but indirect action on host cells. J Immunol 170:4427–4431

Seliger B, Wollscheid U, Momburg F, Blankenstein T, Huber C (2001) Characterization of the major histocompatibility complex class I deficiencies in B16 melanoma cells. Cancer Res 61:1095–1099

Serre K, Machy P, Grivel JC, Jolly G, Brun N, Barbet J, Leserman L (1998) Efficient presentation of multivalent antigens targeted to various cell surface molecules of dendritic cells and surface Ig of antigen-specific B cells. J Immunol 161:6059–6067

Sha Y, Zmijewski J, Xu Z, Abraham E (2008) HMGB1 develops enhanced proinflammatory activity by binding to cytokines. J Immunol 180:2531–2537

Singh S, Ross SR, Acena M, Rowley DA, Schreiber H (1992) Stroma is critical for preventing or permitting immunological destruction of antigenic cancer cells. J Exp Med 175:139–146

Sinha P, Okoro C, Foell D, Freeze HH, Ostrand-Rosenberg S, Srikrishna G (2008) Proinflammatory S100 proteins regulate the accumulation of myeloid-derived suppressor cells. J Immunol 181:4666–4675

Slansky JE, Rattis FM, Boyd LF, Fahmy T, Jaffee EM, Schneck JP, Margulies DH, Pardoll DM (2000) Enhanced antigen-specific antitumor immunity with altered peptide ligands that stabilize the MHC-peptide-TCR complex. Immunity 13:529–538

Smyth MJ, Godfrey DI (2000) NKT cells and tumor immunity – a double-edged sword. Nat Immunol 1:459–460

Sriram V, Cho S, Li P, O'Donnell PW, Dunn C, Hayakawa K, Blum JS, Brutkiewicz RR (2002) Inhibition of glycolipid shedding rescues recognition of a CD1+ T cell hybridoma by natural killer T (NKT) cells. Proc Natl Acad Sci USA 99:8197–8202

Steinman RM, Turley S, Mellman I, Inaba K (2000) The induction of tolerance by dendritic cells that have captured apoptotic cells. J Exp Med 191:411–416

Stolina M, Sharma S, Lin Y, Dohadwala M, Gardner B, Luo J, Zhu L, Kronenberg M, Miller PW, Portanova J, Lee JC, Dubinett SM (2000) Specific inhibition of cyclooxygenase 2 restores antitumor reactivity by altering the balance of IL-10 and IL-12 synthesis. J Immunol 164:361–370

Sugiyama H (2008) Editorial overview. Curr Opinion Immunol 20:208–210

Tato CM, Cua DJ (2008) Alternative lifestyles of T cells. Nat Immunol 9:1323–1325

Toscano MA, Bianco GA, Ilarregui JM, Croci DO, Correale J, Hernandez JD, Zwirner NW, Poirier F, Riley EM, Baum LB, Rabinovich GA (2007) Differential glycosylation of Th1, Th2 and Th17 effector cells selectively regulates susceptibility to cell death. Nat Immunol 8: 825–834

van Elsas A, Sutmuller RPM, Hurwitz AA, Ziskin J, Villasenor J, Medema JP, Overwijk WW, Restifo NP, Melief CJM, Offringa R, Allison JP (2001) Elucidating the autoimmune and antitumor effector mechanisms of a treatment based on cytotoxic T lymphocyte antigen-4 blockade in combination with a B16 melanoma vaccine: comparison of prophylaxis and therapy. J Exp Med 194:481–489

van Stipdonk MJB, Hardenberg G, Bijker MS, Lemmens E, Droin NM, Green DR, Schoenberger SP (2003) Dynamic programming of CD8$^+$ T lymphocyte responses. Nat Immunol 4:361–365

Vantourout P, Martinez LO, Fabre A, Collet X, Champagne E (2008) Ecto-F1-ATPase and MHCI close association on cell membranes. Mol Immunol 45:485–492

Vignali DAA, Collison LW, Workman CJ (2008) How regulatory T cells work. Nat Rev Immunol 8:523–532

Vivier E, Anfossi N (2004) Inhibitory NK-cell receptors on T cells: witness of the past, actors of the future. Nat Rev Immunol 4:190–198

Wang T, Niu G, Kortylewski M, Burdelya L, Shain K, Zhang S, Bhattacharya R, Gabrilivich D, Heller R, Coppola D, Dalton W, Jove R, Pardoll D, Yu H (2004) Regulation of the innate and adaptive immune responses by stat-3 signaling in tumor cells. Nat Med 10:48–54

Wierzbicki A, Gil M, Ciesielski M, Fenstermaker RA, Kaneko Y, Rotika H, Lau JT, Kozbor D (2008) Immunization with a mimotope of GD2 ganglioside induces $CD8^+$ T cells that recognize cell adhesion molecules on tumor cells. J Immunol 181:6644–6653

Wu DY, Segal NH, Sidobre S, Kronenberg M, Chapman PB (2003) Cross-presentation of disialoganglioside GD3 to natural killer T cells. J Exp Med 198:173–181

Xue W, Zender L, Miething C, Dickins RA, Hernando E, Krizhanovsky V, Cordon-Cardo C, Lowe SW (2007) Senescence and tumor clearance is triggered by p53 restoration in murine liver carcinomas. Nature 445:656–660

Yamasaki S, Ishikawa E, Sakuma M, Hara H, Ogata K, Saito T (2008) Mincle is an ITAM-coupled activating receptor that senses damaged cells. Nat Immunol 9:1179–1188

Yamazaki S, Dudziak D, Heidkamp GF, Fiorese C, Bonito AJ, Inaba K, Nussenzweig MN, Steinman RM (2008) $CD8^+CD205^+$ splenic dendritic cells are specialized to induce $Foxp3^+$ regulatory T cells. J Immunol 181:6923–6933

Yingling JM, Blanchard KL, Sawyer JS (2004) Development of TGFβ signaling inhibitors for cancer therapy. Nat Rev Drug Discov 3:1011–1022

Yu P, Lee Y, Liu W, Chin RK, Wang J, Wang Y, Schietinger A, Philip M, Schreiber H, Fu YX (2004) Priming of naive T cells inside tumors leads to eradication of established tumors. Nat Immunol 5:141–149

Zhang B, Bowerman NA, Salama JK, Schmidt H, Spiotto MT, Schietinger A, Yu P, Fu YX, Weichelbaum RR, Rowley DA, Kranz DM, Schreiber H (2007) Induced sensitization of tumor stroma leads to eradication of established cancer by T cells. J Exp Med 204:49–55

Zitvogel L, Apetoh L, Ghiringhelli F, Kroemer G (2008) Immunological aspects of cancer chemotherapy. Nat Rev Immunol 8:59–73

Zou W (2005) Immunosuppressive networks in the tumor environment and their therapeutic relevance. Nat Rev Cancer 5:263–274

Zou W (2006) Regulatory T cells, tumor immunity and immunotherapy. Nat Rev Immunol 6: 295–307

Angiogenesis and the Tumor Vasculature as Antitumor Immune Modulators: The Role of Vascular Endothelial Growth Factor and Endothelin

Lana E. Kandalaft, Gregory T. Motz, Johanna Busch, and George Coukos

Contents

1 Introduction 130
2 Angiogenesis and Cancer 131
3 Vascular Endothelial Growth Factor 132
4 Direct Effects of VEGF on Leukocytes 133
 4.1 Dendritic Cell Defects in Cancer Patients and Mouse Models: A Role for VEGF 133
 4.2 Effects of VEGF on T Cells 135
5 VEGF, the Tumor Vascular Endothelium, and Immune Evasion 137
 5.1 The Vascular Endothelium 137
 5.2 VEGF and Adhesion Molecule Expression 137
6 The Tumor Endothelium and VEGF Crosstalk: A Role for the Endothelin System 138
 6.1 The Endothelin System 138
 6.2 Endothelin and Tumor Angiogenesis 139
 6.3 ET_BR and the Tumor Endothelial Barrier to T Cell Homing 140
7 Concluding Statements 141
References 142

Abstract Cancer immunotherapies have yielded promising results in recent years, but new approaches must be utilized if more patients are to experience the benefits of these therapies. Angiogenesis and the tumor endothelium confer unique immune privilege to a growing tumor, with significant effects on diverse immunological processes such as hematopoietic cell maturation, antigen presentation, effector T cell differentiation, cytokine production, adhesion, and T cell homing and extravasation. Here, we review the role of angiogenesis and the tumor endothelium on regulation of the antitumor immune response. We place particular emphasis on the role of vascular endothelial growth factor (VEGF) in the suppression of numerous immunological processes that control tumor progression. Further, we

L.E. Kandalaft, G.T. Motz, J. Busch, and G. Coukos (✉)
Ovarian Cancer Research Center, University of Pennsylvania, Philadelphia, PA 19104, USA
e-mail: gcks@mail.med.upenn.edu

G. Dranoff (ed.), *Cancer Immunology and Immunotherapy*,
Current Topics in Microbiology and Immunology 344, DOI 10.1007/82_2010_95

describe the unique crosstalk between the VEGF and endothelin systems, and how their interactions may shape the antitumor immune response. These insights establish new targets for combinatorial approaches to modify existing cancer immunotherapies.

Abbreviations

ACT	Adoptive cell transfer
APC	Antigen-presenting cell
CD	Cluster of differentiation
CTLA-4	Cytotoxic T-lymphocyte antigen-4
DC	Dendritic cell
ECE	Endothelin-converting enzymes
EDB^{+} FN	Extra domain-B containing fibronectin
ET	Endothelin
$ET_{A}R$	Endothelin receptor A
$ET_{B}R$	Endothelin receptor B
GM-CSF	Granulocyte macrophage colony stimulating factor
GPCR	G protein-coupled receptors
HUVEC	Human umbilical vascular endothelial cell
ICAM-1	Intercellular adhesion molecule-1
IFN-γ	Interferon-gamma
IL	Interleukin
NF-κB	Nuclear factor-kappa B
NO	Nitric oxide
PD-1	Programmed death-1
PlGF	Placenta growth factor
TGF-β	Transforming growth factor-beta
Th	T helper
TIL	Tumor-infiltrating lymphocyte
TNF-α	Tumor necrosis factor-alpha
Treg	Regulatory T cell
VCAM-1	Vascular cell adhesion molecule-1
VEGF	Vascular endothelial growth factor
VEGF-R	Vascular endothelial growth factor receptor

1 Introduction

In recent years, cancer immunotherapy has had promising successes, resulting in objective clinical responses in patients with melanoma and other tumors (a historical perspective of cancer immunotherapy has been reviewed in detail by Rosenberg et al. 2008 and Gattinoni et al. 2006b). Conventionally, investigational approaches have centered on nonspecific immune modulation capitalizing on intrinsic tumor immunogenicity (e.g., therapeutic use of interleukin-2 [IL-2] or blocking antibody against cytotoxic T-lymphocyte antigen-4 [CTLA-4]) (Phan et al. 2003; Rosenberg et al. 1985, 1998), cancer vaccines (using tumor antigens or tumor antigen-pulsed antigen-presenting cells) (Chiang et al. 2010), or adoptive cell therapy (ACT) using expanded, autologous tumor-infiltrating lymphocytes (TILs) (Gattinoni et al. 2006a; Rosenberg et al. 2008). Several of these therapies have yielded substantial results (particularly ACT), while other strategies have been less successful (cancer vaccines), or have produced significant adverse effects (severe autoimmunity in anti-CTLA-4 treated patients) (Phan et al. 2003). Therefore, new combinatorial approaches toward cancer immunotherapy must be considered to improve the clinical outcome for all patients.

Although generating more effective antitumor immune response is extremely pertinent to the success of future immune therapies, a major obstacle impeding the success of cancer immunotherapy is the tumor microenvironment itself. The tumor microenvironment consists of the tumor cells, blood vessels, stromal cells, immune cells, extracellular matrix components, cytokines, and proteases (Hanahan and Weinberg 2000). The tumor microenvironment can impede the success of immune-based therapies through the suppression of homing, extravasation, and effector functions of effector lymphocytes (Witz 2008). In this review, we describe the underappreciated role of tumor angiogenesis, and vascular endothelial growth factor (VEGF) in particular, in modulating the antitumor response. Additionally, we review the crosstalk between VEGF and the endothelin signaling pathways, and its relationship to antitumor immunity.

2 Angiogenesis and Cancer

Proposed in 1971 by Judah Folkman (Folkman 1971) as an important mechanism for tumor growth, angiogenesis is now a well-established facet of tumor biology and is key to the progression of cancer. Angiogenesis is important for the supply of oxygen, nutrients, growth factors, and additional survival factors necessary for the cellular function and subsistence of tumors. Angiogenesis is considered a balance between pro- and antiangiogenic forces, and the "switch" to a proangiogenic phenotype is one of the hallmarks of malignant processes involved in cancer (Hanahan and Weinberg 2000). Importantly, increased vascularization and the expression of proangiogenic factors are commonly associated with an advanced tumor stage and a poor prognosis in cancer patients (Dvorak et al. 1995; Hicklin and Ellis 2005).

Angiogenesis is a multistep, complex process that begins with the recruitment of sprouting vessels from the existing vasculature and incorporation of endothelial progenitor cells into the newly developing vascular bed (Hicklin and Ellis 2005; Rafii et al. 2002). Endothelial cells proliferate, migrate, and invade the new area forming functional tubular structures that mature into fully formed vessels. Although the development and maturation of new vessel growth is multifaceted, requiring the precise and coordinated activation of a multitude of ligands and receptors (e.g., PDGF, Tie-1, Tie-2), the most pivotal regulator in both physiologic and pathologic angiogenesis is the VEGF and VEGF-receptor (VEGF-R) system (Hicklin and Ellis 2005; Rafii et al. 2002). VEGF signaling remains a critical rate-limiting agent in angiogenesis with pleiotropic effects controlling a multitude of angiogenic processes (Ferrara 2004).

VEGF overexpression is associated with tumorigenesis and a poor prognosis in a multitude of cancers, including gastric carcinoma (Maeda et al. 1996), colorectal carcinoma (Lee et al. 2000; Takahashi et al. 1995), lung cancer (Fontanini et al. 1997), melanoma (Gorski et al. 2003), prostate cancer (George et al. 2001), breast (Berns et al. 2003), and ovarian carcinoma (Paley et al. 1997). VEGF is upregulated in cancer cells *in vivo* by hypoxia and starvation (Zhang et al. 2002), and also by oncogene activation, which drives constitutive VEGF overexpression (Zhang et al. 2003b). VEGF directly promotes tumor angiogenesis through multiple mechanisms such as endothelial cell proliferation and survival, endothelial cell migration, vessel destabilization via Tie-2 (Zhang et al. 2003c), and enhancing chemotaxis of bone marrow-derived vascular precursor cells (e.g., endothelial cells, pericytes, vascular leukocytes) (Conejo-Garcia et al. 2004; Ellis and Hicklin 2008). In addition, VEGF promotes tumorigenesis through autocrine signaling, regulating tumor cell functions and driving tumor metastases (Ellis and Hicklin 2008). Important for cancer immunotherapy, VEGF has significant roles in modulation of the immune system and tuning the vascular endothelium, leading to the immune evasion by the tumor.

3 Vascular Endothelial Growth Factor

The mammalian VEGF family is comprised of five proteins: VEGF-A, VEGF-B, VEGF-C, VEGF-D, and placenta growth factor (PlGF). The most well-studied family member is VEGF-A (frequently referred to as simply VEGF) (Ellis and Hicklin 2008; Hicklin and Ellis 2005). Alternative splicing of VEGF leads to the expression of multiple functional isoforms of the VEGF protein containing 121, 165, 189, and 206 amino acids. $VEGF_{165}$ is the predominant functional isoform (Ellis and Hicklin 2008; Hicklin and Ellis 2005). The VEGF ligands bind and activate three structurally similar receptors, tyrosine kinases, VEGF-R1 (also referred to as FLT1), VEGF-R2 (or KDR), and VEGF-R3 (or FTL4). The different VEGF ligands have unique binding specificities for each of these receptors, leading to a complex diversity of function following ligation (Ferrara 2004). In addition, neuropilins (NP-1 and -2) act as coreceptors, increasing the binding affinity of VEGF for VEGF-Rs (Soker et al. 1998). It has been proposed that NPs may signal independently of VEGF-Rs, but this has not been definitively demonstrated.

Ligation of the VEGF-Rs initiates multiple signal transduction cascades unique to each individual VEGF-R, and is responsible for activating the appropriate gene networks (Kowanetz and Ferrara 2006). VEGF-R2 is expressed primarily in the vasculature, and is the key mediator of VEGF-induced angiogenesis. VEGF-R1 is also expressed on the vasculature, and can also be found on other cell types. Although VEGF-R1 has a higher binding affinity relative to VEGF-R2, it induces less activation than VEGF-R2 (Waltenberger et al. 1994). Therefore, VEGF-R1 may act as a functional inhibitor of VEGF-R2 mediated angiogenesis through competitive binding (Hiratsuka et al. 1998). VEGF-R3 primarily binds VEGF-C and -D, and has important roles in cardiovascular development as well as lymphangiogenesis (Ellis and Hicklin 2008; Kukk et al. 1996).

4 Direct Effects of VEGF on Leukocytes

4.1 Dendritic Cell Defects in Cancer Patients and Mouse Models: A Role for VEGF

Dendritic cells (DCs) are central to the generation of an antitumor response. As professional antigen-presenting cells (APC), they present tumor antigens to both B cells and T cells, generating an antigen-specific antitumor response. Defective DC function, combined with a failure of DC maturation, is frequently observed in cancer patients and in tumor-bearing mice. These defects occur in DCs found in the blood, tumor tissue, or draining lymph nodes (Almand et al. 2000; Gabrilovich et al. 1996a, b, 1997; Nestle et al. 1997). The effects of defective DC function (i.e., defective antigen presentation) on the antitumor response are somewhat clear; lack of tumor antigen presentation means lack of effective antitumor response or even worse, active tolerance. Indeed, it has been speculated that immature or incompletely matured DCs may mediate tumor tolerance, inducing T cell anergy or the expansion of regulatory T cells (Tregs) (Lutz and Schuler 2002; Mahnke et al. 2002).

The clinical significance of DC dysfunction has been demonstrated in a study of patients with breast, neck/head, and lung cancer (Almand et al. 2000); DCs isolated from cancer patients were functionally impaired in a mixed leukocyte reaction, and this functional impairment corresponded to a more severe cancer diagnosis (higher stage) (Almand et al. 2000). Further, both the percentage and the total number of DCs were significantly reduced in the peripheral blood of cancer patients, and this observation correlated with an increase in the total number of immature hematopoietic cells. The increase of immature cells in the blood was closely correlated to serum VEGF levels, but not transforming growth factor-beta (TGF-β), IL-6, or granulocyte macrophage colony stimulating factor (GM-CSF) (Almand et al. 2000). Importantly, these aberrations in DCs were somewhat corrected following chemotherapy and anti-VEGF therapy (Almand et al. 2000).

DC defects can be induced by tumor-derived TGF-β (Geissmann et al. 1999) and IL-10 (Steinbrink et al. 1999). However, VEGF plays a significant role in the suppression of DC maturation and function. Although DC defects in cancer patients and tumor-bearing mice had been appreciated for several years prior, Gabrilovich and colleagues were the first to identify a soluble factor, released from tumor cells, that was capable of impairing both DC function and DC maturation from CD34+ hematopoietic precursors (Gabrilovich et al. 1996a). By using neutralizing blocking antibodies, the tumor-derived soluble factor was discovered to be VEGF, and antibodies against IL-10 or TGF-β were unable to reverse the suppression (Gabrilovich et al. 1996a). Similar observations of defective DCs in cancer patients, with a dependence or association with VEGF, have since been made (Della Porta et al. 2005; Takahashi et al. 2004; Yang and Carbone 2004). Experimentally, these finding have been recapitulated in the mouse, suggesting a common mechanism and inherent role for VEGF in the antitumor response. In particular, Ishida and colleagues demonstrated that tumor-bearing mice displayed defects in DC numbers as well as function, and that VEGF blocking antibody reversed these defects (Ishida et al. 1998).

Although several mechanisms may be involved in the generation of DC defects, VEGF can exert its immunosuppressive effects through the disruption of normal hematopoiesis. VEGF continually infused in mice, at levels commonly associated with cancer pathology, resulted not only in defects of DC maturation and function, but also in widespread changes in the differentiation of multiple hematopoietic lineages. For example, VEGF infusion induced a significant increase in B cells and Gr-1+ immature myeloid cells (Della Porta et al. 2005; Gabrilovich et al. 1996a, 1998; Ishida et al. 1998; Ohm and Carbone 2001; Ohm et al. 1999; Takahashi et al. 2004; Yang and Carbone 2004). It has been discovered that VEGF mediates the suppression of DC maturation through the impairment of normal nuclear factor-kappa B (NF-κB) signaling during hematopoiesis (Oyama et al. 1998), mediated through VEGF-R1 signaling on CD34+ hematopoietic progenitor cells (Dikov et al. 2005).

The effects of VEGF on DC maturation and function can be partially reversed through VEGF blockade. Treatment of patients with the VEGF blocking antibody, Bevacizumab, has been shown to partially reverse some of the DC defects. In an initial study by Almand et al., cancer patients receiving anti-VEGF antibody demonstrated a reversal of maturation defects of their DCs, and this observation has also been observed by others (Almand et al. 2000; Fricke et al. 2007; Osada et al. 2008). These observations have also been recapitulated experimentally in mouse tumor models (Gabrilovich et al. 1999; Nair et al. 2003; Roland et al. 2009). Therefore, VEGF blockade may be critical to the success of any cancer immunotherapeutic strategy.

VEGF likely exerts effects on the immune system beyond its role in the suppression of hematopoiesis. B7-H1 is expressed on tumor cells, but it is also highly expressed on tumor-associated myeloid DCs in ovarian cancer patients (Curiel et al. 2003). Interestingly, incubation of blood myeloid DCs with VEGF induced robust expression of B7-H1 on the cell surface (Curiel et al. 2003). B7-H1 is a cell surface protein belonging to the B7 family of costimulatory molecules. B7-H1 may inhibit T cell growth by ligation of the programmed death-1 (PD-1) receptor, as well as promote programmed cell death of effector T cells through an unknown mechanism (Curiel et al. 2003). Therefore, expression of B7-H1 is associated with suppression of T cell effector functions. Thus, VEGF has potential roles in multiple aspects of immunosuppression mediated through DCs.

4.2 Effects of VEGF on T Cells

In the context of cancer immunotherapy, T cells have a well-appreciated role in the antitumor response, and cancer immunotherapies rely on the use of autologous, tumor-reactive T cells to mediate tumor regression (Rosenberg et al. 2008). In ovarian cancer, our lab has demonstrated that the presence of intratumoral T cells (also called intraepithelial T cells) was significantly associated with an increase in the five-year overall survival rate (Zhang et al. 2003a). Specifically, the five-year overall survival rate was 38% for patients with intratumoral T cells, and only 4.5% in patients whose tumor islets contained no T cells (Zhang et al. 2003a). This observation is not unique to ovarian cancer as the infiltration of T cells into tumors has been associated with positive clinical outcomes in breast (Marrogi et al. 1997), prostate (Vesalainen et al. 1994), esophageal (Schumacher et al. 2001), and colorectal cancers (Naito et al. 1998). The effects of VEGF extend to many cell types in the hematopoietic system, and are not exclusive to DCs (Gabrilovich et al. 1998; Huang et al. 2007). VEGF-Rs are expressed on many additional cell types, notably T cells. Interestingly, we observed that ovarian tumors expressing high levels of VEGF were rarely associated with intratumoral T cells (Zhang et al. 2003a). Whether this observation is mediated by VEGF through direct or indirect action on T cells remains to be determined.

Thymic atrophy is a common characteristic of cancer patients (Ohm et al. 2003). Although most cancer patients tend to be older, premature thymic atrophy occurs in many childhood cancers, which is partially reversible upon treatment (Ohm et al. 2003). Further, thymic involution occurs in tumor-bearing mice, suggesting a common mechanism (Ohm et al. 2003). In addition to negative effects on DC maturation, VEGF is also believed to suppress proper T cell development (Huang et al. 2007; Ohm et al. 2003). Treatment of mice with pathologic levels of VEGF, comparable to that seen in cancer patients, induced a robust thymic atrophy, and a significant reduction in CD4+ and CD8+ T cells (Ohm et al. 2003). Further, VEGF blockade in tumor-bearing mice partially reversed the thymic atrophy (Ohm et al. 2003). The immunosuppressive effects of VEGF on T cells occurred on bone marrow precursors, as VEGF did not appreciably disrupt maturation of T cells already in the thymus (Ohm et al. 2003). These effects likely occur through VEGF-R2 signaling on bone marrow precursor cells (Huang et al. 2007). Although pathologic levels of VEGF clearly influence the proper development of T cells, the relevance of these findings and their impact on the antitumor response remain undefined.

Tregs control peripheral tolerance through the suppression of autoreactivity, but are believed to also suppress antitumor immunity. CD4+CD25+Foxp3+ Tregs isolated from tumors were recently demonstrated to suppress tumor-specific T cell immunity both *in vitro* and *in vivo*, and importantly, an accumulation of tumor Tregs was associated with reduced survival and a high death hazard (Curiel et al. 2004). However, the precise mechanisms controlling the activation and accumulation of Tregs into tumors remain poorly defined. NP-1, a coreceptor that interacts with VEGF-R1 and -R2, has been detected on CD4+CD25+ Tregs (Sarris et al. 2008). Enhanced activation of NP-1 increased CD4+CD25+ Treg interactions with DCs in preference to T helper (Th) cells (Sarris et al. 2008). Although not specifically demonstrated, enhanced VEGF signaling, in conjunction with NP-1, may enhance Treg activation, creating a tolerogenic environment and tumor evasion. Additionally, VEGF treatment of mouse splenocytes during T cell stimulation has been demonstrated to induce IL-10 production from T cells while suppressing IFN-γ production (Shin et al. 2009). This immunosuppressive effect was attributed to VEGF-R1 expressed on T cells (Shin et al. 2009). Therefore, although it remains to be specifically demonstrated, direct VEGF signaling on T cells may enhance T cell regulatory functions, contributing to an immunosuppressive environment.

In contrast to the observations above, it has been suggested that direct VEGF signaling on T cells may enhance T cell functions (Mor et al. 2004). Coincubation with VEGF of concanavalin A or antigen-stimulated T cells supported Th1 differentiation, enhanced IFN-γ production, and suppressed IL-10 production (Mor et al. 2004). Further, VEGF treatment of T cells during peptide stimulation enhanced the severity of an adoptive transfer model of experimental allergic encephalomyelitis (Mor et al. 2004). In addition, both VEGF-R1 and -R2 were expressed in memory phenotype CD4+CD45RO+ cells in human T cells, but not naïve cells (Basu et al. 2010). VEGF treatment of these cells activated the MAPK and the PI3K-Akt pathways and enhanced IFN-γ production. Further, VEGF was chemotactic for the CD4+CD45RO+ T cells (Basu et al. 2010).

Clearly, the direct effects of VEGF on T cell functions remain inconclusive. However, insights into the roles of VEGF on the T cell antitumor response, either direct or indirect, can be gleaned from studies using VEGF blocking antibodies. In one single-arm clinical trial of a tumor vaccine combined with anti-VEGF therapy (Bevacizumab), it has been shown that the combination is associated with a high rate of T cell specific immune response, characterized by increased IFN-γ levels and T cell proliferation following stimulation with antigen (Rini et al. 2006). Supporting this observation, VEGF-R2 blockade in mice using an anti-VEGF-R2 antibody has been demonstrated to induce a de novo T cell-mediated antitumor response in mice (Manning et al. 2007). VEGF-R2 blockade resulted in spontaneous infiltration of CD4+ and CD8+ T cells that produced IFN-γ, and VEGF-R2 blockade protected against subsequent tumor challenge in a tumor vaccine model (Manning et al. 2007). However, VEGF-R2 blockade resulted in a substantial increase in serum VEGF levels. Therefore, it is unknown whether the antitumor T cell response was generated through blockade of tumorigenic angiogenesis, or increased serum VEGF enhanced activation of T cells through VEGF-R1 signaling.

On the other hand, consistent with a role for VEGF signaling in CD4+CD25+ Tregs, VEGF-R2 blockade in this study enhanced T cell effector functions in a tolerized mouse tumor model system (Manning et al. 2007). This observation is supported by the demonstration that anti-VEGF treatment in mice reduced the number of Tregs, decreased Foxp3 expression, enhanced cytotoxic lymphocyte (CTL) induction, and increased tumor vaccine efficacy (Li et al. 2006). In conclusion, VEGF or VEGF-R blockade predominantly enhances T cell antitumor immunity, an effect most consistent with the concept that VEGF has direct immunosuppressive functions on T cells.

5 VEGF, the Tumor Vascular Endothelium, and Immune Evasion

5.1 The Vascular Endothelium

The tumor vascular endothelium presents a significant challenge to the success of immune therapy, as it provides a physical barrier through which tumor-reactive T cells must extravasate, recognize tumors, and exert their cytotoxic effects. The vascular endothelial barrier, frequently prohibitive to tumor-reactive T cells, is maintained by locally expressed cytokines, growth factors, and the nature and quantity of adhesion molecules expressed by the endothelium (Zitvogel et al. 2006). In many of the T cell immune therapies that have been conducted, it has been noted that while activated T cells could be found in the periphery, they often failed to infiltrate the tumor itself (Boon et al. 2006; Dudley et al. 2002; Lurquin et al. 2005). Thus, successful transmigration through the tumor endothelial barrier is required for activated or administered lymphocytes to execute their effector functions, resulting in tumor regression. Precisely how the tumor vasculature establishes immune privilege is not well known, but the ongoing processes of angiogenesis may participate in immune escape. Specifically, tumor-derived VEGF may play a pivotal role in reducing leukocyte homing to and extravasation through the vascular endothelium.

5.2 VEGF and Adhesion Molecule Expression

T cells extravasate through the endothelium to the tumor in a multistep process that includes binding to adhesion molecules expressed on endothelial cells, and is followed by diapedesis. VEGF has been demonstrated to increase the expression of many endothelial cell adhesion molecules (CAMs), particularly in the context of angiogenesis (reviewed in detail by Francavilla et al. 2009). In agreement with this observation, VEGF-induced enhancement of CAM expression has been associated with increased leukocyte adhesion both *in vitro* and *in vivo* (Detmar et al. 1998; Min et al. 2005). However, understanding the role of VEGF in leukocyte adhesion is complicated by reports that demonstrate VEGF may actually inhibit adhesion molecule expression on endothelial cells (Bouzin et al. 2007; Detmar et al. 1998; Dirkx et al. 2003; Griffioen et al. 1996a,b; Min et al. 2005).

Although the role of VEGF signaling and leukocyte adhesion may be difficult to discern, in the context of a proinflammatory environment the emerging concept is that angiogenic growth factors impair immune cell adhesion (Bouzin et al. 2007; Griffioen et al. 1996a, b). For example, Griffioen and colleagues demonstrated reduced expression of adhesion molecules intercellular adhesion molecule-1 (ICAM-1) and vascular cell adhesion molecule (VCAM-1) after treatment of tumor necrosis factor-alpha (TNF-α) stimulated HUVEC with basic fibroblast growth factor (bFGF) or VEGF (Griffioen et al. 1996a). In a similar manner, Bouzin and colleagues observed reductions in ICAM-1 and VCAM-1 expression in TNF-α stimulated HUVECs as early as 2 h after VEGF addition (Bouzin et al. 2007). Although these effects on adhesion molecule expression were transient, longer treatment times demonstrated a disruption of adhesion molecule organization and clustering on the cell surface (Bouzin et al. 2007). This response was associated with a perturbation of the spatial organization and clustering of ICAM-1, and was dependent on caveolin-1 and nitric oxide (Bouzin et al. 2007).

6 The Tumor Endothelium and VEGF Crosstalk: A Role for the Endothelin System

6.1 The Endothelin System

Members of the endothelin system have been identified in a broad array of tissue types, including neuronal, renal, and vascular tissues, and regulate a number of critical physiological processes including reproduction, embryonic development, and cardiovascular homeostasis (Grant et al. 2003; Kedzierski and Yanagisawa 2001; Meidan and Levy 2007; Yanagisawa et al. 1998). The endothelin system has well-known roles in regulating vasoconstriction and mediates both cardiovascular and renal disorders (Bagnato and Rosano 2008; Nelson et al. 2003). Particularly, the endothelin system is an important regulator of physiologic and pathogenic angiogenesis, and VEGF signaling is intimately involved in dynamic crosstalk with the endothelin system (Bagnato and Rosano 2008; Nelson et al. 2003).

The endothelin system is comprised of four endothelin (ET) peptide ligands, ET-1, ET-2, ET-3, and ET-4 (Saida et al. 1989; Yanagisawa and Masaki 1989) that signal through their two G protein-coupled receptors (GPCR), ET_AR and ET_BR (Frommer and Muller-Ladner 2008; Meidan and Levy 2007). Biologically active ETs are derived from precursor proteins following cleavage by membrane-bound metalloproteinases termed endothelin-converting enzymes (ECE) (Valdenaire et al.

1995). Amongst the four endothelin ligands, ET-1 is the most potent ligand and is widely expressed in multiple cells types, notably endothelial cells (Luscher and Barton 2000). Binding of the ET_AR and ET_BR by ET peptides triggers downstream signal transduction pathways, including, but not limited to, the RAF/MEK/MAPK pathway and PI3K/AKT pathway (Nelson et al. 2003).

The endothelin axis has been speculated to play significant roles in tumorigenesis. Endothelin or the endothelin receptors or both are upregulated in a number of cancers including ovarian, breast, renal, colon, and prostate cancer (Bagnato and Rosano 2008; Nelson et al. 2003). Importantly, the use of specific endothelin receptor antagonists has been demonstrated to slow tumor growth in patients, or prevent tumor growth in mouse models (Bagnato and Rosano 2008; Nelson et al. 2003). In addition to its role in angiogenesis described in more detail below, the endothelin axis is believed to activate autocrine/paracrine loops that promote proliferation, protection from apoptosis, immune evasion, vasculogenesis, and invasion and metastatic dissemination of tumors (Bagnato and Rosano 2008; Nelson et al. 2003).

6.2 Endothelin and Tumor Angiogenesis

The interactions between endothelin and VEGF regulate multiple aspects of angiogenesis including endothelial cell proliferation, migration, invasion, vessel formation, and neovascularization (Nelson et al. 2003). Further, endothelin and VEGF signaling influence the regulation of vascular permeability (Nelson et al. 2003). In the context of angiogenesis, ET-1 upregulates the expression of the extra domain-B containing fibronectin (EDB^+ FN) in human vascular endothelial cells (Bagnato and Spinella 2003; Khan et al. 2005). EDB^+ FN has been suggested as a marker of angiogenesis in human cancers and is believed to control ocular neovascularization in patients with proliferative diabetic retinopathy (Bagnato and Spinella 2003; Khan et al. 2005). Additionally, the expression of endothelins, or their receptors, correlates with high expression of VEGF in a multitude of tumor types (Boldrini et al. 2006; Salani et al. 2000a; Wulfing et al. 2004), and elevated expression of ET-1 and VEGF was associated with lymphatic vessel invasion and poor outcomes in invasive ductal breast carcinoma (Gasparini et al. 1994).

ET-1 induces the expression of VEGF in cancer cell lines *in vitro* (Rosano et al. 2003; Salani et al. 2000b; Spinella et al. 2002, 2007). ET-1 increases VEGF production through HIF-1α (Salani et al. 2000b) by ovarian cancer cells via ET_AR activation (Spinella et al. 2004). Additionally, ovarian tumor growth in nude mice was inhibited after treatment with the ET_AR-selective antagonist ABT-627, an effect associated with reduced VEGF expression (Spinella et al. 2004). ET_BR activation counters ET-1/ET_AR activity by increasing production of nitric oxide, promoting ET-1 clearance, triggering apoptotic pathways, and blocking cell growth. However, it is unclear whether this antagonism occurs in tumor cells (Lalich et al. 2007). As such, there may also be role for ET_BR in tumor angiogenesis and cancer development (Bagnato and Rosano 2008). ET-1 has been shown to directly promote tumor angiogenesis by inducing endothelial cell survival, proliferation, and invasion in an ET_BR-dependent manner (Salani et al. 2000b). ET_BR may promote angiogenesis indirectly by upregulating VEGF production in the vasculature (Jesmin et al. 2006). Furthermore, there is a strong correlation between ET_BR and VEGF expression in a number of different tumor specimens (Kato et al. 2001). In summary, the interaction of the endothelin system and angiogenesis, and VEGF in particular, may be a significant regulator of tumorigenesis.

6.3 ET_BR and the Tumor Endothelial Barrier to T Cell Homing

ET_BR is overexpressed in melanoma and is associated with aggressive tumor phenotype (Bachmann-Brandt et al. 2000). Highlighting the role of ET_BR in melanoma, the receptor antagonist BQ-788 inhibited the growth of human melanoma cell lines and reduced human melanoma tumor growth in a nude mouse model (Lahav 2005; Lahav et al. 1999). ET_BR is also overexpressed in ovarian cancer, Kaposi's sarcoma, glioblastoma, and breast cancer (Bagnato et al. 2004; Egidy et al. 2000; Kefford et al. 2007; Rosano 2003). Interestingly, ET_BR upregulation predicts poor outcome in both breast and ovarian cancers (Grimshaw et al. 2004; Wulfing et al. 2003), and ET_BR overexpression has even been proposed as tumor progression marker (Demunter et al. 2001).

Our laboratory has recently demonstrated a novel role for ET_BR in tumor immunotherapy (Buckanovich et al. 2008). Microarray analysis was conducted using the endothelial cells isolated using laser capture microdissection. ET_BR was discovered as one of the few genes overexpressed in the endothelial cells of tumors lacking TILs (Buckanovich et al. 2008). Immunohistochemical staining of ovarian cancer tumors confirmed this result, and ET_BR was localized to the endothelium and the stroma. Importantly, ET_BR overexpression was associated with poor survival, likely due to lack of TILs, which was previously demonstrated as an indicator of a good prognosis (Zhang 2003). Further, recombinant human ET-1 blocked the adhesion of activated T cells to human umbilical vein endothelial cells (HUVECs) *in vitro* (Buckanovich et al. 2008). This effect was reversed if HUVECs were treated with the specific ET_BR antagonist, BQ-788. ET-1 signaling through ET_BR was discovered to block T cell adhesion to the endothelium through suppression of ICAM-1 expression. ET_BR blockade upregulated ICAM-1, promoted ICAM-1 clustering, and restored T cell adhesion (Buckanovich et al. 2008). Thus, these data provide a mechanistic link between the observations made in ovarian cancer patients.

TNF-α is a major inflammatory cytokine implicated in carcinogenesis, tumor angiogenesis, and progression; and it is upregulated in ovarian cancer (Merogi et al. 1997). It has been previously reported that the overall TNF-α mRNA levels are similar in ovarian tumors with or without intraepithelial T cells (Zhang et al. 2003a). This was counterintuitive, as TNF-α is a major factor activating endothelium and promoting adhesion of T cells. It has now been found that ET-1 efficiently blocks adhesion of T cells to endothelial cells even when endothelial cells are activated with TNF-α (Buckanovich et al. 2008). This observation explains the paradox of how tumors may exhibit inflammation yet be prohibitive to T cell infiltration, thus establishing immune privilege even in the face of inflammation.

Based on the above data, the effectiveness of ET_BR blockade, using the receptor antagonist BQ-788, was determined using a tumor vaccine therapy that controls tumor growth very poorly. In this context, the tumor vaccine had little effect on tumor growth, but ET_BR blockade significantly enhanced the antitumor effect by permitting the infiltration of tumor antigen-specific T cells into the tumor site (Buckanovich et al. 2008). The benefits of ET_BR blockade were attenuated with the use of an ICAM-1 neutralizing antibody, indicating that adhesion molecule interactions between the endothelium and T cells were responsible for the antitumor effects of ET_BR blockade (Buckanovich et al. 2008). Thus, in tumors there is likely a hyperactivation of ET-1/ET_BR signaling that is responsible for the suppression of T cell homing. Furthermore, these results establish a vascular mechanism of tumor immune evasion mediated by the endothelium, and also present a new opportunity to target the ET_BR to prevent tumor growth and enhance cancer immunotherapy.

7 Concluding Statements

The mechanisms regulating the overexpression of ET_BR on the tumor endothelium are unknown. However, the overexpression of ET_BR may participate in a feed-forward loop of autocrine/paracrine ET-1 production and ET receptor signaling between the tumor and the vascular endothelium. Thus, enhanced ET-1 signaling in tumor and endothelial cells through ET_BR would lead to enhanced NO and HIF-1α production, followed by increased VEGF production by tumor cells. In the context of inflammation, ET_BR and VEGF signaling on endothelial cells would shut down the capacity of T cells to extravasate through the endothelium to attack the tumor through a reduction in adhesion molecule expression, particularly ICAM-1. Further, enhanced VEGF production would support ongoing maturation defects in DCs and possibly T cells, while enhancing Treg activation, leading to reduced antigen presentation and immune evasion.

If this hypothesis is correct, targeted therapies to break the cyclical enhancement of VEGF, ET-1, and NO production should be the key components of any cancer immunotherapy. The use of ET_BR receptor antagonists combined with anti-VEGF antibody administration may function synergistically to sanction the tumor environment to attack by the immune system. Thus, new complimentary approaches to existing cancer immunotherapies may enhance the existing therapies and extend their benefits to more patients.

Acknowledgments This work was supported by NIH R01-CA098951; NIH P50-CA083638 Ovarian Cancer SPORE; and NIH R01-CA112162.

References

Almand B, Resser JR, Lindman B, Nadaf S, Clark JI, Kwon ED, Carbone DP, Gabrilovich DI (2000) Clinical significance of defective dendritic cell differentiation in cancer. Clin Cancer Res 6:1755–1766

Bachmann-Brandt S, Bittner I, Neuhaus P, Frei U, Schindler R (2000) Plasma levels of endothelin-1 in patients with the hepatorenal syndrome after successful liver transplantation. Transpl Int 13:357–362

Bagnato A, Rosano L (2008) The endothelin axis in cancer. Int J Biochem Cell Biol 40:1443–1451

Bagnato A, Spinella F (2003) Emerging role of endothelin-1 in tumor angiogenesis. Trends Endocrinol Metab 14:44–50

Bagnato A, Rosano L, Spinella F, Di Castro V, Tecce R, Natali PG (2004) Endothelin B receptor blockade inhibits dynamics of cell interactions and communications in melanoma cell progression. Cancer Res 64:1436–1443

Basu A, Hoerning A, Datta D, Edelbauer M, Stack MP, Calzadilla K, Pal S, Briscoe DM (2010) Cutting edge: Vascular endothelial growth factor-mediated signaling in human CD45RO+ CD4+ T cells promotes Akt and ERK activation and costimulates IFN-gamma production. J Immunol 184:545–549

Berns EM, Klijn JG, Look MP, Grebenchtchikov N, Vossen R, Peters H, Geurts-Moespot A, Portengen H, van Staveren IL, Meijer-van Gelder ME, Bakker B, Sweep FC, Foekens JA (2003) Combined vascular endothelial growth factor and TP53 status predicts poor response to tamoxifen therapy in estrogen receptor-positive advanced breast cancer. Clin Cancer Res 9:1253–1258

Boldrini L, Pistolesi S, Gisfredi S, Ursino S, Ali G, Pieracci N, Basolo F, Parenti G, Fontanini G (2006) Expression of endothelin 1 and its angiogenic role in meningiomas. Virchows Arch 449:546–553

Boon T, Coulie PG, Van den Eynde BJ, van der Bruggen P (2006) Human T cell responses against melanoma. Annu Rev Immunol 24:175–208

Bouzin C, Brouet A, De Vriese J, Dewever J, Feron O (2007) Effects of vascular endothelial growth factor on the lymphocyte-endothelium interactions: identification of caveolin-1 and nitric oxide as control points of endothelial cell anergy. J Immunol 178:1505–1511

Buckanovich RJ, Facciabene A, Kim S, Benencia F, Sasaroli D, Balint K, Katsaros D, O'Brien-Jenkins A, Gimotty PA, Coukos G (2008) Endothelin B receptor mediates the endothelial barrier to T cell homing to tumors and disables immune therapy. Nat Med 14:28–36

Chiang CL-L, Benencia F, Coukos G (2010) Whole tumor antigen vaccines. Semin Immunol 22:132–143

Conejo-Garcia JR, Benencia F, Courreges MC, Kang E, Mohamed-Hadley A, Buckanovich RJ, Holtz DO, Jenkins A, Na H, Zhang L, Wagner DS, Katsaros D, Caroll R, Coukos G (2004) Tumor-infiltrating dendritic cell precursors recruited by a beta-defensin contribute to vasculogenesis under the influence of Vegf-A. Nat Med 10:950–958

Curiel TJ, Wei S, Dong H, Alvarez X, Cheng P, Mottram P, Krzysiek R, Knutson KL, Daniel B, Zimmermann MC, David O, Burow M, Gordon A, Dhurandhar N, Myers L, Berggren R,

Hemminki A, Alvarez RD, Emilie D, Curiel DT, Chen L, Zou W (2003) Blockade of B7-H1 improves myeloid dendritic cell-mediated antitumor immunity. Nat Med 9:562–567

Curiel TJ, Coukos G, Zou L, Alvarez X, Cheng P, Mottram P, Evdemon-Hogan M, Conejo-Garcia JR, Zhang L, Burow M, Zhu Y, Wei S, Kryczek I, Daniel B, Gordon A, Myers L, Lackner A, Disis ML, Knutson KL, Chen L, Zou W (2004) Specific recruitment of regulatory T cells in ovarian carcinoma fosters immune privilege and predicts reduced survival. Nat Med 10:942–949

Della Porta M, Danova M, Rigolin GM, Brugnatelli S, Rovati B, Tronconi C, Fraulini C, Russo Rossi A, Riccardi A, Castoldi G (2005) Dendritic cells and vascular endothelial growth factor in colorectal cancer: correlations with clinicobiological findings. Oncology 68:276–284

Demunter A, De Wolf-Peeters C, Degreef H, Stas M, van den Oord JJ (2001) Expression of the endothelin-B receptor in pigment cell lesions of the skin. Evidence for its role as tumor progression marker in malignant melanoma. Virchows Arch 438:485–491

Detmar M, Brown LF, Schon MP, Elicker BM, Velasco P, Richard L, Fukumura D, Monsky W, Claffey KP, Jain RK (1998) Increased microvascular density and enhanced leukocyte rolling and adhesion in the skin of VEGF transgenic mice. J Invest Dermatol 111:1–6

Dikov MM, Ohm JE, Ray N, Tchekneva EE, Burlison J, Moghanaki D, Nadaf S, Carbone DP (2005) Differential roles of vascular endothelial growth factor receptors 1 and 2 in dendritic cell differentiation. J Immunol 174:215–222

Dirkx AE, Oude Egbrink MG, Kuijpers MJ, van der Niet ST, Heijnen VV, Bouma-ter Steege JC, Wagstaff J, Griffioen AW (2003) Tumor angiogenesis modulates leukocyte-vessel wall interactions *in vivo* by reducing endothelial adhesion molecule expression. Cancer Res 63:2322–2329

Dudley ME, Wunderlich JR, Robbins PF, Yang JC, Hwu P, Schwartzentruber DJ, Topalian SL, Sherry R, Restifo NP, Hubicki AM, Robinson MR, Raffeld M, Duray P, Seipp CA, Rogers-Freezer L, Morton KE, Mavroukakis SA, White DE, Rosenberg SA (2002) Cancer regression and autoimmunity in patients after clonal repopulation with antitumor lymphocytes. Science 298:850–854

Dvorak HF, Brown LF, Detmar M, Dvorak AM (1995) Vascular permeability factor/vascular endothelial growth factor, microvascular hyperpermeability, and angiogenesis. Am J Pathol 146:1029–1039

Egidy G, Eberl LP, Valdenaire O, Irmler M, Majdi R, Diserens AC, Fontana A, Janzer RC, Pinet F, Juillerat-Jeanneret L (2000) The endothelin system in human glioblastoma. Lab Invest 80:1681–1689

Ellis LM, Hicklin DJ (2008) VEGF-targeted therapy: mechanisms of anti-tumour activity. Nat Rev Cancer 8:579–591

Ferrara N (2004) Vascular endothelial growth factor: basic science and clinical progress. Endocr Rev 25:581–611

Folkman J (1971) Tumor angiogenesis: therapeutic implications. N Engl J Med 285:1182–1186

Fontanini G, Lucchi M, Vignati S, Mussi A, Ciardiello F, De Laurentiis M, De Placido S, Basolo F, Angeletti CA, Bevilacqua G (1997) Angiogenesis as a prognostic indicator of survival in non-small-cell lung carcinoma: a prospective study. J Natl Cancer Inst 89:881–886

Francavilla C, Maddaluno L, Cavallaro U (2009) The functional role of cell adhesion molecules in tumor angiogenesis. Semin Cancer Biol 19:298–309

Fricke I, Mirza N, Dupont J, Lockhart C, Jackson A, Lee JH, Sosman JA, Gabrilovich DI (2007) Vascular endothelial growth factor-trap overcomes defects in dendritic cell differentiation but does not improve antigen-specific immune responses. Clin Cancer Res 13:4840–4848

Frommer KW, Muller-Ladner U (2008) Expression and function of ETA and ETB receptors in SSc. Rheumatology (Oxford) 47(Suppl 5):v27–v28

Gabrilovich DI, Chen HL, Girgis KR, Cunningham HT, Meny GM, Nadaf S, Kavanaugh D, Carbone DP (1996a) Production of vascular endothelial growth factor by human tumors inhibits the functional maturation of dendritic cells. Nat Med 2:1096–1103

Gabrilovich DI, Ciernik IF, Carbone DP (1996b) Dendritic cells in antitumor immune responses. I. Defective antigen presentation in tumor-bearing hosts. Cell Immunol 170:101–110

Gabrilovich DI, Corak J, Ciernik IF, Kavanaugh D, Carbone DP (1997) Decreased antigen presentation by dendritic cells in patients with breast cancer. Clin Cancer Res 3:483–490

Gabrilovich D, Ishida T, Oyama T, Ran S, Kravtsov V, Nadaf S, Carbone DP (1998) Vascular endothelial growth factor inhibits the development of dendritic cells and dramatically affects the differentiation of multiple hematopoietic lineages *in vivo*. Blood 92:4150–4166

Gabrilovich DI, Ishida T, Nadaf S, Ohm JE, Carbone DP (1999) Antibodies to vascular endothelial growth factor enhance the efficacy of cancer immunotherapy by improving endogenous dendritic cell function. Clin Cancer Res 5:2963–2970

Gasparini G, Weidner N, Bevilacqua P, Maluta S, Dalla Palma P, Caffo O, Barbareschi M, Boracchi P, Marubini E, Pozza F (1994) Tumor microvessel density, p53 expression, tumor size, and peritumoral lymphatic vessel invasion are relevant prognostic markers in node-negative breast carcinoma. J Clin Oncol 12:454–466

Gattinoni L, Powell DJ Jr, Rosenberg SA, Restifo NP (2006) Adoptive immunotherapy for cancer: building on success. Nat Rev Immunol 6:383–393

Geissmann F, Revy P, Regnault A, Lepelletier Y, Dy M, Brousse N, Amigorena S, Hermine O, Durandy A (1999) TGF-beta 1 prevents the noncognate maturation of human dendritic Langerhans cells. J Immunol 162:4567–4575

George DJ, Halabi S, Shepard TF, Vogelzang NJ, Hayes DF, Small EJ, Kantoff PW (2001) Prognostic significance of plasma vascular endothelial growth factor levels in patients with hormone-refractory prostate cancer treated on Cancer and Leukemia Group B 9480. Clin Cancer Res 7:1932–1936

Gorski DH, Leal AD, Goydos JS (2003) Differential expression of vascular endothelial growth factor-A isoforms at different stages of melanoma progression. J Am Coll Surg 197:408–418

Grant K, Loizidou M, Taylor I (2003) Endothelin-1: a multifunctional molecule in cancer. Br J Cancer 88:163–166

Griffioen AW, Damen CA, Blijham GH, Groenewegen G (1996a) Tumor angiogenesis is accompanied by a decreased inflammatory response of tumor-associated endothelium. Blood 88:667–673

Griffioen AW, Damen CA, Martinotti S, Blijham GH, Groenewegen G (1996b) Endothelial intercellular adhesion molecule-1 expression is suppressed in human malignancies: the role of angiogenic factors. Cancer Res 56:1111–1117

Grimshaw MJ, Hagemann T, Ayhan A, Gillett CE, Binder C, Balkwill FR (2004) A role for endothelin-2 and its receptors in breast tumor cell invasion. Cancer Res 64:2461–2468

Hanahan D, Weinberg RA (2000) The hallmarks of cancer. Cell 100:57–70

Hicklin DJ, Ellis LM (2005) Role of the vascular endothelial growth factor pathway in tumor growth and angiogenesis. J Clin Oncol 23:1011–1027

Hiratsuka S, Minowa O, Kuno J, Noda T, Shibuya M (1998) Flt-1 lacking the tyrosine kinase domain is sufficient for normal development and angiogenesis in mice. Proc Natl Acad Sci USA 95:9349–9354

Huang Y, Chen X, Dikov MM, Novitskiy SV, Mosse CA, Yang L, Carbone DP (2007) Distinct roles of VEGFR-1 and VEGFR-2 in the aberrant hematopoiesis associated with elevated levels of VEGF. Blood 110:624–631

Ishida T, Oyama T, Carbone DP, Gabrilovich DI (1998) Defective function of Langerhans cells in tumor-bearing animals is the result of defective maturation from hemopoietic progenitors. J Immunol 161:4842–4851

Jesmin S, Miyauchi T, Goto K, Yamaguchi I (2006) Down-regulated VEGF expression in the diabetic heart is normalized by an endothelin ETA receptor antagonist. Eur J Pharmacol 542:184–185

Kato T, Kameoka S, Kimura T, Soga N, Abe Y, Nishikawa T, Kobayashi M (2001) Angiogenesis as a predictor of long-term survival for 377 Japanese patients with breast cancer. Breast Cancer Res Treat 70:65–74

Kedzierski RM, Yanagisawa M (2001) Endothelin system: the double-edged sword in health and disease. Annu Rev Pharmacol Toxicol 41:851–876

Kefford R, Beith JM, Van Hazel GA, Millward M, Trotter JM, Wyld DK, Kusic R, Shreeniwas R, Morganti A, Ballmer A, Segal E, Nayler O, Clozel M (2007) A phase II study of bosentan, a dual endothelin receptor antagonist, as monotherapy in patients with stage IV metastatic melanoma. Invest New Drugs 25:247–252

Khan ZA, Chan BM, Uniyal S, Barbin YP, Farhangkhoee H, Chen S, Chakrabarti S (2005) EDB fibronectin and angiogenesis – a novel mechanistic pathway. Angiogenesis 8:183–196

Kowanetz M, Ferrara N (2006) Vascular endothelial growth factor signaling pathways: therapeutic perspective. Clin Cancer Res 12:5018–5022

Kukk E, Lymboussaki A, Taira S, Kaipainen A, Jeltsch M, Joukov V, Alitalo K (1996) VEGF-C receptor binding and pattern of expression with VEGFR-3 suggests a role in lymphatic vascular development. Development 122:3829–3837

Lahav R (2005) Endothelin receptor B is required for the expansion of melanocyte precursors and malignant melanoma. Int J Dev Biol 49:173–180

Lahav R, Heffner G, Patterson PH (1999) An endothelin receptor B antagonist inhibits growth and induces cell death in human melanoma cells *in vitro* and *in vivo*. Proc Natl Acad Sci USA 96:11496–11500

Lalich M, McNeel DG, Wilding G, Liu G (2007) Endothelin receptor antagonists in cancer therapy. Cancer Invest 25:785–794

Lee JC, Chow NH, Wang ST, Huang SM (2000) Prognostic value of vascular endothelial growth factor expression in colorectal cancer patients. Eur J Cancer 36:748–753

Li B, Lalani AS, Harding TC, Luan B, Koprivnikar K, Huan Tu G, Prell R, VanRoey MJ, Simmons AD, Jooss K (2006) Vascular endothelial growth factor blockade reduces intratumoral regulatory T cells and enhances the efficacy of a GM-CSF-secreting cancer immunotherapy. Clin Cancer Res 12:6808–6816

Lurquin C, Lethe B, De Plaen E, Corbiere V, Theate I, van Baren N, Coulie PG, Boon T (2005) Contrasting frequencies of antitumor and anti-vaccine T cells in metastases of a melanoma patient vaccinated with a MAGE tumor antigen. J Exp Med 201:249–257

Luscher TF, Barton M (2000) Endothelins and endothelin receptor antagonists: therapeutic considerations for a novel class of cardiovascular drugs. Circulation 102:2434–2440

Lutz MB, Schuler G (2002) Immature, semi-mature and fully mature dendritic cells: which signals induce tolerance or immunity? Trends Immunol 23:445–449

Maeda K, Chung YS, Ogawa Y, Takatsuka S, Kang SM, Ogawa M, Sawada T, Sowa M (1996) Prognostic value of vascular endothelial growth factor expression in gastric carcinoma. Cancer 77:858–863

Mahnke K, Schmitt E, Bonifaz L, Enk AH, Jonuleit H (2002) Immature, but not inactive: the tolerogenic function of immature dendritic cells. Immunol Cell Biol 80:477–483

Manning EA, Ullman JG, Leatherman JM, Asquith JM, Hansen TR, Armstrong TD, Hicklin DJ, Jaffee EM, Emens LA (2007) A vascular endothelial growth factor receptor-2 inhibitor enhances antitumor immunity through an immune-based mechanism. Clin Cancer Res 13:3951–3959

Marrogi AJ, Munshi A, Merogi AJ, Ohadike Y, El-Habashi A, Marrogi OL, Freeman SM (1997) Study of tumor infiltrating lymphocytes and transforming growth factor-beta as prognostic factors in breast carcinoma. Int J Cancer 74:492–501

Meidan R, Levy N (2007) The ovarian endothelin network: an evolving story. Trends Endocrinol Metab 18:379–385

Merogi AJ, Marrogi AJ, Ramesh R, Robinson WR, Fermin CD, Freeman SM (1997) Tumor-host interaction: analysis of cytokines, growth factors, and tumor-infiltrating lymphocytes in ovarian carcinomas. Hum Pathol 28:321–331

Min JK, Lee YM, Kim JH, Kim YM, Kim SW, Lee SY, Gho YS, Oh GT, Kwon YG (2005) Hepatocyte growth factor suppresses vascular endothelial growth factor-induced expression of endothelial ICAM-1 and VCAM-1 by inhibiting the nuclear factor-kappaB pathway. Circ Res 96:300–307

Mor F, Quintana FJ, Cohen IR (2004) Angiogenesis-inflammation cross-talk: vascular endothelial growth factor is secreted by activated T cells and induces Th1 polarization. J Immunol 172:4618–4623

Nair S, Boczkowski D, Moeller B, Dewhirst M, Vieweg J, Gilboa E (2003) Synergy between tumor immunotherapy and antiangiogenic therapy. Blood 102:964–971

Naito Y, Saito K, Shiiba K, Ohuchi A, Saigenji K, Nagura H, Ohtani H (1998) CD8+ T cells infiltrated within cancer cell nests as a prognostic factor in human colorectal cancer. Cancer Res 58:3491–3494

Nelson J, Bagnato A, Battistini B, Nisen P (2003) The endothelin axis: emerging role in cancer. Nat Rev Cancer 3:110–116

Nestle FO, Burg G, Fah J, Wrone-Smith T, Nickoloff BJ (1997) Human sunlight-induced basal-cell-carcinoma-associated dendritic cells are deficient in T cell co-stimulatory molecules and are impaired as antigen-presenting cells. Am J Pathol 150:641–651

Ohm JE, Carbone DP (2001) VEGF as a mediator of tumor-associated immunodeficiency. Immunol Res 23:263–272

Ohm JE, Shurin MR, Esche C, Lotze MT, Carbone DP, Gabrilovich DI (1999) Effect of vascular endothelial growth factor and FLT3 ligand on dendritic cell generation *in vivo*. J Immunol 163:3260–3268

Ohm JE, Gabrilovich DI, Sempowski GD, Kisseleva E, Parman KS, Nadaf S, Carbone DP (2003) VEGF inhibits T-cell development and may contribute to tumor-induced immune suppression. Blood 101:4878–4886

Osada T, Chong G, Tansik R, Hong T, Spector N, Kumar R, Hurwitz HI, Dev I, Nixon AB, Lyerly HK, Clay T, Morse MA (2008) The effect of anti-VEGF therapy on immature myeloid cell and dendritic cells in cancer patients. Cancer Immunol Immunother 57:1115–1124

Oyama T, Ran S, Ishida T, Nadaf S, Kerr L, Carbone DP, Gabrilovich DI (1998) Vascular endothelial growth factor affects dendritic cell maturation through the inhibition of nuclear factor-kappa B activation in hemopoietic progenitor cells. J Immunol 160:1224–1232

Paley PJ, Staskus KA, Gebhard K, Mohanraj D, Twiggs LB, Carson LF, Ramakrishnan S (1997) Vascular endothelial growth factor expression in early stage ovarian carcinoma. Cancer 80:98–106

Phan GQ, Yang JC, Sherry RM, Hwu P, Topalian SL, Schwartzentruber DJ, Restifo NP, Haworth LR, Seipp CA, Freezer LJ, Morton KE, Mavroukakis SA, Duray PH, Steinberg SM, Allison JP, Davis TA, Rosenberg SA (2003) Cancer regression and autoimmunity induced by cytotoxic T lymphocyte-associated antigen 4 blockade in patients with metastatic melanoma. Proc Natl Acad Sci USA 100:8372–8377

Rafii S, Lyden D, Benezra R, Hattori K, Heissig B (2002) Vascular and haematopoietic stem cells: novel targets for anti-angiogenesis therapy? Nat Rev Cancer 2:826–835

Rini BI, Weinberg V, Fong L, Conry S, Hershberg RM, Small EJ (2006) Combination immunotherapy with prostatic acid phosphatase pulsed antigen-presenting cells (provenge) plus bevacizumab in patients with serologic progression of prostate cancer after definitive local therapy. Cancer 107:67–74

Roland CL, Lynn KD, Toombs JE, Dineen SP, Udugamasooriya DG, Brekken RA (2009) Cytokine levels correlate with immune cell infiltration after anti-VEGF therapy in preclinical mouse models of breast cancer. PLoS One 4:e7669

Rosano L, Spinella F, Salani D, Di Castro V, Venuti A, Nicotra MR, Natali PG, Bagnato A (2003) Therapeutic targeting of the endothelin a receptor in human ovarian carcinoma. Cancer Res 63:2447–2453

Rosenberg SA, Lotze MT, Muul LM, Leitman S, Chang AE, Ettinghausen SE, Matory YL, Skibber JM, Shiloni E, Vetto JT et al (1985) Observations on the systemic administration of autologous lymphokine-activated killer cells and recombinant interleukin-2 to patients with metastatic cancer. N Engl J Med 313:1485–1492

Rosenberg SA, Yang JC, White DE, Steinberg SM (1998) Durability of complete responses in patients with metastatic cancer treated with high-dose interleukin-2: identification of the antigens mediating response. Ann Surg 228:307–319

Rosenberg SA, Restifo NP, Yang JC, Morgan RA, Dudley ME (2008) Adoptive cell transfer: a clinical path to effective cancer immunotherapy. Nat Rev Cancer 8:299–308

Saida K, Mitsui Y, Ishida N (1989) A novel peptide, vasoactive intestinal contractor, of a new (endothelin) peptide family. Molecular cloning, expression, and biological activity. J Biol Chem 264:14613–14616

Salani D, Di Castro V, Nicotra MR, Rosano L, Tecce R, Venuti A, Natali PG, Bagnato A (2000a) Role of endothelin-1 in neovascularization of ovarian carcinoma. Am J Pathol 157: 1537–1547

Salani D, Taraboletti G, Rosano L, Di Castro V, Borsotti P, Giavazzi R, Bagnato A (2000b) Endothelin-1 induces an angiogenic phenotype in cultured endothelial cells and stimulates neovascularization *in vivo*. Am J Pathol 157:1703–1711

Sarris M, Andersen KG, Randow F, Mayr L, Betz AG (2008) Neuropilin-1 expression on regulatory T cells enhances their interactions with dendritic cells during antigen recognition. Immunity 28:402–413

Schumacher K, Haensch W, Roefzaad C, Schlag PM (2001) Prognostic significance of activated CD8(+) T cell infiltrations within esophageal carcinomas. Cancer Res 61:3932–3936

Shin JY, Yoon IH, Kim JS, Kim B, Park CG (2009) Vascular endothelial growth factor-induced chemotaxis and IL-10 from T cells. Cell Immunol 256:72–78

Soker S, Takashima S, Miao HQ, Neufeld G, Klagsbrun M (1998) Neuropilin-1 is expressed by endothelial and tumor cells as an isoform-specific receptor for vascular endothelial growth factor. Cell 92:735–745

Spinella F, Rosano L, Di Castro V, Natali PG, Bagnato A (2002) Endothelin-1 induces vascular endothelial growth factor by increasing hypoxia-inducible factor-1alpha in ovarian carcinoma cells. J Biol Chem 277:27850–27855

Spinella F, Rosano L, Di Castro V, Nicotra MR, Natali PG, Bagnato A (2004) Inhibition of cyclooxygenase-1 and -2 expression by targeting the endothelin a receptor in human ovarian carcinoma cells. Clin Cancer Res 10:4670–4679

Spinella F, Rosano L, Di Castro V, Decandia S, Nicotra MR, Natali PG, Bagnato A (2007) Endothelin-1 and endothelin-3 promote invasive behavior via hypoxia-inducible factor-1alpha in human melanoma cells. Cancer Res 67:1725–1734

Steinbrink K, Jonuleit H, Muller G, Schuler G, Knop J, Enk AH (1999) Interleukin-10-treated human dendritic cells induce a melanoma-antigen-specific anergy in CD8(+) T cells resulting in a failure to lyse tumor cells. Blood 93:1634–1642

Takahashi Y, Kitadai Y, Bucana CD, Cleary KR, Ellis LM (1995) Expression of vascular endothelial growth factor and its receptor, KDR, correlates with vascularity, metastasis, and proliferation of human colon cancer. Cancer Res 55:3964–3968

Takahashi A, Kono K, Ichihara F, Sugai H, Fujii H, Matsumoto Y (2004) Vascular endothelial growth factor inhibits maturation of dendritic cells induced by lipopolysaccharide, but not by proinflammatory cytokines. Cancer Immunol Immunother 53:543–550

Valdenaire O, Rohrbacher E, Mattei MG (1995) Organization of the gene encoding the human endothelin-converting enzyme (ECE-1). J Biol Chem 270:29794–29798

Vesalainen S, Lipponen P, Talja M, Syrjanen K (1994) Histological grade, perineural infiltration, tumour-infiltrating lymphocytes and apoptosis as determinants of long-term prognosis in prostatic adenocarcinoma. Eur J Cancer 30A:1797–1803

Waltenberger J, Claesson-Welsh L, Siegbahn A, Shibuya M, Heldin CH (1994) Different signal transduction properties of KDR and Flt1, two receptors for vascular endothelial growth factor. J Biol Chem 269:26988–26995

Witz IP (2008) Tumor-microenvironment interactions: dangerous liaisons. Adv Cancer Res 100:203–229

Wulfing P, Diallo R, Kersting C, Wulfing C, Poremba C, Rody A, Greb RR, Bocker W, Kiesel L (2003) Expression of endothelin-1, endothelin-A, and endothelin-B receptor in human breast cancer and correlation with long-term follow-up. Clin Cancer Res 9:4125–4131

Wulfing P, Kersting C, Tio J, Fischer RJ, Wulfing C, Poremba C, Diallo R, Bocker W, Kiesel L (2004) Endothelin-1-, endothelin-A-, and endothelin-B-receptor expression is correlated with

vascular endothelial growth factor expression and angiogenesis in breast cancer. Clin Cancer Res 10:2393–2400
Yanagisawa M, Masaki T (1989) Molecular biology and biochemistry of the endothelins. Trends Pharmacol Sci 10:374–378
Yanagisawa H, Hammer RE, Richardson JA, Williams SC, Clouthier DE, Yanagisawa M (1998) Role of Endothelin-1/Endothelin-A receptor-mediated signaling pathway in the aortic arch patterning in mice. J Clin Invest 102:22–33
Yang L, Carbone DP (2004) Tumor-host immune interactions and dendritic cell dysfunction. Adv Cancer Res 92:13–27
Zhang L, Conejo-Garcia J-R, Yang N, Huang W, Mohamed-Hadley A, Yao W, Benencia F, Coukos G (2002) Different effects of glucose starvation on expression and stability of VEGF mRNA isoforms in murine ovarian cancer cells. Biochem Biophys Res Commun 292:860–868
Zhang L, Conejo-Garcia JR, Katsaros D, Gimotty PA, Massobrio M, Regnani G, Makrigiannakis A, Gray H, Schlienger K, Liebman MN, Rubin SC, Coukos G (2003a) Intratumoral T cells, recurrence, and survival in epithelial ovarian cancer. N Engl J Med 348:203–213
Zhang L, Yang N, Katsaros D, Huang W, Park J-W, Fracchioli S, Vezzani C, Rigault de la Longrais IA, Yao W, Rubin SC, Coukos G (2003b) The Oncogene Phosphatidylinositol 3'-Kinase Catalytic Subunit alpha Promotes Angiogenesis via Vascular Endothelial Growth Factor in Ovarian Carcinoma. Cancer Res 63:4225–4231
Zhang L, Yang N, Park J-W, Katsaros D, Fracchioli S, Cao G, O'Brien-Jenkins A, Randall TC, Rubin SC, Coukos G (2003c) Tumor-derived vascular endothelial growth factor up-regulates angiopoietin-2 in host endothelium and destabilizes host vasculature, supporting angiogenesis in ovarian cancer. Cancer Res 63:3403–3412
Zitvogel L, Tesniere A, Kroemer G (2006) Cancer despite immunosurveillance: immunoselection and immunosubversion. Nat Rev Immunol 6:715–727

Adoptive Cellular Therapy

Stephan A. Grupp and Carl H. June

Contents

1 Introduction 150
2 Finding the Right Tool for the Job 151
3 Considerations of Cell Culture Technology 153
3.1 General Approaches for Cell Manufacturing 154
3.2 Artificial APC 155
3.3 Moving to the Dark Side: Culture Systems for Tregs 156
4 Engineering T Cells 157
4.1 Introduction of Transgenic TCRs 157
4.2 Creation of MHC-Independent T Cells with Chimeric Antigen Receptors 158
4.3 Issues Facing the Field with Gene-Modified ACT 159
5 Post-Transplant ACT 160
5.1 ACT for Hematologic Malignancies 162
5.2 ACT for Neuroblastoma 164
6 Concluding Remarks 165
References 166

Abstract Cell-based therapies with various lymphocytes and antigen-presenting cells are promising approaches for cancer immunotherapy. The transfusion of T lymphocytes, also called adoptive cell therapy (ACT), is an effective treatment for viral infections, has induced regression of cancer in early stage clinical trials, and may be a particularly important and efficacious modality in the period following

---

S.A. Grupp
Division of Oncology and Department of Pathology and Laboratory Medicine, Children's Hospital of Philadelphia; and the Department of Pediatrics, University of Pennsylvania School of Medicine, Philadelphia, PA, USA

C.H. June (✉)
Abramson Family Cancer Research Institute and the Department of Pathology and Laboratory Medicine, University of Pennsylvania, 554 Biomedical Research Building II/III, 421 Curie Blvd., Philadelphia, PA, USA
e-mail: cjune@exchange.upenn.edu

G. Dranoff (ed.), *Cancer Immunology and Immunotherapy*,
Current Topics in Microbiology and Immunology 344, DOI 10.1007/82_2010_94

hematopoietic stem cell transplantation (HSCT). Immune reconstitution post-SCT is often slow and incomplete, which in turn leads to an increased risk of infection and may impact relapse risk in patients with malignant disease. Immunization post-HSCT is frequently unsuccessful, due to the prolonged lymphopenia, especially of CD4 T cells, seen following transplant. ACT has the potential to enhance antitumor and overall immunity, and augment vaccine efficacy in the post-transplant setting. The ability to genetically engineer lymphocyte subsets has the further potential to improve the natural immune response, correct impaired immunity, and redirect T cells to an antitumor effector response. This chapter focuses on various applications of ACT for cancer immunotherapy, and we discuss some of the latest progress and hurdles in translating these technologies to the clinic.

1 Introduction

The principles of adoptive immunotherapy established in animal models have formed the basis for the testing of therapeutic strategies for human tumors. The primary rationale for the use of T cells for adoptive therapy is their ability to specifically target tumor cells that express small peptides, even if the intact target protein itself is not expressed on the cell surface. A second attraction is the potentially long clonal lifespan of memory T cell subsets, so that both therapeutic and immunoprophylactic therapies can be envisioned. A third feature is that T cells are well suited for genetic manipulation, so that the adoptive transfer of engineered T cells with enhanced antitumor properties is being tested in pilot clinical trials. Finally, there is a prospect for significant expansion of therapeutic T cells in vivo, if the appropriate methods are used to culture and expand T cells, and if the host is conditioned to promote homeostatic expansion.

The infusion of various mature lymphocyte subsets into patients with the goal of treating cancer or correcting immunodeficiency is an old concept that has recently gained momentum in the clinic (Fig. 1). Both allogeneic and autologous lymphocytes have been used over the years. In studies later criticized for ethical concerns (Lerner 2004), Southam and colleagues demonstrated that the subcutaneous growth of human tumor autografts to patients bearing advanced cancers was inhibited by cotransfer of autologous leukocytes in about half of the patients (Southam et al. 1966), suggesting that lymphocytes with a specific inhibitory effect on the implantation and growth of cancer cells were present in many patients. Perhaps the most potent therapeutic benefit yet realized with unmodified lymphocytes is due to the allogeneic effect, a term referring to the tumoricidal activity following an infusion of allogeneic lymphocytes. It was only retrospectively appreciated that the powerful and durable antitumor effects of bone marrow transplantation can largely be ascribed to allogeneic T cell transfer (Weiden et al. 1979).

Interest in genetically modifying lymphocytes has increased dramatically in recent years, as a number of basic and translational scientists have concluded that the modification of autologous lymphocytes should enable the creation of

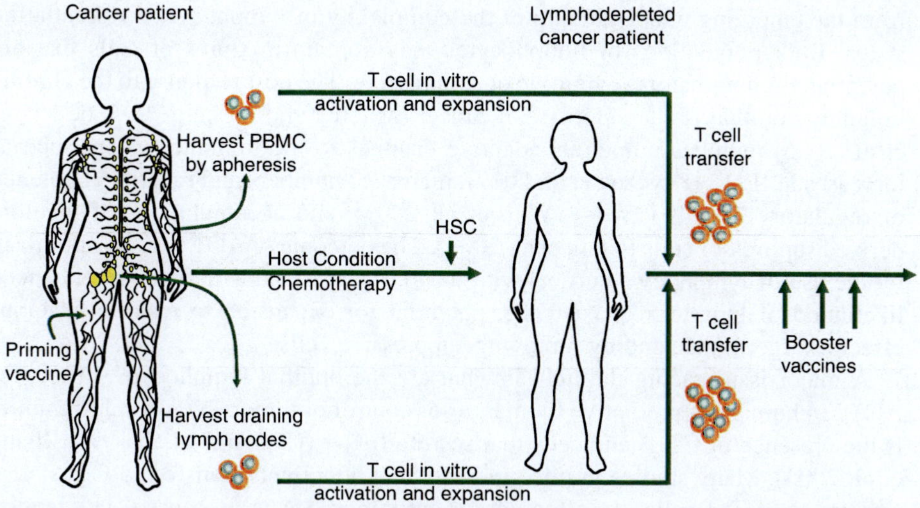

Fig. 1 General schema for adoptive transfer strategies. For melanoma, input lymphocytes are obtained from tumor, and tumor infiltrating lymphocytes (TIL) propagated. For other cancers, input lymphocytes are obtained from peripheral blood and expanded. The activated lymphocytes are returned to the patient, often after iatrogenic immunosuppression induced by chemotherapy or other means, including hematopoietic stem cell transplantation (HSCT)

pharmacologically enhanced immune systems that are more potent and have a larger therapeutic window than allogeneic T cell transfer. In 1990, the first study using gene-modified T cell infusions in patients with cancer reported retrovirus-mediated insertion of the neomycin phosphotransferase gene into the genome of lymphocytes (Rosenberg et al. 1990). The goal of these studies was to mark but not pharmacologically alter the function of the infused T cells in order to track tumor infiltration following infusion. The study was a clinical success in that there was no significant toxicity; however, scientifically there was much room for improvement in that at 1 week after infusion barely 0.01% of transferred T cells remained in the circulation. Significant progress has been achieved since then, and in this chapter we provide an overview of adoptive cell transfer therapy and discuss some of the issues and challenges currently facing the field.

2 Finding the Right Tool for the Job

Until recently, mature T cells were thought to be comprised primarily of CD4+ helper cells and CD8+ killer cells, and for several decades most investigators focused adoptive cell therapy (ACT) on approaches that used CD8+ cytotoxic T lymphocytes (CTLs). However, a series of recent discoveries from developmental immunologists indicates that mature lymphocytes have a bewildering and complex set of differentiation choices (Zhou et al. 2009). There are a number of implications from the emerging understanding of the complexity of lymphocyte differentiation states. Bulk populations of lymphocytes may contain mixtures of cells that are potentially inflammatory, cytotoxic or suppressive. The host response to the chronic inflammation that is characteristic of cancer (Mueller and Fusenig 2004; de Visser et al. 2006) includes numerous adaptive changes to the immune system such as increases in IL-17 (Kryczek et al. 2009), increased numbers and functional potency of regulatory T cells (Tregs) (Woo et al. 2001), and accumulations of myeloid derived suppressor cells (Clark et al. 2007). The outcome of ACT may be optimized by the use of lymphocyte subsets with desired properties of trafficking, enhanced likelihood of long-term persistence, potential for expansion to reach efficacious effector:target ratios, and by removing suppressive cells.

A major issue facing the field is what are the optimal lymphocyte subsets for ACT? In humans, a predictive biomarker of control of tumors by natural immunity is the presence of CTLs and cells that secrete IFN-γ (Clemente et al. 1998; Zhang et al. 2003). Many studies in mice indicate that adoptively transferred CTLs, also referred to as Tc1 cells, are effective for antitumor effects. Because CTLs require cytokines and other signals from CD4 cells to maintain function, there is an increasing use of cell populations that contain CD4+ Th1 cells to provide help to the infused CD8+ effector cells (June 2007).

In addition to Th1 and Th2 cells, a third subset of effector Th cells has recently been described in mice and humans, and termed Th17. Th17 cells produce IL-17, IL-17F, IL-21, IL-22, and induce the recruitment of neutrophils and macrophages to tissues (Korn et al. 2009). Based on previous studies, Th1 and Tc1 cells (CTLs) have been widely considered to be the optimal cells for ACT. However, recent studies report that Th17-polarized cells were more effective in mediating regression of B16 melanoma than Th0 (unpolarized) or Th1-polarized cells (Muranski et al. 2008; Martin-Orozco et al. 2009). CD8 cells that secrete IL-17 (Tc17 cells) also are effective as a form of ACT for cancer in preclinical models (Hinrichs et al. 2009). It should be noted that IL-17 and IL-23 can promote tumor growth through tissue remodeling and other mechanisms (Langowski et al. 2006; Lin and Karin 2007), and that the potential use of Th17 cells for ACT is distinct from their potential roles in the pathogenesis of inflammation leading to cancer. Preclinical models indicate that it is the IFN-γ secreted by Th17 cells that promotes tumor rejection, and that the IL-17 secretion is not sustained by the Th17 cells after adoptive transfer (Muranski et al. 2008).

T cells with highly active and specific effector function can be engineered in a variety of ways (see below). The central issues that must be addressed to achieve clinical efficacy of ACT are the related issues of expansion and persistence of therapeutic cells after infusion. Expansion is required to achieve an adequate effector:target ratio, persistence may be needed to achieve full cytoreduction of tumor, and, if long-term immunosurveillance is desired, long-term persistence is necessary. Well-defined subsets of memory T cells appear to be the key to understanding and optimizing persistence and expansion. Two subsets of memory cells, "effector memory" (T_{EM}) and "central memory" (T_{CM}), were originally identified on the basis of tissue homing molecules and effector function (Sallusto et al. 2004).

T_{CM} were described as CCR7+ cells that home to lymph nodes and have relatively low immediate effector function and a higher replicative capacity. T_{EM} were defined as CCR7 cells that preferentially home to peripheral tissues and inflammatory sites and possess relatively high immediate effector function. In mice with acute lymphocytic choriomeningitis virus infection, the adoptive transfer of T_{CM} was highly effective (Barber et al. 2003). Retrospective studies in melanoma patients indicate that, on a per cell basis, adoptive transfer of tumor infiltrating lymphocytes (TIL) cells with extensive replicative capacity resulted in both improved engraftment and antitumor effects compared with patients infused with terminally differentiated effector cells that have a more potent cytotoxic effector function (Zhou et al. 2005). This paradox is likely explained by the ability of T_{CM} to expand and self renew as well as differentiate into effector T cells in vivo, while T_{EM} have limited renewal and expansion capacity (Lanzavecchia and Sallusto 2005; Seder et al. 2008).

A controversy has arisen in the field as to how best to achieve the dual goals of persistence/expansion and a high effector:target ratio. One approach is to isolate T_{CM} cells with the desired specificity in vitro by sorting or other means of physical separation, engineer the desired specificity, expand and then infuse the T_{CM} cells (Berger et al. 2009). We have proposed that specific costimulation of bulk T cell culture conditions can enrich and maintain T_{CM} cells, obviate the need for cell sorting procedures, while providing a streamlined process yielding a higher number of T cells for ACT in the clinical setting. Our group and others have found that cell culture conditions that augment CD28 and CD137 (4-1BB) costimulation in vitro promote the maintenance of T_{CM} cells in vitro (Levine et al. 1997; Maus et al. 2004; Bondanza et al. 2006) and in vivo (Pulle et al. 2006; Zhang et al. 2007; Zhu et al. 2007).

Several laboratories have described the existence of mature CD8+ T cells that have characteristics of stem cells in the mouse (Fearon et al. 2001; Zhang et al. 2005) and in humans (Turtle et al. 2009). The use of memory stem T cells for ACT has significant potential; however, the developmental relationship of these cells in the murine and primate immune systems remains unknown. For many principles of ACT therapy, the conserved nature of T cell biology has meant that approaches developed in the mouse are often predictive of results seen in the human clinical setting. However, caution in this area is warranted because of fundamental differences in mechanisms of immunosenescence between mice and humans (Weng 2006) and in the regulation of CD28 expression on CD8+ cells (Azuma et al. 1993) that have important implications for adoptive T cell transfer therapeutics and in the optimal selection of lymphocyte subsets for cancer therapy.

3 Considerations of Cell Culture Technology

Currently, most oncologists have a bias that ACT as an example of personalized medicine will always remain on the sidelines as a "boutique" treatment rather than a mainstream therapy for oncology. At present, the only form of adoptive cellular therapy routinely used in the practice of medicine is allogeneic bone marrow or peripheral blood stem cell transplantation (Thomas 1999). In this setting, donor leukocyte infusions mediate various potent antitumor effects (Barrett and Jiang 2000). The adoptive transfer of activated donor (allogeneic) T cells has promise to augment this effect (Fowler et al. 2006; Porter et al. 2006). However, for most patients, comorbidity, increasing age, and the challenges in finding a suitably matched allogeneic donor mean that effective autologous approaches would be preferred. Therefore, a central issue for the development of widely available clinical ACT strategies has been the development of efficient and robust culture systems in order to produce adequate numbers of T cells for autologous therapy. An emerging principle is that cell culture conditions must be optimized for the propagation of desired lymphocyte subsets; the one size fits all approach does not apply to lymphocyte cell culture.

3.1 General Approaches for Cell Manufacturing

An overview of cell culture approaches used for various lymphocyte subsets that have been tested in human trials is shown in Fig. 2. The basic principles of T cell

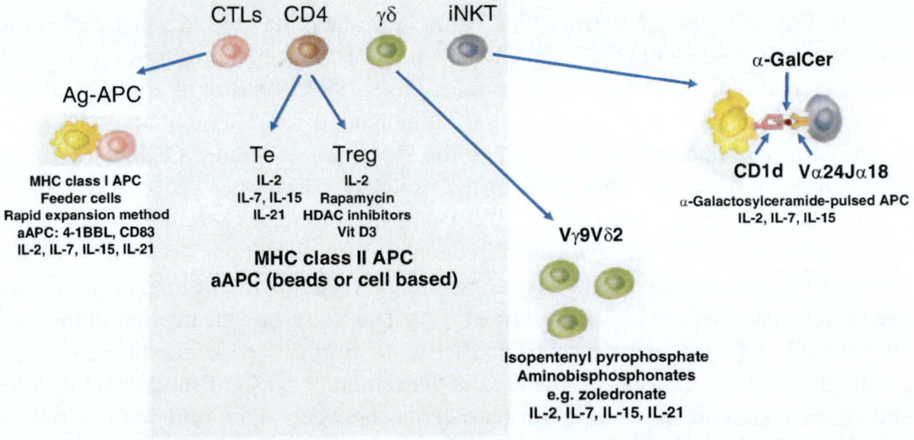

Fig. 2 Cell culture approaches for adoptive transfer of lymphocyte subsets. Culture conditions required for distinct lymphocyte subsets vary, depending on the activation and costimulatory requirements. CTLs express αβ TCRs and are stimulated by APCs that express MHC class I. CTLs require 4-1BB stimulation for optimal expansion and have been expanded by the addition of feeder cells or artificial APC that express the costimulatory ligands. CD4 T cells are stimulated by APC that express peptide loaded MHC class II. The dominant costimulatory molecule for CD4 cells is CD28. Effector CD4 cells can be stimulated by beads or cell based aAPC in the presence of various cytokines. Regulatory CD4 T cells (Tregs) require culture in IL-2, and the addition of number of reagents to the culture may enhance the suppressive functions of ex vivo expanded Tregs. CD1d-restricted Vα24 iNKTs are stimulated by α-GalCer. Cells expressing γδ TCRs are stimulated by APC that present exogenous isopentenyl pyrophosphate or other endogenous ligands stimulated by aminobisphosphonates such as zoledronate

biology can be used for a bottom-up approach to engineer efficient culture processes using engineered cells or synthetic substrates. The first approach has been to isolate and activate antigen-specific T cells from peripheral blood or tumor specimens in vitro, and then to use repetitive stimulation with antigen-presenting cells (APCs) or feeder cells to clonally expand the antigen-specific cells in vitro by various approaches. The most appropriate methods of ex vivo T cell culture mimic the physiologic processes whereby dendritic cells (DCs) generate a constellation of antigen-specific and costimulatory signals in the T cells. The best results to date have been with the rapid expansion method developed by Riddell and coworkers, which uses irradiated allogeneic peripheral blood mononuclear cells as feeder cells to expand CTLs for adoptive transfer (Riddell and Greenberg 1990). The main limitation of this approach is in scale-up because FDA-mandated requirements for the validation and qualification of allogeneic feeder cells can be tedious and expensive. Schultze and coworkers have shown that CD40-stimulated B cells, which have an extensive replicative potential, are an efficient means to propagate antigen-specific T cells (Schultze et al. 1997). Thus, while previous effective but unwieldy tissue culture approaches have provided proof-of-concept for adoptive therapy, a current priority is to develop alternative approaches that can support large scale trials required for FDA approval and wider clinical application.

3.2 Artificial APC

To generate antigen-specific T cells, clonal cell lines and even beads can be engineered as artificial antigen-presenting cells (aAPCs) and avoid the need to use autologous APCs for patient-specific cultures (reviewed in Kim et al. 2004). General approaches have been to produce aAPCs, either by coating beads with CD3-specific antibody or peptide–MHC complexes or by transfecting cells that lack endogenous MHC molecules with MHC molecules and costimulatory molecules. Enhanced polyclonal T cell activation and proliferation results when cells are stimulated through the TCR and CD28 (Levine et al. 1997). In addition, CD28 stimulation maintains telomere length in human T cells, and this is associated with improved engraftment and the persistence of the adoptively transferred T cells (Weng et al. 1997; Zhou et al. 2005). This culture system has been adapted for clinical use, and starting with an initial apheresis product, it is possible to generate a number of mature T cells equivalent to the entire T cell mass of an adult (10^{12} cells) within about 2 weeks of ex vivo culture (Kalamasz et al. 2004).

Magnetic beads coated with recombinant MHC class I dimeric molecules loaded with specific peptide have been used to elicit antigen-specific T cell propagation (Oelke et al. 2003). Following isolation and expansion, cell populations generated using such beads specifically kill antigen-expressing target cells in vitro and display antiviral therapeutic effects in rodents (Luxembourg et al. 1998). Others have used nonmagnetic microspheres coated with complexes of recombinant peptide–loaded MHC molecules to successfully generate CTLs ex vivo from naïve precursors (Lone et al. 1998).

Sadelain and colleagues have engineered APCs that could be used to stimulate T cells of many patients expressing a specific HLA allele (Latouche and Sadelain 2000). Mouse fibroblasts were retrovirally transduced with a single HLA class I complex along with the human accessory molecules CD80 (also known as B7-1), CD54 (also known as ICAM-1), and CD58 (also known as LFA-3). A panel of these aAPCs consistently selected and expanded relevant CTLs from most patients with many common HLA alleles (Hasan et al. 2009). K562 cells are particularly attractive for use as aAPCs, as we were able to obtain simultaneous expression of up to seven transgenes (costimulatory molecules, HLA alleles, and cytokines) in a single aAPC (Suhoski et al. 2007). aAPCs that express 4-1BB ligand efficiently expand human CD8+ T_{CM} cells that have potent cytolytic function (Maus et al. 2002, 2004), and have a specialized ability to expand human T_{EM} cells that no longer express CD28 (Suhoski et al. 2007). Others have shown that CD83 expression on aAPCs enhances the generation of CTLs (Hirano et al. 2006).

3.3 *Moving to the Dark Side: Culture Systems for Tregs*

Tregs are essential for maintaining tolerance in healthy individuals, and in cancer there is often a "gain of function" of Tregs, in which a relative or absolute increase in Tregs can be demonstrated in the tumor microenvironment (Curiel 2007), which may supply one mechanism of immune evasion. CD28 costimulation is essential for the development of Tregs in mice (Salomon et al. 2000), and in humans CD28 costimulation is essential for ex vivo expansion and to maintain suppressive function of Tregs (Golovina et al. 2008). In mice, adoptive transfer of ex vivo expanded Tregs can prevent lethal graft-versus-host disease (GVHD) (Taylor et al. 2002). Based on these findings, a clinical trial testing the safety and feasibility of ex vivo expanded cord blood Tregs to prevent GVHD in adults with hematologic malignancies has just been completed at the University of Minnesota. Current issues regarding Treg cell biology and the status of clinical trials with adoptively transferred Treg cells have been reviewed recently (Riley et al. 2009). Ex vivo culture approaches to alter the ratio of effector T cells, and Tregs have the potential to decrease the risk of GVHD while preserving antitumor effects (Edinger et al. 2003). In future, infusions of Tregs may be used to prevent or treat GVHD that may occur with the adoptive transfer of allogeneic T cells (donor leukocyte infusions), or for more specialized purposes, such as to induce tolerance to transgenes that are incorporated into ACT protocols using autologous engineered lymphocytes.

4 Engineering T Cells

Mature T cells are among the most suitable cells for modification, and stable modification has been achieved using a number of approaches. The efficiency of mature lymphocyte modification has been consistently higher than with hematopoietic stem cells (HSCs), such that with current technologies, transgene delivery and expression in adoptively transferred T cells are not limiting (June et al. 2009). Immunotherapy with engineered T cells is attractive for several reasons, including significantly improved persistence that has been demonstrated in humans following adoptive transfer (Muul et al. 2003). A major advantage of ACT is that the therapeutic effects can be augmented by isolating the lymphocytes with desired effector or regulatory properties, while removing the cells that may have antagonistic effects. Clinical studies with effector T cells are most mature and have progressed to a Phase III clinical trial testing the efficacy of T cells that are transduced to express a herpes simplex virus thymidine kinase (HSV-TK) conditional "safety switch" in the setting of haploidentical stem cell transplantation for high-risk acute leukemia in remission (Ciceri et al. 2009). In this approach, allogeneic T cells can mediate antitumor effects in the context of allogeneic stem cell transplantation, and in the event of significant GVHD, the cells can be ablated by administration of the antiviral drug gancyclovir.

4.1 Introduction of Transgenic TCRs

At present, there is considerable enthusiasm for adoptive transfer of engineered CD8+ CTLs. The transfer of MHC class I-restricted TCRs can "convert" a population of polyclonal CD8+ T cells to CTLs with a monoclonal TCR specificity (Cooper et al. 2000). This approach is attractive because high-affinity CTLs of appropriate specificity are generally lacking in patients with advanced cancer or chronic infections. Thus, the introduction of TCRs with higher affinity or even a supraphysiological affinity has the potential to increase recognition and killing of tumor cells that have low expression of cognate peptide–MHC class I complexes. In the case of exogenous antigens, high-affinity TCRs seem to have an improved ability to control viral infection and to delay the appearance of escape virus mutants (Varela-Rohena et al. 2008). Clinical trials testing the adoptive transfer of engineered TCRs for self antigens in cancer patients have been reported with promising clinical results and acceptable tissue-specific "on-target" toxicity (Johnson et al. 2009).

The expression of additional TCR chains in T cells can lead to the generation of T cells with potentially novel specificity, due to the formation of mixed dimers between the endogenous and introduced TCR chains (Schumacher 2002), as the endogenous TCR does not undergo allelic exclusion as a result of expression of the introduced TCR. One approach to mitigate the possibility of forming mixed dimers is to incorporate an additional disulfide bond between the introduced TCR chains by cysteine modification of the transgenic TCR chains (Boulter et al. 2003). This may facilitate matched pairing of the introduced TCR chains. Another approach is the use of γδ T cells, which can be engineered to express αβ TCRs (van der Veeken et al. 2009). Cell-based therapies with γδ T cells may provide a significant safety feature over the use of TCR-engineered αβ T cells, taking advantage of the finding that αβ TCRs cannot pair with γδ TCRs. The open questions regarding engineered γδ T cells are whether the adoptively transferred cells will home to tumor or sites of inflammation, and if so, what is the best source of γδ T cells? Blood-derived Vγ9Vδ2+ T cells are the most convenient cells to harvest and are cytotoxic for a variety of tumors (Thedrez et al. 2007), but Vγ9Vδ2 T cells derived from tissues may be preferable as they may have longer persistence and improved homing capacity, especially for patients with tumors located in the skin and intestines, sites that are preferentially targeted by γδ T cells.

4.2 Creation of MHC-Independent T Cells with Chimeric Antigen Receptors

Since the development of chimeric antigen receptors (CARs) was first reported in mice more than two decades previously (Gross et al. 1989), the transfer of CD8+ T cells engineered to express MHC-unrestricted CARs is now rapidly advancing in human trials. CARs have the potential to serve as an "off the shelf" reagent to redirect T cells with cytotoxic or regulatory functions to desired cell surface ligands in a variety of tumor, stromal, and viral targets (Sadelain et al. 2009). Because CARs bind to target antigens in an HLA-unrestricted manner, they are resistant to many of the immune evasion mechanisms of tumor, such as downregulation of HLA class I molecules or failure to process or present proteins. Our previous studies showed that infusions of autologous T cells expressing the CD4ζ CAR in patients with HIV infection were safe. In addition, the use of a CD3/CD28 costimulated activated T cell product in which the CAR was expressed resulted in prolonged high level engraftment for up to 6 months (Deeks et al. 2002).

The first report of CAR-modified T cells specific for neuroblastoma was published in 2001 (Rossig et al. 2001), and research since that time has led to an early-phase clinical trial published in 2007 (Park et al. 2007). To safely redirect T cells against a tumor, the CAR must target a tumor-specific antigen that is minimally expressed on normal tissues. In the Park trial, the authors targeted a potential neuroblastoma antigen, the L1 cell-adhesion molecule (L1-CAM). While outcome was not a primary measure of the trial, there was at least one patient with a complete response. An important 2008 study from the Brenner group used an approach to address problems of persistence of infused cells, engineering Epstein–Barr virus-specific cytotoxic T lymphocytes (EBV-CTLs) to express a first-generation CAR recognizing the well-characterized neuroblastoma disialoganglioside antigen GD2 and using the TCRζ domain to provide an activation signal in a 11-patient clinical trial. This trial used improved methods of cell culture that were shown to contribute to enhanced persistence of the adoptively transferred CAR-modified T cells. In specific, the study demonstrated much better persistence of the EBV-CTLs compared to CD3-activated T cells, and clinical responses were seen in four patients (Pule et al. 2008). More advanced vector designs incorporating lentiviral vector technology and multiple costimulatory domains are now entering clinical trials at various centers (Maher et al. 2002; Carpenito et al. 2009; Milone et al. 2009).

4.3 Issues Facing the Field with Gene-Modified ACT

The major issues with engineered T cell therapies in cancer patients relate to the low levels of persistence in the trials reported to date, and to potential toxicity. Again, issues of persistence and expansion have limited the efficacy of CAR therapy. There are two cell engineering considerations that may apply. First is the T cell product used for CAR introduction and means by which the T cells are expanded ex vivo. Second, there may be an impact of CAR design on persistence related to nonphysiologic signal transduction that occurs as a result of the structure of the CAR and the signaling domains that are included in the signal transduction portion of the CAR. Our group has shown that incorporation of the signaling domain from the TNF family molecule CD137 (4-1BB) can enhance persistence (Carpenito et al. 2009), and others have shown that other TNF family members such as Ox40 can have similar effects (Pule et al. 2005). Similarly, modifications of the CD28 signaling domain to remove the dileucine motif can improve CAR function in mouse T cells (Nguyen et al. 2003).

One approach to improve the survival of CAR T cells is to engineer them into central memory cells, cells that presumably have already been selected for long-term survival. For example, it has been shown that endogenous cytotoxic CD4+ T cells specific for varicella zoster virus (VZV) can be engineered to express tumor-specific CARs, and that the VSV-specific T cells can be expanded in vivo by stimulation of their native receptor by administration of VZV vaccine, while retaining the ability of the VZV-CAR CD4+ T cells to recognize and lyse tumor targets in a MHC-independent manner (Landmeier et al. 2007). Together, these results are important because tumor cells often have decreased expression of antigen-loaded MHC molecules, and low levels of stimulation in the context of the immunosuppressive tumor microenvironment will promote loss of function of the T cells, or to poor persistence.

Recently, serious adverse events (SAEs) were reported in two subjects enrolled in trials containing CARs, raising concerns about this form of T cell therapy. The first event occurred in a patient with advanced chronic lymphocytic leukemia who died following infusion of a CD19-specific CAR that contained CD28 signaling domain (Brentjens et al. 2010). The second case occurred in a patient with widely metastatic colon cancer who died shortly after treatment with a CAR targeting HER2/neu containing CD28 and 4-1BB signaling domains after intensive lymphodepletion (Morgan et al. 2010). In both cases, elevated cytokine levels were seen in the serum and the cause of death was not clear at necropsy. The first adverse event appeared to result from "on-target" toxicity, as there was evidence of tumor lysis syndrome in a patient with a high tumor burden, while in the case of the HER2/neu CAR, the toxicity was most likely due to "on-target off-organ" toxicity triggered by low level expression of HER2/neu in the cardiopulmonary tissues, rather than by CAR signaling triggered by the HER2/neu overexpressed on tumor tissues. Similar but manageable toxicities have been reported previously in a trial of patients treated with a CAR specific for carbonic anhydrase IX expressed on renal cell carcinoma cells, and later found to be expressed on biliary tract epithelium after patients developed significant liver toxicity (Lamers et al. 2006). A number of strategies are being tested to ameliorate or prevent toxicity from CARs (Sadelain et al. 2009), but in the short term the key is selection of a tumor antigen target with limited normal tissue expression. Finally, another potential toxicity concern in the use of genetically engineered T cells expressing CARs or exogenous TCRs relates to genotoxicity. This concern is raised by the T cell leukemias that have occurred in patients given genetically modified HSC to correct IL-2R γ chain deficiency, a syndrome in males termed X-linked severe combined immunodeficiency-X1 (Hacein-Bey-Abina et al. 2008). However, none of the clinical trials carried out so far using mature T cells genetically modified using gammaretrovirus or lentivirus vectors have reported adverse events due to insertional mutagenesis (June et al. 2009).

5 Post-Transplant ACT

In addition to compromising the ability of hematopoietic stem cell transplantation (HSCT) patients to mount effective antitumor immune responses, post-transplant immune suppression clearly increases the risk for serious infections with VZV, cytomegalovirus (CMV), and *Streptococcus pneumoniae* (Hoyle and Goldman 1994). Late infectious complications are common after autologous and allogeneic HSCT, particularly cord blood HSCT (Hamza et al. 2004). Early recovery of lymphocytes and lymphocyte function has been linked to improved survival following both auto- and allotransplantation (Porrata et al. 2001; Ege et al. 2008). In the immediate post-transplant period, lymphocyte restoration is achieved by expansion of mature T cells present in the graft and not de novo production from the thymus or bone marrow (Roux et al. 1996; Hakim et al. 1997). CD4+ T cell regeneration occurs by a thymus-dependent mechanism, while CD8+ T cell regeneration occurs by a thymus-independent pathway (Mackall et al. 1997). Therefore, after transplant, there is a prolonged deficiency of CD4+ compared to CD8+ T cells, particularly in older patients, secondary to limited thymic regenerative capacity and impaired homeostatic proliferation in vivo. Increased homeostatic proliferation in the post-SCT setting is due at least in part to compensatorily elevated levels of IL-7 as a result of severe lymphopenia. In addition, the inflammatory milieu seen in the immediate post-SCT may augment homeostatic proliferation (Rapoport et al. 2009). However, IL-7 signaling on IL-7 receptor-α–positive DCs in lymphopenic settings paradoxically diminishes the homeostatic proliferation of CD4+ T cells. Chronically elevated systemic IL-7 levels diminish the capacity for IL-7 receptor-α DCs to support CD4 homeostatic expansion, at least in part via IL-7 mediated downregulation of MHC II expression (Guimond et al. 2009). While younger patients eventually recover thymic output, the thymic deficiency seen post-transplant often fails to fully correct in older patients (Storek et al. 2001, 2004).

The post-transplant setting is an ideal platform for ACT strategies to capitalize on homeostatic T cell proliferation (Surh and Sprent 2008), in which naive T cells begin to proliferate and differentiate into memory-like T cells when total numbers of naive T cells are reduced below a certain threshold. Host lymphodepletion may enhance the effectiveness of adoptively transferred T cells (Dummer et al. 2002). Homeostatic T cell proliferation can result in the induction of autoimmunity (King et al. 2004), providing a clue to improved antitumor strategies. T cells can undergo up to seven rounds of cell division after being deprived of contact with APC (Kaech and Ahmed 2001). This homeostatic response of T cells is directed largely to self antigens (Ernst et al. 1999). The use of ACT in the setting of homeostatic expansion was first tested clinically in patients with relapsed or refractory non-Hodgkin's lymphoma after autologous HSCT (Laport et al. 2003). In these studies, a high rate of clinical disease regression was observed in patients who received a lymphodepleting conditioning regimen prior to adoptive transfer of costimulated autologous T cells.

The CD4+ T cell deficiency noted after transplant is particularly significant, as several studies have demonstrated the importance of these cells in the stimulation of CD8+ T cells and the enhancement of antibody production by B cells. CD8+ T cells that engage antigen in the absence of CD4+ T cells develop normally but do not proliferate well and do not persist, becoming so-called helpless T cells (Janssen et al. 2003). In addition to providing a critical stimulus for CD8+ T cells, CD4+ T cells are required for maximal antibody production. The importance of CD4+ T cells has been demonstrated in humans where responses to immunization and severity of infection have been correlated with CD4 counts (Kroon et al. 1994).

Humoral immunity recovers more quickly than cellular immunity in the immediate post-transplant period; however, immunoglobulin subset levels are often suppressed such that protective immunity is compromised and response to vaccination remains a significant problem in HSCT patients (Avigan et al. 2001). In the setting of allogeneic HSCT, immunization of the donor has led to increased titers of *Haemophilus influenzae* type B (HiB) and tetanus toxoid antibodies (Molrine et al. 1996; Storek et al. 2003). In this age when so many promising tumor vaccines are in clinical trials, strategies to optimize responses in HSCT patients to vaccination have become increasingly important.

5.1 *ACT for Hematologic Malignancies*

We have completed three phase I/II trials in patients transplanted for hematologic malignancies using ex vivo activated and expanded autologous T cells stimulated by coculture with immunomagnetic beads to which anti-CD3 and anti-CD28 monoclonal antibodies had been conjugated to form aAPCs (Levine et al. 1995) using the general trial design shown in Fig. 3. In the first trial, patients with relapsed or refractory non-Hodgkin's lymphoma were treated with CD34+-selected HSCT followed by infusion of up to 1×10^{10} CD3+ autologous T cells at day 14 after transplant (Laport et al. 2003). Infusion of autologous costimulated T cells resulted in a rapid, dose-dependent reconstitution of lymphocyte counts. Importantly, the expanded cells were functionally superior to those obtained directly from the patients, as determined by interferon-γ secretion. Complete or partial responses were observed in eight of the 17 patients infused, although it was not possible to discriminate antitumor effects of the ACT from the transplant itself.

In a second phase I/II trial, we examined the role of pre-transplant immunization and costimulated/activated ACT in autologous transplantation for multiple myeloma (Rapoport et al. 2005). All patients received two doses of Prevnar®, the seven-valent pneumococcal conjugate vaccine (PCV), beginning 1 month after transplant. Half of the patients received an additional PCV vaccine 2 weeks prior to a steady-state leukapheresis. The harvested T cells were expanded in vitro using the beads described above. Patients received a standard, non-lymphocyte–depleted, autologous HSCT after melphalan conditioning, and then received approximately 1×10^{10} autologous, CD3/CD28 bead expanded CD3+ T cells based on

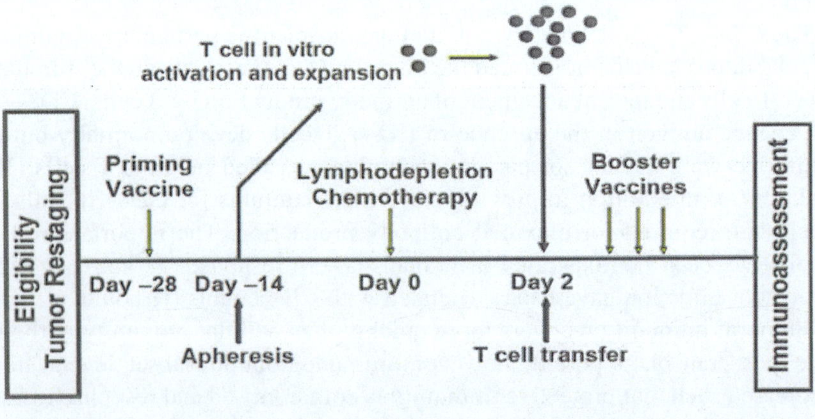

Fig. 3 Approach for combination vaccine and adoptive transfer strategies. For vaccine prime boost strategies, patients are primed with vaccine after protocol enrollment, followed by lymphocyte harvest several weeks later. The autologous T cells undergo polyclonal in vitro activation and expansion and are reinfused on day 2 after lymphodepleting chemotherapy; Tregs may be depleted during the expansion procedure. Antigen-specific immune function is measured after the administration of booster vaccines

randomization to either 14 days or 100 days post-transplant. Consistent with our initial experience with this T cell product, early T cell recovery was observed in both patient groups that received the day 14 T cell add-back while the day 100 add-back groups remained significantly lymphopenic. We also found that only those individuals who received PCV-primed T cells early after transplant developed and maintained protective levels of antipneumococcal antibodies, as well as PCV-specific CD4 responses. Notably, T cell responses to antigens not included in the vaccine were also improved in this group. These data demonstrated that combination immunotherapy consisting of a single early post-transplant infusion of antigen-primed, ex vivo costimulated autologous T cells followed by post-transplant booster immunizations improved the severe immunodeficiency associated with high-dose chemotherapy, and led to clinically relevant immunity in adults within a month following transplantation.

The above studies together with the studies in neuroblastoma described below provide "proof-of-concept" that immunosuppressed patients can be vaccinated and rapidly develop potent responses against foreign antigens. However, with the exception of virally induced tumors such as cervical cancer and some EBV-induced lymphomas, human tumors such as myeloma do not have foreign antigens. Instead, the tumors express weaker self antigens to which some degree of tolerance exists and that tend to induce T cells with lower avidity TCRs. To begin to establish whether the combined vaccine and adoptive transfer approach could augment antitumor immunity, a two arm trial in which the HLA-A2+ patients were vaccinated with a multipeptide vaccine to hTERT and survivin was recently completed. This was designed as a pilot study to determine whether combined vaccines and vaccine-primed T cell infusions generate antitumor/antiself responses in the setting of an autologous HSCT. The main differences between this trial and the earlier trials were that: (1) this trial incorporated the multipeptide peptide tumor vaccine; (2) the T cell infusions were given on day +2 post-HSCT rather than day +12; and (3) the dose of T cells was increased from 1×10^{10} to 5×10^{10}. Clinically, the day +2 T cell transfers were well tolerated with the most common adverse effects being chills/rigors, nausea, and low-grade fevers. Immune reconstitution was rapid and robust, as a relative and absolute lymphocytosis developed in the week following the ACT, which persisted in many cases throughout the transplant period (Rapoport et al. 2009). The lymphocytosis was comprised of CD3+ T cells that have markers consistent with T_{CM} cells. It is intriguing to note that the lymphocytosis was not observed in earlier trials when the T cell infusions were given later after chemotherapy and HSCT. The T cell lymphocytosis is remarkable in that patients were not treated with exogenous cytokines such as IL-2 or IL-7. In addition to the accelerated immune reconstitution, a subset of patients developed a T cell "engraftment syndrome" characterized by diarrhea, fever, rash, and colitis that was clinically and histopathologically indistinguishable from acute GVHD. The mechanism of the T cell lymphocytosis is under investigation, and in part, may be attributed to a relative paucity of Tregs after day 2 ACT. The engraftment syndrome does not appear to be specifically related to myeloma and the high levels of IL-6 that are characteristic of myeloma

(Bataille et al. 1989), because a similar syndrome has been observed in our trials of neuroblastoma (described below). It is intriguing to note that the survival of patients with multiple myeloma after unmodified HSCT directly correlates both with lymphocyte counts early (on day 15) after HSCT (Porrata et al. 2001). Furthermore, the survival of newly diagnosed MM patients is strongly correlated with the lymphocyte count at presentation (Ege et al. 2008).

5.2 ACT for Neuroblastoma

Neuroblastoma is the most common extracranial solid tumor of childhood and an important cause of childhood cancer mortality. High-risk neuroblastoma has proven refractory to conventional treatment modalities (Matthay et al. 1999; Grupp et al. 2000b; Maris et al. 2007), although some improvements in outcome have been achieved through chemotherapeutic dose escalation (Cheung and Heller 1991). This concept has reached a practical limit with the use of tandem stem cell transplantation approaches, which have achieved potentially promising results (Grupp et al. 2000a, b; Kletzel et al. 2002; George et al. 2006). Having reached an effective limit in chemotherapeutic intensity with tandem transplant, any further improvement of survival in children with high-risk neuroblastoma will have to come from novel therapeutic approaches. The most immediate hope for an effective and distinct treatment modality lies in immunotherapy. There is already data suggesting a potential benefit of antineuroblastoma monoclonal antibodies (Cheung et al. 2001; Simon et al. 2004), strengthening the case appropriately-targeted for cell-based therapy in neuroblastoma.

EBV lymphoproliferative disease has been seen among patients treated on the largest published tandem transplant study for neuroblastoma (Powell et al. 2004). EBV lymphoproliferative disease is associated with significant immunosuppression, is usually uncommon following autologous HSCT, and these cases suggest that immunosuppression induced by autologous HSCT is extremely important when considering immunotherapeutic approaches to treating high-risk neuroblastoma. ACT, possibly paired with a cancer vaccine, represents a major area to explore novel treatments. However, the limitations are clear: ACT, which may have antitumor efficacy, is almost certainly best deployed at the point of minimal residual disease rather than treating bulk disease. In neuroblastoma, this point is reached after chemotherapy, surgery, radiation, and HSCT. Immunotherapy and/or tumor vaccines should be deployed as quickly as possible after completion of conventional therapy, but this is also a point where numbers of T cells and effector function are minimal to absent. One solution to this problem is to provide activated polyclonal T cells to the patient in an attempt to speed immunological recovery, based on the improved ability of costimulated/activated T cells to engraft. This also has the potential to harness a profoundly lymphopenic environment supportive of homeostatic expansion. Unfortunately, the passenger T cells provided with a PBSC product, although large in number, do not provide this solution, as recovery of cellular immunity after standard autologous HSCT takes many months, and many T cells fail to persist due to increased rates of apoptosis (Hakim et al. 1997).

We have recently tested an alternative approach in studies at the University of Pennsylvania and Children's Hospital of Philadelphia. Again, the cell product used is ex vivo costimulated autologous T cells cultured on anti CD3/CD28 beads. This GMP cell manufacturing process produces a highly activated polyclonal T cell population, with a T cell repertoire representative of the full repertoire of the cells input into the culture. In ongoing studies, we have tested costimulated/activated ACT in patients with high-risk neuroblastoma (S. Grupp, unpublished data). In a series of studies, we are assessing the impact of activated ACT on immune reconstitution in these profoundly immunodeficient patients. These patients are an interesting group to study ACT, as the need for HSCT is known at diagnosis and T cells may thus be collected prior to exposure to any immunosuppressive chemotherapy. While patients getting a CD34-selected PBSC product have recovery of CD4+ T cells that may take 4–6 months, we have seen that both CD4 and CD8 recovery is significantly and strikingly improved after activated T cells are given on d + 12 after PBSC infusion. Interestingly, CD4 recovery is even more rapid when the infusion time is moved to d + 2, with supranormal lymphocyte and T cell counts apparent as soon at 10 days after costimulated/activated T cell infusion. Among patients receiving d + 2 ACT, we have observed lymphocyte counts on d + 12 post-HSCT as high at 10,000/μL. Four of these patients experienced a GVHD-like engraftment syndrome similar to that seen in the myeloma study (Rapoport, et al. 2009). In addition, protective antibody responses emerge as early as d + 30 following a d + 12 immunization with a PCV (S. Grupp, unpublished data). This experience supports the hypothesis that activated ACT could be used to support an anticancer immunization strategy early after HSCT.

6 Concluding Remarks

Progress in the understanding of the biology of T cell mediated antitumor effects have opened up real opportunities to ACT for clinical benefit in cancer patients. While clear proof of principle has been demonstrated, substantial work is needed to optimize these therapies and enhance the effectiveness of tumor-directed therapies. For the first time, improved culture technology is permitting randomized controlled studies. A humbling observation is that though adoptive T cell therapy of rodent malignancies was first reported in 1955 (Mitchison 1955), there are as yet no forms of FDA-approved ACT available after more than 60 years of research into adoptive immunity for tumors. However, the first autologous cellular vaccine for prostate cancer has just been approved by the FDA, initiating the era of clinical personalized cell therapies. There is increasing optimism that the scientific barriers preventing clinically effective adoptive immunotherapy have been addressed. Advances in the understanding of the T cell biology and T cell engineering have provided multiple novel adoptive transfer strategies that are now poised for translation into clinical trials. Finally, it is likely that adoptive immunotherapy will not be used alone, but rather in combination with other forms of immunotherapy and chemotherapy, to maximize both passive and active immunity.

Acknowledgments This work was supported by National Institutes of Health Public Health Service grant 1R01CA120409 and 5P01-CA-066726 to C.H.J and R21CA110516 to S.G. Additional support provided by the Weinberg Foundation and W.W. Smith Charitable Trust to S.G.

References

Avigan D, Pirofski L, Lazarus H (2001) Vaccination against infectious disease following hematopoietic stem cell transplantation. Biol Blood Marrow Transplant 7:171–183

Azuma M, Phillips JH, Lanier LL (1993) CD28- T lymphocytes. Antigenic and functional properties. J Immunol 150:1147–1159

Barber DL, Wherry EJ, Ahmed R (2003) Cutting edge: rapid in vivo killing by memory CD8 T cells. J Immunol 171:27–31

Barrett J, Jiang YZ (2000) Allogeneic immunotherapy for malignant diseases. Marcel Dekker, New York

Bataille R, Jourdan M, Zhang X, Klein B (1989) Serum levels of interleukin 6, a potent myeloma cell growth factor, as a reflect of disease severity in plasma cell dyscrasias. J Clin Invest 84:2008–2011

Berger C, Turtle CJ, Jensen MC, Riddell SR (2009) Adoptive transfer of virus-specific and tumor-specific T cell immunity. Curr Opin Immunol 21:224–232

Bondanza A, Valtolina V, Magnani Z, Ponzoni M, Fleischhauer K, Bonyhadi M, Traversari C, Sanvito F, Toma S, Radrizzani M, La Seta-Catamancio S, Ciceri F, Bordignon C, Bonini C (2006) Suicide gene therapy of graft-versus-host disease induced by central memory human T lymphocytes. Blood 107:1828–1836

Boulter JM, Glick M, Todorov PT, Baston E, Sami M, Rizkallah P, Jakobsen BK (2003) Stable, soluble T cell receptor molecules for crystallization and therapeutics. Protein Eng 16:707–711

Brentjens R, Yeh R, Bernal Y, Riviere I, Sadelain M (2010) Treatment of chronic lymphocytic leukemia with genetically targeted autologous T cells: case report of an unforeseen adverse event in a phase I clinical trial. Mol Ther 18:666–668

Carpenito C, Milone MC, Hassan R, Simonet JC, Lakhal M, Suhoski MM, Varela-Rohena A, Haines KM, Heitjan DF, Albelda SM, Carroll RG, Riley JL, Pastan I, June CH (2009) Control of large, established tumor xenografts with genetically retargeted human T cells containing CD28 and CD137 domains. Proc Natl Acad Sci USA 106:3360–3365

Cheung NK, Kushner BH, Kramer K (2001) Monoclonal antibody-based therapy of neuroblastoma. Hematol Oncol Clin North Am 15:853–866

Cheung NV, Heller G (1991) Chemotherapy dose intensity correlates strongly with response, median survival, and median progression-free survival in metastatic neuroblastoma. J Clin Oncol 9:1050–1058

Ciceri F, Bonini C, Stanghellini MTL, Bondanza A, Traversari C, Salomoni M, Turchetto L, Colombi S, Bernardi M, Peccatori J (2009) Infusion of suicide-gene-engineered donor lymphocytes after family haploidentical haemopoietic stem-cell transplantation for leukaemia (the TK007 trial): a non-randomised phase I–II study. Lancet Oncol 10:489–500

Clark CE, Hingorani SR, Mick R, Combs C, Tuveson DA, Vonderheide RH (2007) Dynamics of the immune reaction to pancreatic cancer from inception to invasion. Cancer Res 67:9518–9527

Clemente C, Mihm M Jr, Bufalino R, Zurrida S, Collini P, Cascinelli N (1998) Prognostic value of tumor infiltrating lymphocytes in the vertical growth phase of primary cutaneous melanoma. Cancer 77:1303–1310

Cooper LJ, Kalos M, Lewinsohn DA, Riddell SR, Greenberg PD (2000) Transfer of specificity for human immunodeficiency virus type 1 into primary human T lymphocytes by introduction of T cell receptor genes. J Virol 74:8207–8212

Curiel T (2007) Tregs and rethinking cancer immunotherapy. J Clin Invest 117:1167–1174

de Visser K, Eichten A, Coussens L (2006) Paradoxical roles of the immune system during cancer development. Nat Rev Cancer 6:24–37

Deeks SG, Wagner B, Anton PA, Mitsuyasu RT, Scadden DT, Huang C, Macken C, Richman DD, Kwok S, June CH, Lazar R, Broad DF, Jalali S, Hege KM (2002) A phase II randomized study of HIV-specific T cell gene therapy in subjects with undetectable plasma viremia on combination anti-retroviral therapy. Mol Ther 5:788–797

Dummer W, Niethammer AG, Baccala R, Lawson BR, Wagner N, Reisfeld RA, Theofilopoulos AN (2002) T cell homeostatic proliferation elicits effective antitumor autoimmunity. J Clin Invest 110:185–192

Edinger M, Hoffmann P, Ermann J, Drago K, Fathman CG, Strober S, Negrin RS (2003) CD4+CD25+ regulatory T cells preserve graft-versus-tumor activity while inhibiting graft-versus-host disease after bone marrow transplantation. Nat Med 9:1144–1150

Ege H, Gertz MA, Markovic SN, Lacy MQ, Dispenzieri A, Hayman SR, Kumar SK, Porrata LF (2008) Prediction of survival using absolute lymphocyte count for newly diagnosed patients with multiple myeloma: a retrospective study. Br J Haematol 141:792–798

Ernst B, Lee DS, Chang JM, Sprent J, Surh CD (1999) The peptide ligands mediating positive selection in the thymus control T cell survival and homeostatic proliferation in the periphery. Immunity 11:173–181

Fearon DT, Manders P, Wagner SD (2001) Arrested differentiation, the self-renewing memory lymphocyte, and vaccination. Science 293:248–250

Fowler DH, Odom J, Steinberg SM, Chow CK, Foley J, Kogan Y, Hou J, Gea-Banacloche J, Sportes C, Pavletic S, Leitman S, Read EJ, Carter C, Kolstad A, Fox R, Beatty GL, Vonderheide RH, Levine BL, June CH, Gress RE, Bishop MR (2006) Phase I clinical trial of costimulated, IL-4 polarized donor CD4+ T cells as augmentation of allogeneic hematopoietic cell transplantation. Biol Blood Marrow Transplant 12:1150–1160

George RE, Li S, Medeiros-Nancarrow C, Neuberg D, Marcus K, Shamberger RC, Pulsipher M, Grupp SA, Diller L (2006) High-risk neuroblastoma treated with tandem autologous peripheral-blood stem cell-supported transplantation: long-term survival update. J Clin Oncol 24:2891–2896

Golovina TN, Mikheeva T, Suhoski MM, Aqui NA, Tai VC, Shan X, Liu R, Balcarcel RR, Fisher N, Levine BL, Carroll RC, Warner N, Blazar BR, June CH, Riley JL (2008) CD28 costimulation is essential for human T regulatory expansion and function. J Immunol 181:2855–2868

Gross G, Waks T, Eshhar Z (1989) Expression of immunoglobulin-T cell receptor chimeric molecules as functional receptors with antibody-type specificity. Proc Natl Acad Sci USA 86:10024–10028

Grupp SA, Stern JW, Bunin N, Nancarrow C, Adams R, Gorlin JB, Griffin G, Diller L (2000a) Rapid-sequence tandem transplant for children with high-risk neuroblastoma. Med Pediatr Oncol 35:696–700

Grupp SA, Stern JW, Bunin N, Nancarrow C, Ross AA, Mogul M, Adams R, Grier HE, Gorlin JB, Shamberger R, Marcus K, Neuberg D, Weinstein HJ, Diller L (2000b) Tandem high-dose therapy in rapid sequence for children with high-risk neuroblastoma. J Clin Oncol 18:2567–2575

Guimond M, Veenstra R, Grindler D, Zhang H, Cui Y, Murphy R, Kim S, Na R, Hennighausen L, Kurtulus S (2009) Interleukin 7 signaling in dendritic cells regulates the homeostatic proliferation and niche size of CD4+ T cells. Nat Immunol 10:149–157

Hacein-Bey-Abina S, Garrigue A, Wang GP, Soulier J, Lim A, Morillon E, Clappier E, Caccavelli L, Delabesse E, Beldjord K, Asnafi V, Macintyre E, Dal CL, Radford I, Brousse N, Sigaux F, Moshous D, Hauer J, Borkhardt A, Belohradsky BH, Wintergerst U, Velez MC, Leiva L, Sorensen R, Wulffraat N, Blanche S, Bushman FD, Fischer A, Cavazzana-Calvo M (2008)

Insertional oncogenesis in 4 patients after retrovirus-mediated gene therapy of SCID-X1. J Clin Invest 118:3132–3142

Hakim F, Cepeda R, Kaimei S, Mackall C, McAtee N, Zujewski J, Cowan K, Gress R (1997) Constraints on CD4 recovery postchemotherapy in adults: thymic insufficiency and apoptotic decline of expanded peripheral CD4 cells. Blood 90:3789–3798

Hamza N, Lisgaris M, Yadavalli G, Nadeau L, Fox R, Fu P, Lazarus H, Koc O, Salata R, Laughlin M (2004) Kinetics of myeloid and lymphocyte recovery and infectious complications after unrelated umbilical cord blood versus HLA-matched unrelated donor allogeneic transplantation in adults. Br J Haematol 124:488–498

Hasan A, Kollen W, Trivedi D, Selvakumar A, Dupont B, Sadelain M, O'Reilly R (2009) A panel of artificial APCs Expressing prevalent HLA alleles permits generation of cytotoxic T cells specific for both dominant and subdominant viral epitopes for adoptive therapy. J Immunol 183:2837–2850

Hinrichs C, Kaiser A, Paulos C, Cassard L, Sanchez-Perez L, Heemskerk B, Wrzesinski C, Borman Z, Muranski P, Restifo N (2009) Type 17 CD8+ T cells display enhanced antitumor immunity. Blood 114:596–599

Hirano N, Butler MO, Xia Z, Ansen S, von Bergwelt-Baildon MS, Neuberg D, Freeman GJ, Nadler LM (2006) Engagement of CD83 ligand induces prolonged expansion of CD8+ T cells and preferential enrichment for antigen specificity. Blood 107:1528–1536

Hoyle C, Goldman JM (1994) Life-threatening infections occurring more than 3 months after BMT. Bone Marrow Transplant 14:247–252

Janssen EM, Lemmens EE, Wolfe T, Christen U, von Herrath MG, Schoenberger SP (2003) CD4+ T cells are required for secondary expansion and memory in CD8+ T lymphocytes. Nature 421:852–856

Johnson LA, Morgan RA, Dudley ME, Cassard L, Yang JC, Hughes MS, Kammula US, Royal RE, Sherry RM, Wunderlich JR, Lee CC, Restifo NP, Schwarz SL, Cogdill AP, Bishop RJ, Kim H, Brewer CC, Rudy SF, Vanwaes C, Davis JL, Mathur A, Ripley RT, Nathan DA, Laurencot CM, Rosenberg SA (2009) Gene therapy with human and mouse T cell receptors mediates cancer regression and targets normal tissues expressing cognate antigen. Blood 114:535–546

June CH (2007) Principles of adoptive T cell cancer therapy. J Clin Invest 117:1204–1212

June CH, Blazar BR, Riley JL (2009) Engineering lymphocyte subsets: tools, trials and tribulations. Nat Rev Immunol 9:704–716

Kaech SM, Ahmed R (2001) Memory CD8+ T cell differentiation: initial antigen encounter triggers a developmental program in naive cells. Nat Immunol 2:415–422

Kalamasz D, Long SA, Taniguchi R, Buckner JH, Berenson RJ, Bonyhadi M (2004) Optimization of human T cell expansion exvivo using magnetic beads conjugated with anti-CD3 and Anti-CD28 antibodies. J Immunother 27:405–418

Kim JV, Latouche JB, Riviere I, Sadelain M (2004) The ABCs of artificial antigen presentation. Nat Biotechnol 22:403–410

King C, Ilic A, Koelsch K, Sarvetnick N (2004) Homeostatic expansion of T cells during immune insufficiency generates autoimmunity. Cell 117:265–277

Kletzel M, Katzenstein HM, Haut PR, Yu AL, Morgan E, Reynolds M, Geissler G, Marymount MH, Liu D, Kalapurakal JA, Shore RM, Bardo DM, Schmoldt J, Rademaker AW, Cohn SL (2002) Treatment of high-risk neuroblastoma with triple-tandem high-dose therapy and stem-cell rescue: results of the Chicago Pilot II Study. J Clin Oncol 20:2284–2292

Korn T, Bettelli E, Oukka M, Kuchroo VK (2009) IL-17 and Th17 Cells. Annu Rev Immunol 27:485–517

Kroon F, van Dissel J, de Jong J, van Furth R (1994) Antibody response to influenza, tetanus and pneumococcal vaccines in HIV-seropositive individuals in relation to the number of CD4+ lymphocytes. Aids 8:469–476

Kryczek I, Banerjee M, Cheng P, Vatan L, Szeliga W, Wei S, Huang E, Finlayson E, Simeone D, Welling T (2009) Phenotype, distribution, generation, and functional and clinical relevance of Th17 cells in the human tumor environments. Blood 114:1141–1149

Lamers CH, Sleijfer S, Vulto AG, Kruit WH, Kliffen M, Debets R, Gratama JW, Stoter G, Oosterwijk E (2006) Treatment of metastatic renal cell carcinoma with autologous T-lymphocytes genetically retargeted against carbonic anhydrase IX: first clinical experience. J Clin Oncol 24:e20–e22

Landmeier S, Altvater B, Pscherer S, Eing BR, Kuehn J, Rooney CM, Juergens H, Rossig C (2007) Gene-engineered varicella-zoster virus reactive CD4+ cytotoxic T cells exert tumor-specific effector function. Cancer Res 67:8335–8343

Langowski JL, Zhang XQ, Wu LL, Mattson JD, Chen TY, Smith K, Basham B, McClanahan T, Kastelein RA, Oft M (2006) IL-23 promotes tumour incidence and growth. Nature 442:461–465

Lanzavecchia A, Sallusto F (2005) Understanding the generation and function of memory T cell subsets. Curr Opin Immunol 17:326–332

Laport GG, Levine BL, Stadtmauer EA, Schuster SJ, Luger SM, Grupp S, Bunin N, Strobl FJ, Cotte J, Zheng Z, Gregson B, Rivers P, Vonderheide RH, Liebowitz DN, Porter DL, June CH (2003) Adoptive transfer of costimulated T cells induces lymphocytosis in patients with relapsed/refractory non-Hodgkin's lymphoma following CD34-selected hematopoietic cell transplantation. Blood 102:2004–2013

Latouche JB, Sadelain M (2000) Induction of human cytotoxic T lymphocytes by artificial antigen-presenting cells. Nat Biotechnol 18:405–409

Lerner B (2004) Sins of omission–cancer research without informed consent. N Engl J Med 351:628

Levine B, Bernstein W, Connors M, Craighead N, Lindsten T, Thompson C, June C (1997) Effects of CD28 costimulation on long-term proliferation of CD4+ T cells in the absence of exogenous feeder cells. J Immunol 159:5921–5930

Levine BL, Ueda Y, Craighead N, Huang ML, June CH (1995) CD28 ligands CD80 (B7-1) and CD86 (B&-2) induce long-term autocrine growth of CD4+ T cells and induce similar patterns of cytokine secretion in vitro. Int Immunol 7:891–904

Lin W, Karin M (2007) A cytokine-mediated link between innate immunity, inflammation, and cancer. J Clin Invest 117:1175–1183

Lone YC, Motta I, Mottez E, Guilloux Y, Lim A, Demay F, Levraud JP, Kourilsky P, Abastado JP (1998) In vitro induction of specific cytotoxic T lymphocytes using recombinant single-chain MHC class I/peptide complexes. J Immunother 21:283–294

Luxembourg AT, Borrow P, Teyton L, Brunmark AB, Peterson PA, Jackson MR (1998) Biomagnetic isolation of antigen-specific CD8+ T cells usable in immunotherapy. Nat Biotechnol 16:281–285

Mackall CL, Fleisher TA, Brown MR, Andrich MP, Chen CC, Feuerstein IM, Magrath IT, Wexler LH, Dimitrov DS, Gress RE (1997) Distinctions between CD8+ and CD4+ T cell regenerative pathways result in prolonged T cell subset imbalance after intensive chemotherapy. Blood 89:3700–3707

Maher J, Brentjens RJ, Gunset G, Riviere I, Sadelain M (2002) Human T-lymphocyte cytotoxicity and proliferation directed by a single chimeric TCRzeta /CD28 receptor. Nat Biotechnol 20:70–75

Maris JM, Hogarty MD, Bagatell R, Cohn SL (2007) Neuroblastoma. Lancet 369:2106–2120

Martin-Orozco N, Muranski P, Chung Y, Yang X, Yamazaki T, Lu S, Hwu P, Restifo N, Overwijk W, Dong C (2009) T helper 17 cells promote cytotoxic T cell activation in tumor immunity. Immunity 31:787–798

Matthay KK, Villablanca JG, Seeger RC, Stram DO, Harris RE, Ramsay NK, Swift P, Shimada H, Black CT, Brodeur GM, Gerbing RB, Reynolds CP (1999) Treatment of high-risk neuroblastoma with intensive chemotherapy, radiotherapy, autologous bone marrow transplantation, and 13-cis-retinoic acid. Children's Cancer group. N Engl J Med 341:1165–1173

Maus MV, Kovacs B, Kwok WW, Nepom GT, Schlienger K, Riley JL, Allman D, Finkel TH, June CH (2004) Extensive replicative capacity of human central memory T cells. J Immunol 172:6675–6683

Maus MV, Thomas AK, Leonard DG, Allman D, Addya K, Schlienger K, Riley JL, June CH (2002) Ex vivo expansion of polyclonal and antigen-specific cytotoxic T lymphocytes by artificial APCs expressing ligands for the T cell receptor, CD28 and 4-1BB. Nat Biotechnol 20:143–148

Milone MC, Fish JD, Carpenito C, Carroll RG, Binder GK, Teachey D, Samanta M, Lakhal M, Gloss B, net-Desnoyers G, Campana D, Riley JL, Grupp G, June CH (2009) Chimeric receptors containing CD137 signal transduction domains mediate enhanced survival of T cells and increased antileukemic efficacy in vivo. Mol Ther 17:1453–1464

Mitchison NA (1955) Studies on the immunological response to foreign tumor transplants in the mouse I. The role of lymph node cells in conferring immunity by adoptive transfer. J Exp Med 102:157–177

Molrine D, Guinan E, Antin J, Parsons S, Weinstein H, Wheeler C, McGarigle C, Blanding P, Phillips N, Kinsella K (1996) Donor immunization with Haemophilus influenzae type b (HIB)-conjugate vaccine in allogeneic bone marrow transplantation. Blood 87:3012–3018

Morgan R, Yang J, Kitano M, Dudley M, Laurencot C, Rosenberg S (2010) Case report of a serious adverse event following the administration of T cells transduced with a chimeric antigen receptor recognizing ERBB2. Mol Ther 18:843–851

Mueller M, Fusenig N (2004) Friends or foes—bipolar effects of the tumour stroma in cancer. Nat Rev Cancer 4:839–849

Muranski P, Boni A, Antony PA, Cassard L, Irvine KR, Kaiser A, Paulos CM, Palmer DC, Touloukian CE, Ptak K (2008) Tumor-specific Th17-polarized cells eradicate large established melanoma. Blood 112:362–373

Muul LM, Tuschong LM, Soenen SL, Jagadeesh GJ, Ramsey WJ, Long Z, Carter CS, Garabedian EK, Alleyne M, Brown M, Bernstein W, Schurman SH, Fleisher TA, Leitman SF, Dunbar CE, Blaese RM, Candotti F (2003) Persistence and expression of the adenosine deaminase gene for 12 years and immune reaction to gene transfer components: long-term results of the first clinical gene therapy trial. Blood 101:2563–2569

Nguyen P, Moisini I, Geiger T (2003) Identification of a murine CD28 dileucine motif that suppresses single-chain chimeric T cell receptor expression and function. Blood 102:4320

Oelke M, Maus MV, Didiano D, June CH, Mackensen A, Schneck JP (2003) Ex vivo induction and expansion of antigen-specific cytotoxic T cells by HLA-Ig coated artificial antigen presenting cells. Nat Med 9:619–625

Park JR, Digiusto DL, Slovak M, Wright C, Naranjo A, Wagner J, Meechoovet HB, Bautista C, Chang WC, Ostberg JR, Jensen MC (2007) Adoptive transfer of chimeric antigen receptor re-directed cytolytic T lymphocyte clones in patients with neuroblastoma. Mol Ther 15:825–833

Porrata LF, Gertz MA, Inwards DJ, Litzow MR, Lacy MQ, Tefferi A, Gastineau DA, Dispenzieri A, Ansell SM, Micallef IN, Geyer SM, Markovic SN (2001) Early lymphocyte recovery predicts superior survival after autologous hematopoietic stem cell transplantation in multiple myeloma or non-Hodgkin lymphoma. Blood 98:579–585

Porter DL, Levine BL, Bunin N, Stadtmauer EA, Luger SM, Goldstein S, Loren A, Phillips J, Nasta S, Perl A, Schuster S, Tsai D, Sohal A, Veloso E, Emerson SG, June CH (2006) A phase I trial of donor lymphocyte infusions expanded and activated ex-vivo via CD3/CD28 co-stimulation. Blood 107:1325–1331

Powell JL, Bunin NJ, Callahan C, Aplenc R, Griffin G, Grupp SA (2004) An unexpectedly high incidence of Epstein-Barr virus lymphoproliferative disease after CD34+ selected autologous peripheral blood stem cell transplant in neuroblastoma. Bone Marrow Transplant 33:651–657

Pule MA, Straathof KC, Dotti G, Heslop HE, Rooney CM and Brenner MK (2005) A chimeric T cell antigen receptor that augments cytokine release and supports clonal expansion of primary human T cells. Mol Ther 12:933–941

Pule M, Savoldo B, Myers G, Rossig C, Russell H, Dotti G, Huls M, Liu E, Gee A, Mei Z (2008) Virus-specific T cells engineered to coexpress tumor-specific receptors: persistence and anti-tumor activity in individuals with neuroblastoma. Nat Med 14:1264–1270

Pulle G, Vidric M, Watts TH (2006) IL-15-dependent induction of 4-1BB promotes antigen-independent CD8 memory T cell survival. J Immunol 176:2739–2748

Rapoport A, Stadtmauer EA, Aqui N, Badros A, Cotte J, Chrisley L, Veloso EA, Zheng Z, Westphal S, Mair R, Chi N, Ratterree B, Pochran MF, Natt S, Hinkle J, Sickles C, Sohal A, Ruehle K, Lynch C, Zhang L, Porter DL, Luger S, Guo C, Fang HB, Blackwelder W, Hankey K, Mann D, Edelman R, Frasch C, Levine BL, Cross A, June CH (2005) Restoration of immunity in lymphopenic individuals with cancer by vaccination and adoptive T cell transfer. Nat Med 11:1230–1237

Rapoport AP, Stadtmauer EA, Aqui N, Vogl D, Chew A, Fang HB, Janofsky S, Yager K, Veloso E, Zheng Z, Milliron T, Westphal S, Cotte J, Huynh H, Cannon A, Yanovich S, Akpek G, Tan M, Virts K, Ruehle K, Harris C, Philip S, Vonderheide RH, Levine BL, June CH (2009) Rapid immune recovery and graft-versus-host disease-like engraftment syndrome following adoptive transfer of costimulated autologous T cells. Clin Cancer Res 15:4499–4507

Riddell SR, Greenberg PD (1990) The use of anti-CD3 and anti-CD28 monoclonal antibodies to clone and expand human antigen-specific T cells. J Immunol Methods 128:189–201

Riley JL, June CH, Blazar BR (2009) Human T regulatory cell therapy: take a billion and call me in the morning. Immunity 30:656–665

Rosenberg SA, Aebersold P, Cornetta K, Kasid A, Morgan RA, Moen R, Karson EM, Lotze MT, Yang JC, Topalian SL (1990) Gene transfer into humans–immunotherapy of patients with advanced melanoma, using tumor-infiltrating lymphocytes modified by retroviral gene transduction. N Engl J Med 323:570–578

Rossig C, Bollard CM, Nuchtern JG, Merchant DA, Brenner MK (2001) Targeting of G(D2)-positive tumor cells by human T lymphocytes engineered to express chimeric T cell receptor genes. Int J Cancer 94:228–236

Roux E, Helg C, Dumont-Girard F, Chapuis B, Jeannet M, Roosnek E (1996) Analysis of T cell repopulation after allogeneic bone marrow transplantation: significant differences between recipients of T cell depleted and unmanipulated grafts. Blood 87:3984–3992

Sadelain M, Brentjens R, Riviere I (2009) The promise and potential pitfalls of chimeric antigen receptors. Curr Opin Immunol 21:215–223

Sallusto F, Geginat J, Lanzavecchia A (2004) Central memory and effector memory T cell subsets: function, generation, and maintenance. Annu Rev Immunol 22:745–763

Salomon B, Lenschow D, Rhee L, Ashourian N, Singh B, Sharpe A, Bluestone J (2000) B7/CD28 costimulation is essential for the homeostasis of the CD4+ CD25+ immunoregulatory T cells that control autoimmune diabetes. Immunity 12:431–440

Schultze JL, Michalak S, Seamon MJ, Dranoff G, Jung K, Daley J, Delgado JC, Gribben JG, Nadler LM (1997) CD40-activated human B cells: an alternative source of highly efficient antigen presenting cells to generate autologous antigen-specific T cells for adoptive immunotherapy. J Clin Invest 100:2757–2765

Schumacher TN (2002) T cell-receptor gene therapy. Nat Rev Immunol 2:512–519

Seder RA, Darrah PA, Roederer M (2008) T cell quality in memory and protection: implications for vaccine design. Nat Rev Immunol 211:58–66

Simon T, Hero B, Faldum A, Handgretinger R, Schrappe M, Niethammer D, Berthold F (2004) Consolidation treatment with chimeric anti-GD2-antibody ch14.18 in children older than 1 year with metastatic neuroblastoma. J Clin Oncol 22:3549–3557

Southam CM, Brunschwig A, Levin AG, Dizon QS (1966) Effect of leukocytes on transplantability of human cancer. Cancer 19:1743–1753

Storek J, Dawson M, Lim L, Burman B, Stevens-Ayers T, Viganego F, Herremans M, Flowers M, Witherspoon R, Maloney D (2003) Efficacy of donor vaccination before hematopoietic cell transplantation and recipient vaccination both before and early after transplantation. Bone Marrow Transplant 33:337–346

Storek J, Dawson MA, Storer B, Stevens-Ayers T, Maloney DG, Marr KA, Witherspoon RP, Bensinger W, Flowers ME, Martin P, Storb R, Appelbaum FR, Boeckh M (2001) Immune reconstitution after allogeneic marrow transplantation compared with blood stem cell transplantation. Blood 97:3380–3389

Storek J, Zhao Z, Lin E, Berger T, McSweeney P, Nash R, Akatsuka Y, Metcalf M, Lu H, Kalina T (2004) Recovery from and consequences of severe iatrogenic lymphopenia (induced to treat autoimmune diseases). Clin Immunol 113:285–298

Suhoski MM, Golovina T, Aqui NA, Tai VC, Varela R, MiloneMc CRG, Riley JL, June CH (2007) Engineering artificial antigen presenting cells to express a diverse array of co-stimulatory molecules. Mol Ther 15:981–988

Surh C, Sprent J (2008) Homeostasis of naive and memory T cells. Immunity 29:848–862

Taylor PA, Lees CJ, Blazar BR (2002) The infusion of ex vivo activated and expanded CD4(+) CD25(+) immune regulatory cells inhibits graft-versus-host disease lethality. Blood 99: 3493–3499

Thedrez A, Sabourin C, Gertner J, Devilder MC, lain-Maillet S, Fournie JJ, Scotet E, Bonneville M (2007) Self/non-self discrimination by human gammadelta T cells: simple solutions for a complex issue? Immunol Rev 215:123–135

Thomas ED (1999) Bone marrow transplantation: a review. Semin Hematol 36:95–103

Turtle C, Swanson H, Fujii N, Estey E, Riddell S (2009) A distinct subset of self-renewing human memory CD8+ T cells survives cytotoxic chemotherapy. Immunity 31:834–844

van der Veeken LT, Coccoris M, Swart E, Falkenburg JH, Schumacher TN, Heemskerk MH (2009) Alpha beta T cell receptor transfer to gamma delta T cells generates functional effector cells without mixed TCR dimers in vivo. J Immunol 182:164–170

Varela-Rohena A, Molloy PE, Dunn SM, Li Y, Suhoski M, Carroll RG, Milicic A, Mahon T, Suttton DH, Laugel BE, Moysy R, Cameron BJ, Vuidepot A, Prubhoo ME, Cole DK, Philllps RE, June CH, Jakobsen BK, Sewell AK, Riley JL (2008) Control of HIV-1 immune escape by CD8 T cells expressing enhanced T cell receptor. Nat Med 14:1390–1395 [Epub 2008 Nov 1399]

Weiden PL, Flournoy N, Thomas ED, Prentice R, Fefer A, Buckner CD, Storb R (1979) Antileukemic effect of graft-versus-host disease in human recipients of allogeneic-marrow grafts. N Engl J Med 300:1068–1073

Weng NP (2006) Aging of the immune system: How much can the adaptive immune system adapt? Immunity 24:495–499

Weng NP, Levine BL, June CH, Hodes RJ (1997) Regulation of telomerase RNA template expression in human T lymphocyte development and activation. J Immunol 158:3215–3220

Woo EY, Chu CS, Goletz TJ, Schlienger K, Coukos G, Rubin SC, Kaiser LR, June CH (2001) Regulatory CD4+CD25+ T cells in tumors from patients with early-stage non small cell lung cancer and late-stage ovarian cancer. Cancer Res 61:4766–4772

Zhang H, Snyder K, Suhoski MM, Maus MV, Kapoor V, June CH, Mackall CL (2007) 4-1BB is superior to CD28 costimulation for generating CD8+ cytotoxic lymphocytes for adoptive immunotherapy. J Immunol 179:4910–4918

Zhang L, Conejo-Garcia JR, Katsaros D, Gimotty PA, Massobrio M, Regnani G, Makrigiannakis A, Gray H, Schlienger K, Liebman MN, Rubin SC, Coukos G (2003) Intratumoral T cells, recurrence, and survival in epithelial ovarian cancer. N Engl J Med 348:203–213

Zhang Y, Joe G, Hexner E, Zhu J, Emerson SG (2005) Host-reactive CD8+ memory stem cells in graft-versus-host disease. Nat Med 11:1299–1305

Zhou J, Shen X, Huang J, Hodes RJ, Rosenberg SA, Robbins PF (2005) Telomere length of transferred lymphocytes correlates with in vivo persistence and tumor regression in melanoma patients receiving cell transfer therapy. J Immunol 175:7046–7052

Zhou L, Chong M, Littman D (2009) Plasticity of CD4+ T cell lineage differentiation. Immunity 30:646–655

Zhu Y, Zhu G, Luo L, Flies AS, Chen L (2007) CD137 stimulation delivers an antigen-independent growth signal for T lymphocytes with memory phenotype. Blood 109:4882–4889

Dendritic Cell Subsets as Vectors and Targets for Improved Cancer Therapy

Karolina Palucka, Hideki Ueno, Lee Roberts, Joseph Fay, and Jacques Banchereau

Contents

1 Introduction 174
2 Dendritic Cells 175
  2.1 Human Dendritic Cell Subsets 175
  2.2 DCs in Tumor Environment 178
3 Dendritic Cells in Vaccination Against Cancer 180
  3.1 Outcomes of Current DC Vaccination Trials 180
  3.2 The Quality of Elicited Antigen-Specific Immune Responses 180
4 Building on Dendritic Cell Subsets to Improve Cancer Vaccines 181
  4.1 Optimal DCs 181
  4.2 "Ideal" Antigens 182
  4.3 Combining DC Vaccines with Other Therapies 183
5 Concluding Remarks 185
References 186

Abstract Current active immunotherapy trials have shown durable tumor regressions in a fraction of patients. However, the clinical efficacy of current vaccines is limited, possibly because tumors skew the immune system by means of myeloid-derived suppressor cells, inflammatory Type 2 T cells and regulatory T cells (Tregs), all of which prevent the generation of effector cells. To improve the

K. Palucka (✉) and J. Banchereau
Baylor Institute for Immunology Research, 3434 Live Oak, Dallas, TX 75204, USA
Department of Gene and Cell Medicine, Mount Sinai School of Medicine, New York, NY, USA
e-mail: karolinp@baylorhealth.edu

H. Ueno and L. Roberts
Baylor Institute for Immunology Research, 3434 Live Oak, Dallas, TX 75204, USA

J. Fay
Sammons Cancer Center, Baylor University Medical Center, Dallas, TX, USA

G. Dranoff (ed.), *Cancer Immunology and Immunotherapy*,
Current Topics in Microbiology and Immunology 344, DOI 10.1007/82_2010_48

clinical efficacy of cancer vaccines in patients with metastatic disease, we need to design novel and improved strategies that can boost adaptive immunity to cancer, help overcome Tregs and allow the breakdown of the immunosuppressive tumor microenvironment. This can be achieved by exploiting the fast increasing knowledge about the dendritic cell (DC) system, including the existence of distinct DC subsets. Critical to the design of better vaccines is the concept of distinct DC subsets and distinct DC activation pathways, all contributing to the generation of unique adaptive immune responses. Such novel DC vaccines will be used as monotherapy in patients with resected disease and in combination with antibodies and/or drugs targeting suppressor pathways and modulation of the tumor environment in patients with metastatic disease.

1 Introduction

Vaccines against infectious agents demonstrate the power of manipulating the immune system. Vaccines have spared countless numbers of people from polio, measles, tetanus, etc. (Nossal 1997), even though they have not been designed according to immunological principles (Doherty et al. 2006). Immunology has the potential to identify vaccines, i.e., antigen-specific, durable, non-noxious preventions and therapies for infections, cancer, allergy, autoimmunity, transplantation. This has formed a conceptual basis for the development of therapeutic vaccines in cancer. Molecular identification of human cancer antigens has ushered in a new era of antigen specific cancer immunotherapy specifically targeting these antigens. Initial attempts (e.g., peptides, DNA vaccines, viral vectors and first generation dendritic cell (DC)-based vaccines) have thus far met with a limited success in the clinic. However, cancer vaccines are in a renaissance era due to recent clinical trials showing promising immunological data and some clinical benefit to the patients. For example, an active immunotherapy product, sipuleucel-T (APC8015) based on antigen-loaded and GM-CSF activated PBMCs, appears to contribute to prolonged median survival in phase III trials in patients with prostate cancer (Higano et al. 2009). Similarly, a randomized phase II trial of a pox viral-based vaccine targeting PSA (PROSTVAC) in men with metastatic castration-resistant prostate cancer showed improved overall survival in patients who received PROSTVAC compared to those who received control vectors (Kantoff et al. 2010). While these first generation positive randomized phase II/III clinical trials need further analysis and mechanistic studies, they underline the therapeutic potential of the immune system that can be tapped into. Vaccines act through DCs, which induce, regulate and maintain T cell immunity. In this chapter, we summarize our recent studies aimed at a better understanding of the DC system to unravel the pathophysiology of cancer and to design novel cancer vaccines.

2 Dendritic Cells

Generating the right type of immune response can be a matter of life and death. In leprosy, for instance, the tuberculoid form of the disease is characterized by a Type 1 response which keeps the disease in check, while the lepromatous form induces an often fatal Type 2 response (Yamamura et al. 1991). These responses are under the control of DCs (Banchereau and Steinman 1998; Steinman and Banchereau 2007). DCs reside in peripheral tissues and in lymph nodes where they are poised to capture antigens (Ags). DCs present processed protein and lipid Ags to T cells via both classical (MHC class I and class II) and non-classical (CD1 family) antigen presenting molecules (Heath and Carbone 2009) (Fig. 1). In the steady state, non-activated (immature) DCs present self-antigens to T cells, which leads to tolerance (Hawiger et al. 2001; Steinman et al. 2003). DCs induce immune tolerance in a number of ways including (a) T cell deletion (Fairchild and Austyn 1990; Zal et al. 1994; Volkmann et al. 1997); (b) induction of T cell unresponsiveness (Hawiger et al. 2004); and (c) activation of regulatory T cells (Tregs) (Jonuleit et al. 2000; Akbari et al. 2001; Wing and Sakaguchi 2010; Zheng et al. 2010). Once activated (mature), antigen-loaded DCs are geared towards the launching of antigen-specific immunity (Finkelman et al. 1996; Brimnes et al. 2003) leading to the T cell proliferation and differentiation into helper and effector cells. DCs are also important in launching humoral immunity partly due to their capacity to directly interact with B cells (Jego et al. 2005; Qi et al. 2006) and to present unprocessed antigens (Zhong et al. 1997; Wykes et al. 1998; Bergtold et al. 2005; Batista and Harwood 2009).

2.1 Human Dendritic Cell Subsets

To allow resistance to infection and tolerance to self, DCs are endowed with two critical features: subsets and functional plasticity (Steinman and Banchereau 2007). The two major subsets are the myeloid DCs (mDCs) and the plasmacytoid DCs (pDCs). The best studied human mDC subsets are those from skin, where three subsets can be identified. The epidermis hosts only Langerhans Cells (LCs) while the dermis displays two mDC subsets, $CD1a^+$ DCs and $CD14^+$ DCs, as well as macrophages (Zaba et al. 2007; Klechevsky et al. 2008; Merad et al. 2008; Nestle et al. 2009).

2.1.1 Dermal DCs, Antibody Responses and IL-12

In the mid 1990s, we observed that $CD14^+$ DCs derived from $CD34^+$ hematopoietic progenitor cells (HPCs) induce CD40-activated naïve B cells to differentiate into IgM-producing plasma cells through the secretion of IL-6 and IL-12 (Caux et al. 1997).

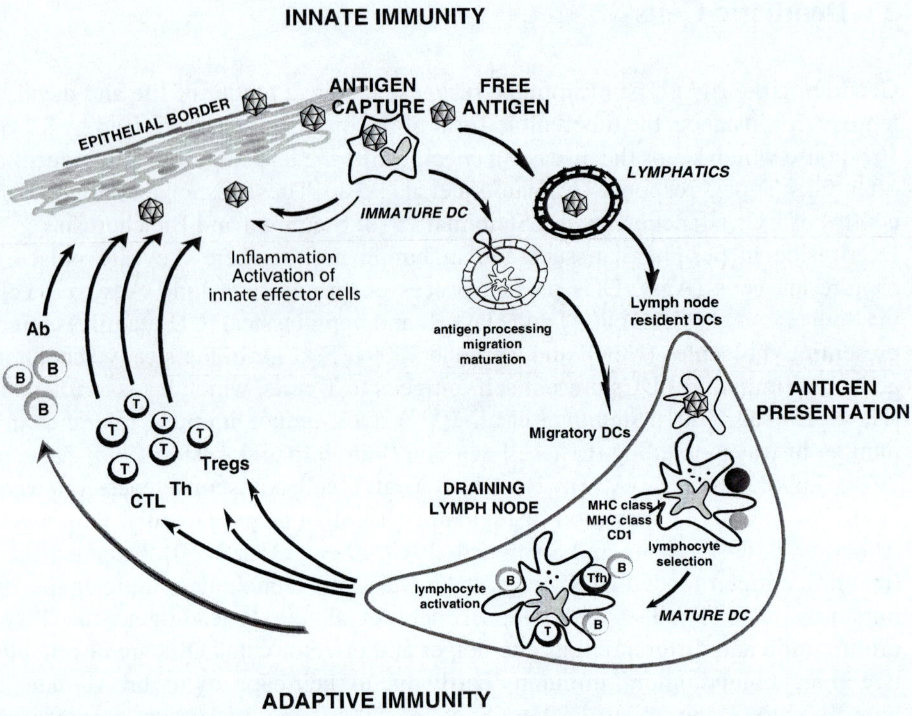

Fig. 1 *Dendritic cells*. DCs reside in the tissue where they are poised to capture antigens (Geissmann et al. 2010). During inflammation, circulating precursor DC enter tissues as immature DC (Geissmann et al. 2010). DCs can encounter pathogens (e.g., viruses) directly, which induce secretion of cytokines (e.g., IFN-α); or indirectly through the pathogen effect on stromal cells. Cytokines secreted by DCs in turn activate effector cells of innate immunity such as eosinophils, macrophages and NK cells. Microbe activation triggers DCs migration towards secondary lymphoid organs and simultaneous activation (maturation). These activated migratory DCs that enter lymphoid organs display antigens in the context of classical MHC class I and class II or non-classical CD1 molecules, which allow selection of rare circulating antigen-specific T lymphocytes. Activated T cells help drive DCs toward their terminal maturation, which allows lymphocyte expansion and differentiation. Activated T lymphocytes traverse inflamed epithelia and reach the injured tissue, where they eliminate microbes and/or microbe-infected cells. B cells, activated by DCs and T cells, migrate into various areas where they mature into plasma cells that produce antibodies that neutralize the initial pathogen. Antigen can also reach draining lymph nodes without involvement of peripheral tissue DCs and be captured and presented by lymph node resident DCs (Itano et al. 2003)

A decade later, we found that CD14$^+$ DCs, but not LCs, induce naïve CD4$^+$ T cells to differentiate into cells with properties of T follicular helper cells (Tfh) (Klechevsky et al. 2008), a CD4$^+$ T cell subset specialized in B cell help (King et al. 2008; Fazilleau et al. 2009). There, CD4$^+$ T cells primed by CD14$^+$ DCs help naïve B cells to produce large amounts of IgM, and switch isotypes towards IgG and IgA. Our recent studies in human indicate that acquisition of Tfh phenotype and function depends on IL-12p70 (Schmitt et al. 2009).

Thus, IL-12 appears to contribute to humoral immunity in humans through a direct path in DC-B interaction, and an indirect path in DC-T cell interaction and induction of Tfh cells. These findings might explain the modest clinical efficacy of systemic IL-12 administration in cancer patients (Motzer et al. 2001; Cheever 2008). Furthermore, the injection of IL-12 into tumor sites of head and neck cancer patients resulted in the activation of B cells in the draining lymph nodes, which was associated with their infiltration into tumor sites and tumor regression (van Herpen et al. 2008).

2.1.2 LCs and CD8$^+$ T Cell Responses

LCs induce a robust proliferation of naïve allogeneic CD8$^+$ T cells when compared to CD14$^+$ DCs (Klechevsky et al. 2008). Furthermore, when pulsed with MHC class I peptides derived from tumor or viral antigens, LCs are far more efficient than CD14$^+$ DCs in the priming of antigen-specific CD8$^+$ T cells. LCs are also efficient in cross-presenting peptides from protein antigens to CD8$^+$ T cells. CD8$^+$ T cells primed by LCs show high avidity in tetramer binding assays and express higher levels of cytotoxic molecules, such as granzymes and perforin. Accordingly, they are remarkably more efficient in killing target cells; in particular tumor cells that express low level of peptide/HLA complexes (Klechevsky et al. 2008). IL-15 might explain the remarkable effects of LCs in the development of Cytotoxic T Lymphocyte (CTL) responses (Mohamadzadeh et al. 2001; Dubsky et al. 2007; Klechevsky et al. 2009). Thus, the two different arms of adaptive immunity, i.e., humoral and cellular arms, might be differentially regulated by the two skin mDC subsets (Fig. 2). Such a framework might be of capital importance for the understanding of the immune alteration in malignancy and for the development of novel and improved vaccination strategies against cancer, as well as chronic infections.

2.1.3 Plasmacytoid DCs

Plasmacytoid DCs (pDCs) are considered as the front line in anti-viral immunity owning to their capacity to rapidly produce high amounts of Type I interferon (Siegal et al. 1999; Liu 2005). Similar to mDCs, pDCs display a remarkable functional plasticity. Thus, pDCs exposed to viruses, such as live influenza virus, are able to launch memory responses by inducing the expansion and differentiation of antigen-specific memory B and T lymphocytes into plasma cells (Jego et al. 2003), and CTLs (Fonteneau et al. 2003; Di Pucchio et al. 2008), respectively. On the contrary, pDCs activated with CpG or IL-3/CD40L induce in vitro IL-10-secreting regulatory CD4$^+$ T cells (Ito et al. 2007) as well as suppressor CD8$^+$ T cells through the expression of ICOS ligand (Gilliet and Liu 2002).

Human pDCs, in fact, are composed of two subsets, distinguished by the expression of CD2 (Matsui et al. 2009). CD2^{high} pDCs are more potent than the CD2^{low} pDCs to induce allogeneic T cell proliferation. These different functional properties of CD2^{high} pDCs and CD2^{low} pDCs are associated with distinct

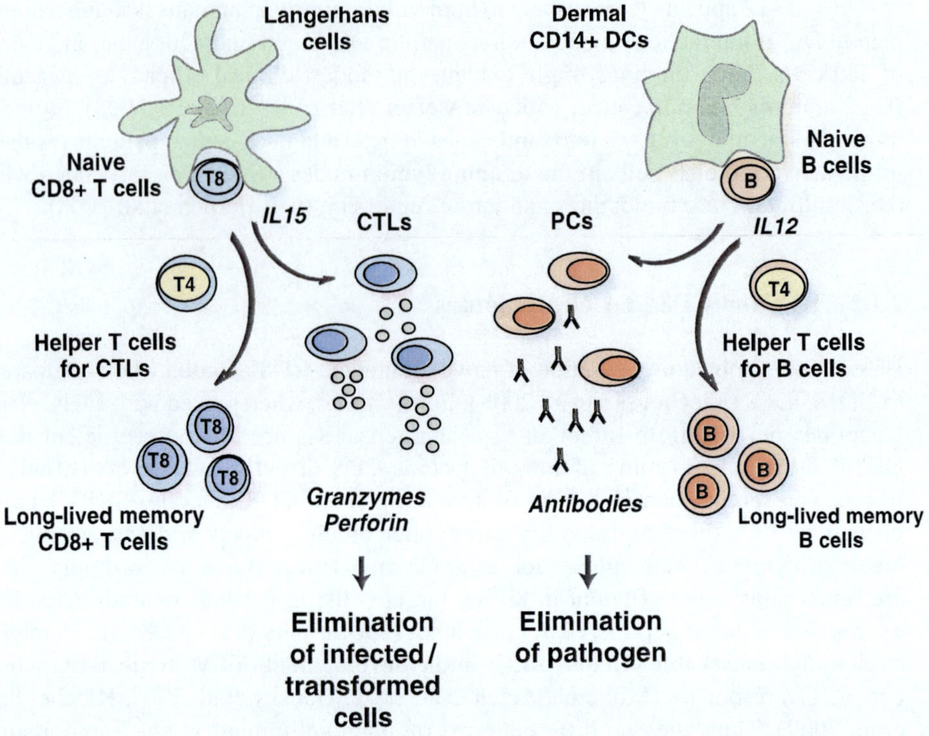

Fig. 2 *DCs as tools for vaccination*. We envision that targeting antigens and activation of distinct mDC subsets, with different specializations, will result in the generation of a broad and long lived immune protection. Thus, the most efficient cancer vaccines might be those that will target LCs thereby allowing the maximal stimulation of cellular immune responses and the generation of long-term memory protection

transcription profiles, differential secretion of IL12 p40 and differential expression of co-stimulatory molecule CD80 on activation. Additional studies will be necessary to understand the biological role of these two pDC subsets.

2.2 *DCs in Tumor Environment*

Numerous studies in humans have concluded that DCs can infiltrate tumors. We found that breast cancer tumor beds are infiltrated with immature DCs. In contrast, mature DCs are found in the peri-tumoral areas in ~60% of cases (Bell et al. 1999). A number of studies have suggested that DCs can contribute to tumor development. Our studies in breast cancer indicate that tumor cells polarize mDCs into a state that drives the differentiation of naïve $CD4^{+}$ T cells into IL-13-secreting T cells (Aspord et al. 2007). These Type 2 T cells in turn facilitate breast tumor development in xenograft model as it can be partly inhibited by administration of IL-13 antagonists (Fig. 3). The role of Th2 cells was further established in a spontaneous mouse breast

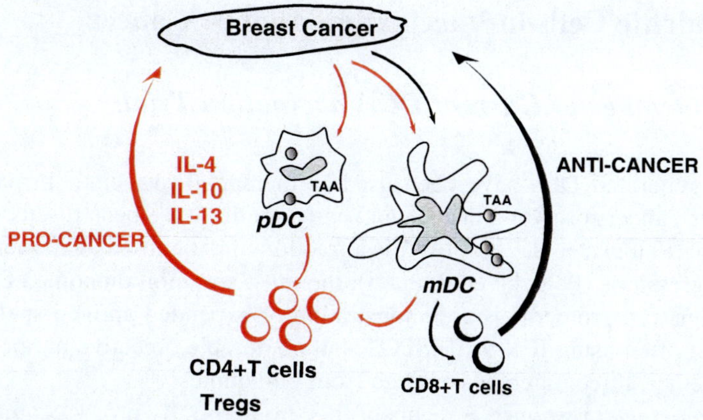

Fig. 3 *DCs as targets for therapy*. Cancer cells attract immature DC possibly through chemokines such as MIP3 alpha and/or SDF-1. The DC can then be either blocked or skewed in their maturation, for example by VEGF, leading to induction of polarized CD4+T cells that promote the expansion of cancer cells (pro-cancer) at the expense of CD8+T cells that can cause tumor regression (anti-cancer). An interesting strategy would be to rewire their molecular pathways from "pro-cancer" DCs into "anti-cancer" DCs for example with antibodies or DC activators

cancer model, where Th2 cells facilitate the development of lung metastasis through macrophage activation (DeNardo et al. 2009). In several other mouse tumor models, IL-13 produced by NKT cells induces myeloid cells to make TGF-β that inhibits CTL functions (Berzofsky and Terabe 2008). Thus, Type 2 cytokines are involved in tumorigenesis through various mechanisms. mDCs can also have direct interactions with tumor cells as shown in multiple myeloma where they directly promote the survival and clonogenicity of tumor cells (Kukreja et al. 2006; Bahlis et al. 2007).

pDCs have been found in approximately 10% of breast carcinomas and are associated with poor prognosis (Treilleux et al. 2004). The infiltrating pDCs produce little Type I IFN upon TLR ligation (Hartmann et al. 2003). This inhibition appears to depend on the ligation of ILT7 on pDCs binding by BST2 expressed on tumor cells (Cao et al. 2009). Likewise, in ovarian carcinoma, tumor-infiltrating pDCs do not induce effector $CD8^+$ T cell responses, but rather promote the differentiation of $IL10^+$ $CCR7^+$ $CD8^+$ Tregs (Wei et al. 2005). Finally, pDCs may promote tumor angiogenesis by the secretion of proangiogenic cytokines (Curiel et al. 2004; Coukos et al. 2005).

DC can fight back tumors at least through two pathways: an indirect one with the induction of potent CTL responses, and a direct one through DC-dependent tumor cytotoxicity. For example, pDCs appear to directly contribute to the anti-tumor activity of in vivo-administered Imiquimod (TLR7 ligand), which is used for the treatment of basal cell carcinoma (Urosevic et al. 2005; Panelli et al. 2007; Stary et al. 2007).

Clearly, understanding the functions of DCs in the tumor bed represents an important area of future investigations and exploitation for therapy. An interesting strategy would be to rewire their molecular pathways from "pro-tumor" DCs into "anti-tumor" DCs.

3 Dendritic Cells in Vaccination Against Cancer

3.1 Outcomes of Current DC Vaccination Trials

Ex vivo-generated DCs have been used as therapeutic vaccines in patients with metastatic cancer for over a decade and early studies have been discussed in detail elsewhere (Palucka et al. 2007). While a fraction of patients can experience durable tumor regressions (Palucka et al. 2006), the most common outcome of the current DC vaccination protocols is a demonstration of expanded antigen-specific immunity, most often using IFN-γ ELISPOT, but no durable objective tumor regression.

Altogether, three outcomes emerge from our studies:

(1) *No immune response*. Patients of this group usually progress quickly. These patients mount immune responses to control antigens such as KLH or viral peptides (Flu-M1 or CMV). In vitro experiments indicated that T cells of several patients can be primed to differentiate into CTLs with specificity for multiple melanoma antigens (Berard et al. 2000). Thus, tumor antigen-specific $CD8^{+}$ T cells are kept anergic rather than deleted. This inability to mount immune responses to tumor antigens in vivo might be at least partly related to the presence of tumor antigen-specific Tregs (Vence et al. 2007; Andrews et al. 2008). Tregs limit the onset of protective immunity through several mechanisms, for example by eliminating DCs in lymph nodes (Boissonnas et al. 2010). As discussed later, the control of Tregs becomes a key target to address first the coming vaccination trials. (2) *Immune response without clinical response*. The most common outcome of current DC vaccination protocols is the induction of immune responses in the absence of clinical responses. This might in part be explained by the quality of the elicited T cells including their capacity to migrate into tumors and penetrate tumor stroma (Gajewski 2007). Improved immunomonitoring is expected to provide insights into the mechanisms of immune efficacy as discussed hereunder (Butterfield et al. 2008; Tahara et al. 2009). (3) *Immune response and clinical response*. Vaccination with DCs can elicit therapeutic immunity. These patients represent a formidable opportunity for the development of cancer immunotherapy. The challenge is twofold: first, establishing the immunological mechanism that allowed tumor eradication and second, finding ways to increase the fraction of patients experiencing durable tumor regression and/or prolonged survival.

3.2 The Quality of Elicited Antigen-Specific Immune Responses

Establishing causative links in clinical studies is a difficult task which often requires large patient cohorts. The current data suggest an association between the tumor-specific $CD8^{+}$ T cell responses and clinical outcomes. In our view, four critical components will determine whether the induced immune response will be therapeutic: (1) the quality of elicited CTLs; (2) the quality of induced $CD4^{+}$ helper

T cells; (3) the elimination and/or non-activation of Tregs; and (4) the breakdown of immunosuppressive tumor microenvironment.

Indeed, the immune responses elicited by the first generation DC vaccines might not be of the quality required to allow the rejection of bulky tumors. For example, the induced T cells might not migrate into the tumor lesions (Appay et al. 2008; Harlin et al. 2009). Furthermore, low avidity T cells might be unable to recognize peptide-MHC class I complexes on tumor cells and/or to kill them (Appay et al. 2008). Finally, the tumor micro-environment might inhibit effector T cell functions, for example by action of myeloid derived suppressor cells and Tregs as summarized in recent reviews, respectively (Gabrilovich and Nagaraj 2009; Menetrier-Caux et al. 2009).

The recent progresses in immunomonitoring of specific immune responses in the blood and at the tumor site should help us address these questions (Palucka et al. 2006; Vence et al. 2007; Butterfield et al. 2008; Janetzki et al. 2009; Tahara et al. 2009). Modern approaches including polychromatic flow cytometry rather than the analysis of a single cytokine (e.g., IFN-γ ELISPOT) and/or frequency of tetramer positive cells will contribute to a better assessment of the quality of the immune responses elicited in the patients (Kammula et al. 1999; Lee et al. 1999). Indeed, several studies, mostly performed in the context of HIV vaccines, have led to the conclusion that a mere measurement of the frequency of IFN-γ secreting $CD8^+$ T cells is insufficient to evaluate the quality of vaccine-elicited immunity (Wille-Reece et al. 2006; Appay et al. 2008; Seder et al. 2008).

4 Building on Dendritic Cell Subsets to Improve Cancer Vaccines

4.1 Optimal DCs

The results summarized above prompted us to hypothesize that DCs with the properties of LCs might prove to be the best ones for the generation of strong cellular immunity (Fig. 2). In line with this, the combination of cytokines used to differentiate monocytes into DCs play a critical role in determining the quality of the elicited T cell responses. For example, DCs generated with GM-CSF and IL-15 display the phenotype and characteristics of LCs. In particular, they are more efficient in priming melanoma-antigen specific $CD8^+$ T cells in vitro than DCs derived with GM-CSF and IL-4 (Mohamadzadeh et al. 2001; Dubsky et al. 2007). Thus, vaccination with IL15-DCs might elicit stronger $CD8^+$ T cell responses that might lead to improved clinical responses. We are currently initiating such a clinical trial in patients with malignant melanoma. The selected method for activating DCs also represents a critical parameter is the DC activation pathway. First, immature (non-activated) DCs induce antigen specific IL-10 producing T cells (Dhodapkar et al. 2001; Dhodapkar and Steinman 2002). Second, IL-4 DCs activated with a cocktail of IFN-α, polyI:C, IL-1β, TNF, and IFN-γ induce up to 40 times more melanoma-specific CTLs in vitro than DCs matured with the "standard" cocktail of IL-1β/TNF/IL-6/prostaglandin E_2 (PGE_2) (Mailliard et al. 2004; Fujita et al. 2009; Giermasz et al. 2009). Additional studies will be necessary to establish the therapeutic value of these newer generation DC vaccines in patients. These studies are critical to the understanding of the human immune system because they permit us to assess *in vivo* the type of immune responses elicited by human DCs generated in different cytokine environments.

This in turn is essential for building a novel approach to vaccination that is based on the delivery of antigens directly to DCs in vivo using chimeric proteins that are made of an anti-DC receptor antibody molecularly fused to a selected antigen (DC targeting). Studies in mice demonstrate that the specific targeting of antigen to DCs in vivo results in considerable potentiation of antigen-specific $CD4^+$ and $CD8^+$ T cell immunity if the DC maturation signal is provided (Hawiger et al. 2001; Bonifaz et al. 2002, 2004). Otherwise, tolerance ensues (Hawiger et al. 2001). Thus, selection of appropriate adjuvant is also a critical parameter for the induction of the immunity of the desired type. Although TLR-ligands are widely considered to promote protective immunity against infectious agents, selecting the appropriate ligand will be critical. For instance, TLR2 ligation, which promotes the induction of Tregs rather than Th1 or Th17 cells (Manicassamy et al. 2009), does not appear to be a preferred option for cancer vaccines.

These pioneering studies have been already extended to demonstrate the targeting of tumor antigens to DCs (Caminschi et al. 2009) and Langerhans cells (LCs) in animal models (Flacher et al. 2008, 2009) and the generation of anti-tumor immunity (Wei et al. 2009). The therapeutic success of these vaccines will build on the recent knowledge and progress in our understanding of the biology of human DC subsets, cutaneous myeloid DCs (mDCs) in particular.

4.2 *"Ideal" Antigens*

Assuming that appropriate solutions are identified to reverse immunosuppression, there is a need for an "ideal" set of target antigens. An "ideal" antigen is one which is necessary for cancer cells to survive and/or for which strong immunity able to reject the tumor and prevent its growth can be elicited.

Candidate tumor antigens include: (a) unique (mutated) antigens; and (b) shared self-antigens including cancer/testis antigens and tissue differentiation antigens (Gilboa 1999; Vlad et al. 2004; Boon et al. 2006; Parmiani et al. 2007). The choice between these types of antigens for vaccination could be viewed as a choice between inducing immunity (mutated antigens) or breaking tolerance and inducing autoimmunity (self antigens). The debate about which type of antigen will be more efficient is still open. Mutated antigens are postulated to present several advantages, for example their specific T cell repertoire should not be deleted as they are not recognized as "self" by immune cells (Parmiani et al. 2007). Shared antigens are attractive as they might allow us to establish "generic" vaccines; however, the enthusiasm for these antigens might be dampened because of (a) their relatively weak immunogenicity due to the negative selection of high affinity auto-reactive cells and (b) the existence of antigen specific Tregs (Hoos et al. 2007).

Perhaps the most compelling evidence of active in vivo tumor antigen-specific immune responses arises from the study of paraneoplastic neurologic disorders (PNDs) that led to the discovery of onconeural antigens (Darnell 1996). PNDs develop as remote effects of systemic malignancies. The discovery of onconeural antibodies led to the proposal that paraneoplastic cerebellar degeneration (PCD), associated to breast and ovarian cancer, is an autoimmune disorder mediated by the humoral arm of the immune system. These antibodies permitted the cloning of the cdr2 antigen, a protein with a coil/leucine zipper domain. It has now been shown that the disease is due to the development of cdr-2 specific $CD8^+$ CTL (Albert et al. 1998). The list of onconeural antigens is growing and, besides cdr2, two other antigens such as Nova and amphiphysin appear as potential targets of the immune system (Floyd et al. 1998; Rosin et al. 1998).

An important shift in the selection of antigen targets might be brought about by the identification of cancer stem cells (Jordan et al. 2006; Polyak and Hahn 2006; Rossi et al. 2008). While a majority of studies have focused on eliminating mature cancer cells with limited proliferation capacity, it seems more efficient to target the self-renewing cancer stem cells. The importance of stem cell associated antigens in malignancy can be best illustrated by the presence of SOX-2-specific immunity in patients with monoclonal gammopathy (Spisek et al. 2007). This immunity is lost in patients who developed multiple myeloma suggesting differential antigenic targets at pre-malignant and malignant stages. In fact, the major factor from the immunization point of view is the linkage between expression of genes associated with pluripotency and those expressed in cancer. Ideal target genes would be those shared between cancer cells and embryonal cells, which are necessary for cancer cell survival but not expressed in adult stem cells (Dhodapkar 2010).

Thus far, all antigenic targets are protein antigens whose peptides can be presented on the cell surface in the form of complexes with classical MHC molecules (Townsend et al. 1985). However, tumors express altered lipids and sugars that can be bound by CD1 molecules on APCs and presented to NKT cells as well as T cells (Beckman et al. 1994; Fujii et al. 2002; Hava et al. 2005). These lipid antigens might possibly be harnessed for improved vaccination.

4.3 *Combining DC Vaccines with Other Therapies*

In view of the remarkable diversity of regulatory/suppressive pathways present in patients with metastatic cancer, any durable clinical response elicited by vaccination with DCs is already a remarkable achievement. However, to improve the outcomes in metastatic disease, DC vaccines need to be combined with other therapies that offset the suppressive environment created by the tumor

(Dougan and Dranoff 2009). Such combination regimens will involve several drugs that target different pathways (Fig. 4).

In particular antibodies, or other soluble antagonists such as engineered receptors, can be exploited for the blockade of suppressive cytokines in the tumor microenvironment such as IL-10 (Moore et al. 2001), IL-13 (Terabe et al. 2000), TGF-β (Li et al. 2005; Terabe et al. 2009) and VEGF (Gabrilovich 2004; Rabinovich et al. 2007). They can also be used to block inhibitory ligand:receptor interactions (Melero et al. 2007) by acting on antigen presenting cells such as tumor or DCs (for example anti-PD-L1) or on lymphocytes as illustrated by anti-CTLA-4 (Peggs et al. 2006, 2009) and/or anti-PD1 (Day et al. 2006; Curran et al. 2010; Pilon-Thomas et al. 2010). In contrast, agonistic antibodies (Gabrilovich 2004; Rabinovich et al. 2007) might further promote co-stimulation of effector T cells as for example with anti-CD137 (Watts 2005), a ligand for 4-1BB (Maus et al. 2002). Just as different tumors are treated with different combinations of cytostatic drugs and targeted therapies, we foresee development of clinical protocols combining DC vaccines with individualized adjunct therapies.

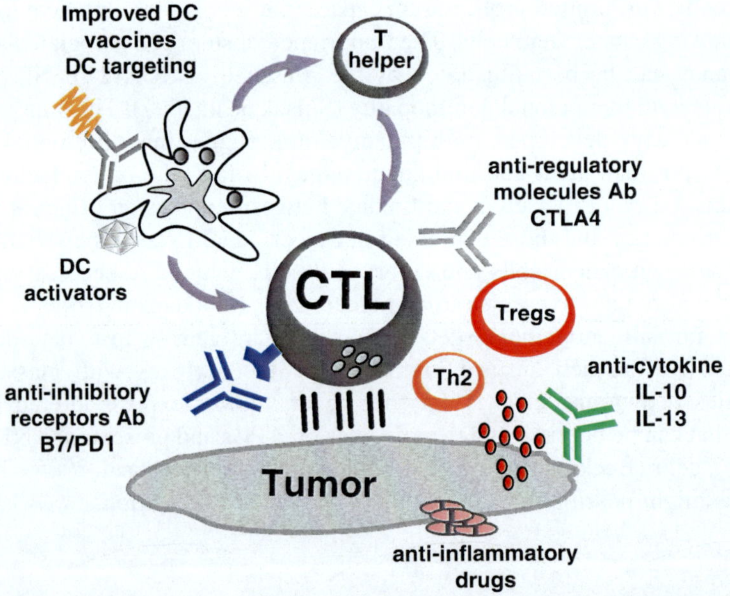

Fig. 4 *DC vaccines in combination therapies*. Current active immunotherapy trials have shown durable tumor regressions in a fraction of patients. However, clinical efficacy of current approaches is limited, possibly because tumors invade the immune system by means of myeloid-derived suppressor cells, inflammatory Type 2 T cells and regulatory T cells (Tregs). To improve the clinical efficacy of immunotherapies, we need to design novel and improved strategies that can boost adaptive immunity to cancer, help overcome Tregs and allow the breakdown of an immunosuppressive tumor microenvironment. This can be achieved by developing combination therapies targeting these three major components

5 Concluding Remarks

The considerable progresses made in the knowledge of DC biology as well as effector/regulatory T cell biology clearly open the avenues for the development of vastly improved clinical protocols. These, optimized vaccines eliciting strong and long-lived antigens-specific CD8+ T cell immunity will be offered to patients in the early stage of the disease. For patients with late stage disease, strategies that combine novel highly immunogenic vaccines and immunomodulatory antibodies will have high impact on enhancing therapeutic immunity in cancer by simultaneously increasing the potency of beneficial immune arms and offsetting immunoregulatory pathways (Fig. 4). These optimized therapeutic strategies will be tailored to the patient and to the specific suppressive pathways that the patient displays (Fig. 5).

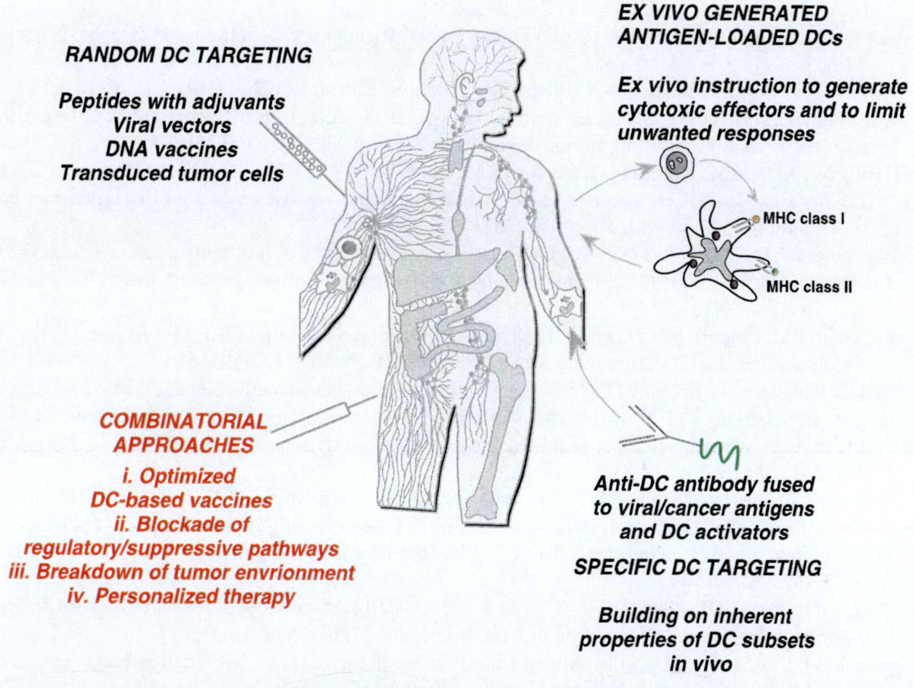

Fig. 5 *Approaches to DC-based immune intervention in cancer*. (1) Vaccines based on antigen with or without adjuvant that target DCs randomly. That might result in vaccine antigens being taken up by a "wrong" type of DCs in the periphery which might lead to "unwanted" type of immune response. Vaccine antigens could also flow to draining lymph nodes where they can be captured by resident DCs; (2) Vaccines based on ex-vivo generated tumor antigen-loaded DCs that are injected back into patients; and (3) specific in vivo DC targeting with anti-DC antibodies fused with antigens and with DC activators. (4) Next generation clinical trials will test optimized DC vaccines combined with patient-adjusted approaches to block Tregs and to breakdown the tumor environment. These therapies will be tested in pre-selected patients thereby leading to personalized therapy

Acknowledgments Dedicated to patients and volunteers who participated in our studies. We thank the former and current members of the Institute for their contributions. Supported by the NIH (P01 CA084514, U19 AIO57234, R01 CA089440 and CA078846), the Dana Foundation, the Susan Komen Foundation, the Baylor Health Care System; the Baylor Health Care System Foundation, the ANRS and the INSERM. KP holds the Michael A. Ramsay Chair for Cancer Immunology Research. JB holds the Caruth Chair for Transplant Immunology Research.

References

Akbari O, DeKruyff RH, Umetsu DT (2001) Pulmonary dendritic cells producing IL-10 mediate tolerance induced by respiratory exposure to antigen. Nat Immunol 2:725–731

Albert ML, Darnell JC, Bender A, Francisco LM, Bhardwaj N, Darnell RB (1998) Tumor-specific killer cells in paraneoplastic cerebellar degeneration. Nat Med 4:1321–1324

Andrews DM, Maraskovsky E, Smyth MJ (2008) Cancer vaccines for established cancer: how to make them better? Immunol Rev 222:242–255

Appay V, Douek DC, Price DA (2008) CD8+ T cell efficacy in vaccination and disease. Nat Med 14:623–628

Aspord C, Pedroza-Gonzalez A, Gallegos M, Tindle S, Burton EC, Su D, Marches F, Banchereau J, Palucka AK (2007) Breast cancer instructs dendritic cells to prime interleukin 13-secreting CD4+ T cells that facilitate tumor development. J Exp Med 204:1037–1047

Bahlis NJ, King AM, Kolonias D, Carlson LM, Liu HY, Hussein MA, Terebelo HR, Byrne GE Jr, Levine BL, Boise LH, Lee KP (2007) CD28-mediated regulation of multiple myeloma cell proliferation and survival. Blood 109:5002–5010

Banchereau J, Steinman RM (1998) Dendritic cells and the control of immunity. Nature 392:245–252

Batista FD, Harwood NE (2009) The who, how and where of antigen presentation to B cells. Nat Rev Immunol 9:15–27

Beckman EM, Porcelli SA, Morita CT, Behar SM, Furlong ST, Brenner MB (1994) Recognition of a lipid antigen by CD1-restricted alpha beta+ T cells. Nature 372:691–694

Bell D, Chomarat P, Broyles D, Netto G, Harb GM, Lebecque S, Valladeau J, Davoust J, Palucka KA, Banchereau J (1999) In breast carcinoma tissue, immature dendritic cells reside within the tumor, whereas mature dendritic cells are located in peritumoral areas. J Exp Med 190:1417–1426

Berard F, Blanco P, Davoust J, Neidhart-Berard EM, Nouri-Shirazi M, Taquet N, Rimoldi D, Cerottini JC, Banchereau J, Palucka AK (2000) Cross-priming of naive CD8 T cells against melanoma antigens using dendritic cells loaded with killed allogeneic melanoma cells. J Exp Med 192:1535–1544

Bergtold A, Desai DD, Gavhane A, Clynes R (2005) Cell surface recycling of internalized antigen permits dendritic cell priming of B cells. Immunity 23:503–514

Berzofsky JA, Terabe M (2008) A novel immunoregulatory axis of NKT cell subsets regulating tumor immunity. Cancer Immunol Immunother 57:1679–1683

Boissonnas A, Scholer-Dahirel A, Simon-Blancal V, Pace L, Valet F, Kissenpfennig A, Sparwasser T, Malissen B, Fetler L, Amigorena S (2010) Foxp3(+) T cells induce perforin-dependent dendritic cell death in tumor-draining lymph nodes. Immunity 32:266–278

Bonifaz L, Bonnyay D, Mahnke K, Rivera M, Nussenzweig MC, Steinman RM (2002) Efficient targeting of protein antigen to the dendritic cell receptor DEC-205 in the steady state leads to antigen presentation on major histocompatibility complex class I products and peripheral CD8+ T cell tolerance. J Exp Med 196:1627–1638

Bonifaz LC, Bonnyay DP, Charalambous A, Darguste DI, Fujii S, Soares H, Brimnes MK, Moltedo B, Moran TM, Steinman RM (2004) In vivo targeting of antigens to maturing dendritic cells via the DEC-205 receptor improves T cell vaccination. J Exp Med 199:815–824

Boon T, Coulie PG, Van den Eynde BJ, van der Bruggen P (2006) Human T cell responses against melanoma. Annu Rev Immunol 24:175–208

Brimnes MK, Bonifaz L, Steinman RM, Moran TM (2003) Influenza virus-induced dendritic cell maturation is associated with the induction of strong T cell immunity to a coadministered, normally nonimmunogenic protein. J Exp Med 198:133–144

Butterfield LH, Disis ML, Fox BA, Lee PP, Khleif SN, Thurin M, Trinchieri G, Wang E, Wigginton J, Chaussabel D, Coukos G, Dhodapkar M, Hakansson L, Janetzki S, Kleen TO, Kirkwood JM, Maccalli C, Maecker H, Maio M, Malyguine A, Masucci G, Palucka AK, Potter DM, Ribas A, Rivoltini L, Schendel D, Seliger B, Selvan S, Slingluff CL Jr, Stroncek DF, Streicher H, Wu X, Zeskind B, Zhao Y, Zocca MB, Zwierzina H, Marincola FM (2008) A systematic approach to biomarker discovery; preamble to "the iSBTc-FDA taskforce on immunotherapy biomarkers". J Transl Med 6:81

Caminschi I, Lahoud MH, Shortman K (2009) Enhancing immune responses by targeting antigen to DC. Eur J Immunol 39:931–938

Cao W, Bover L, Cho M, Wen X, Hanabuchi S, Bao M, Rosen DB, Wang YH, Shaw JL, Du Q, Li C, Arai N, Yao Z, Lanier LL, Liu YJ (2009) Regulation of TLR7/9 responses in plasmacytoid dendritic cells by BST2 and ILT7 receptor interaction. J Exp Med 206:1603–1614

Caux C, Massacrier C, Vanbervliet B, Dubois B, Durand I, Cella M, Lanzavecchia A, Banchereau J (1997) CD34+ hematopoietic progenitors from human cord blood differentiate along two independent dendritic cell pathways in response to granulocyte-macrophage colony-stimulating factor plus tumor necrosis factor alpha: II. Functional analysis. Blood 90:1458–1470

Cheever MA (2008) Twelve immunotherapy drugs that could cure cancers. Immunol Rev 222: 357–368

Coukos G, Benencia F, Buckanovich RJ, Conejo-Garcia JR (2005) The role of dendritic cell precursors in tumour vasculogenesis. Br J Cancer 92:1182–1187

Curiel TJ, Cheng P, Mottram P, Alvarez X, Moons L, Evdemon-Hogan M, Wei S, Zou L, Kryczek I, Hoyle G, Lackner A, Carmeliet P, Zou W (2004) Dendritic cell subsets differentially regulate angiogenesis in human ovarian cancer. Cancer Res 64:5535–5538

Curran MA, Montalvo W, Yagita H, Allison JP (2010) PD-1 and CTLA-4 combination blockade expands infiltrating T cells and reduces regulatory T and myeloid cells within B16 melanoma tumors. Proc Natl Acad Sci USA 107(9):4275–4280

Darnell RB (1996) Onconeural antigens and the paraneoplastic neurologic disorders: at the intersection of cancer, immunity, and the brain. Proc Natl Acad Sci USA 93:4529–4536

Day CL, Kaufmann DE, Kiepiela P, Brown JA, Moodley ES, Reddy S, Mackey EW, Miller JD, Leslie AJ, DePierres C, Mncube Z, Duraiswamy J, Zhu B, Eichbaum Q, Altfeld M, Wherry EJ, Coovadia HM, Goulder PJ, Klenerman P, Ahmed R, Freeman GJ, Walker BD (2006) PD-1 expression on HIV-specific T cells is associated with T-cell exhaustion and disease progression. Nature 443:350–354

DeNardo DG, Barreto JB, Andreu P, Vasquez L, Tawfik D, Kolhatkar N, Coussens LM (2009) CD4(+) T cells regulate pulmonary metastasis of mammary carcinomas by enhancing protumor properties of macrophages. Cancer Cell 16:91–102

Dhodapkar MV (2010) Immunity to stemness genes in human cancer. Curr Opin Immunol 22:245–250

Dhodapkar MV, Steinman RM (2002) Antigen-bearing immature dendritic cells induce peptide-specific CD8(+) regulatory T cells in vivo in humans. Blood 100:174–177

Dhodapkar MV, Steinman RM, Krasovsky J, Munz C, Bhardwaj N (2001) Antigen-specific inhibition of effector T cell function in humans after injection of immature dendritic cells. J Exp Med 193:233–238

Di Pucchio T, Chatterjee B, Smed-Sorensen A, Clayton S, Palazzo A, Montes M, Xue Y, Mellman I, Banchereau J, Connolly JE (2008) Direct proteasome-independent cross-presentation of viral antigen by plasmacytoid dendritic cells on major histocompatibility complex class I. Nat Immunol 9:551–557

Doherty PC, Turner SJ, Webby RG, Thomas PG (2006) Influenza and the challenge for immunology. Nat Immunol 7:449–455

Dougan M, Dranoff G (2009) Immune therapy for cancer. Annu Rev Immunol 27:83–117
Dubsky P, Saito H, Leogier M, Dantin C, Connolly JE, Banchereau J, Palucka AK (2007) IL-15-induced human DC efficiently prime melanoma-specific naive CD8(+) T cells to differentiate into CTL. Eur J Immunol 37:1678–1690
Fairchild PJ, Austyn JM (1990) Thymic dendritic cells: phenotype and function. Int Rev Immunol 6:187–196
Fazilleau N, Mark L, McHeyzer-Williams LJ, McHeyzer-Williams MG (2009) Follicular helper T cells: lineage and location. Immunity 30:324–335
Finkelman FD, Lees A, Birnbaum R, Gause WC, Morris SC (1996) Dendritic cells can present antigen in vivo in a tolerogenic or immunogenic fashion. J Immunol 157:1406–1414
Flacher V, Douillard P, Ait-Yahia S, Stoitzner P, Clair-Moninot V, Romani N, Saeland S (2008) Expression of langerin/CD207 reveals dendritic cell heterogeneity between inbred mouse strains. Immunology 123:339–347
Flacher V, Sparber F, Tripp CH, Romani N, Stoitzner P (2009) Targeting of epidermal Langerhans cells with antigenic proteins: attempts to harness their properties for immunotherapy. Cancer Immunol Immunother 58:1137–1147
Floyd S, Butler MH, Cremona O, David C, Freyberg Z, Zhang X, Solimena M, Tokunaga A, Ishizu H, Tsutsui K, De Camilli P (1998) Expression of amphiphysin I, an autoantigen of paraneoplastic neurological syndromes, in breast cancer. Mol Med 4:29–39
Fonteneau JF, Gilliet M, Larsson M, Dasilva I, Munz C, Liu YJ, Bhardwaj N (2003) Activation of influenza virus-specific CD4+ and CD8+ T cells: a new role for plasmacytoid dendritic cells in adaptive immunity. Blood 101:3520–3526
Fujii S, Shimizu K, Kronenberg M, Steinman RM (2002) Prolonged IFN-gamma-producing NKT response induced with alpha-galactosylceramide-loaded DCs. Nat Immunol 3:867–874
Fujita M, Zhu X, Ueda R, Sasaki K, Kohanbash G, Kastenhuber ER, McDonald HA, Gibson GA, Watkins SC, Muthuswamy R, Kalinski P, Okada H (2009) Effective immunotherapy against murine gliomas using type 1 polarizing dendritic cells–significant roles of CXCL10. Cancer Res 69:1587–1595
Gabrilovich D (2004) Mechanisms and functional significance of tumour-induced dendritic-cell defects. Nat Rev Immunol 4:941–952
Gabrilovich DI, Nagaraj S (2009) Myeloid-derived suppressor cells as regulators of the immune system. Nat Rev Immunol 9:162–174
Gajewski TF (2007) Failure at the effector phase: immune barriers at the level of the melanoma tumor microenvironment. Clin Cancer Res 13:5256–5261
Geissmann F, Manz MG, Jung S, Sieweke MH, Merad M, Ley K (2010) Development of monocytes, macrophages, and dendritic cells. Science 327:656–661
Giermasz AS, Urban JA, Nakamura Y, Watchmaker P, Cumberland RL, Gooding W, Kalinski P (2009) Type-1 polarized dendritic cells primed for high IL-12 production show enhanced activity as cancer vaccines. Cancer Immunol Immunother 58:1329–1336
Gilboa E (1999) The makings of a tumor rejection antigen. Immunity 11:263–270
Gilliet M, Liu Y-J (2002) Generation of human CD8 T regulatory cells by CD40 ligand-activated plasmacytoid dendritic cells. J Exp Med 195:695–704
Harlin H, Meng Y, Peterson AC, Zha Y, Tretiakova M, Slingluff C, McKee M, Gajewski TF (2009) Chemokine expression in melanoma metastases associated with CD8+ T-cell recruitment. Cancer Res 69:3077–3085
Hartmann E, Wollenberg B, Rothenfusser S, Wagner M, Wellisch D, Mack B, Giese T, Gires O, Endres S, Hartmann G (2003) Identification and functional analysis of tumor-infiltrating plasmacytoid dendritic cells in head and neck cancer. Cancer Res 63:6478–6487
Hava DL, Brigl M, van den Elzen P, Zajonc DM, Wilson IA, Brenner MB (2005) CD1 assembly and the formation of CD1-antigen complexes. Curr Opin Immunol 17:88–94
Hawiger D, Inaba K, Dorsett Y, Guo K, Mahnke K, Rivera M, Ravetch JV, Steinman RM, Nussenzweig MC (2001) Dendritic cells induce peripheral T cell unresponsiveness under steady state conditions in vivo. J Exp Med 194:769–780

Hawiger D, Masilamani RF, Bettelli E, Kuchroo VK, Nussenzweig MC (2004) Immunological unresponsiveness characterized by increased expression of CD5 on peripheral T cells induced by dendritic cells in vivo. Immunity 20:695–705

Heath WR, Carbone FR (2009) Dendritic cell subsets in primary and secondary T cell responses at body surfaces. Nat Immunol 10:1237–1244

Higano CS, Schellhammer PF, Small EJ, Burch PA, Nemunaitis J, Yuh L, Provost N, Frohlich MW (2009) Integrated data from 2 randomized, double-blind, placebo-controlled, phase 3 trials of active cellular immunotherapy with sipuleucel-T in advanced prostate cancer. Cancer 115:3670–3679

Hoos A, Parmiani G, Hege K, Sznol M, Loibner H, Eggermont A, Urba W, Blumenstein B, Sacks N, Keilholz U, Nichol G (2007) A clinical development paradigm for cancer vaccines and related biologics. J Immunother 30:1–15

Itano AA, McSorley SJ, Reinhardt RL, Ehst BD, Ingulli E, Rudensky AY, Jenkins MK (2003) Distinct dendritic cell populations sequentially present antigen to CD4 T cells and stimulate different aspects of cell-mediated immunity. Immunity 19:47–57

Ito T, Yang M, Wang YH, Lande R, Gregorio J, Perng OA, Qin XF, Liu YJ, Gilliet M (2007) Plasmacytoid dendritic cells prime IL-10-producing T regulatory cells by inducible costimulator ligand. J Exp Med 204:105–115

Janetzki S, Britten CM, Kalos M, Levitsky HI, Maecker HT, Melief CJ, Old LJ, Romero P, Hoos A, Davis MM (2009) "MIATA"-minimal information about T cell assays. Immunity 31:527–528

Jego G, Palucka AK, Blanck JP, Chalouni C, Pascual V, Banchereau J (2003) Plasmacytoid dendritic cells induce plasma cell differentiation through type I interferon and interleukin 6. Immunity 19:225–234

Jego G, Pascual V, Palucka AK, Banchereau J (2005) Dendritic cells control B cell growth and differentiation. Curr Dir Autoimmun 8:124–139

Jonuleit H, Schmitt E, Schuler G, Knop J, Enk AH (2000) Induction of interleukin 10-producing, nonproliferating CD4(+) T cells with regulatory properties by repetitive stimulation with allogeneic immature human dendritic cells. J Exp Med 192:1213–1222

Jordan CT, Guzman ML, Noble M (2006) Cancer stem cells. N Engl J Med 355:1253–1261

Kammula US, Lee KH, Riker AI, Wang E, Ohnmacht GA, Rosenberg SA, Marincola FM (1999) Functional analysis of antigen-specific T lymphocytes by serial measurement of gene expression in peripheral blood mononuclear cells and tumor specimens. J Immunol 163:6867–6875

Kantoff PW, Schuetz TJ, Blumenstein BA, Glode LM, Bilhartz DL, Wyand M, Manson K, Panicali DL, Laus R, Schlom J, Dahut WL, Arlen PM, Gulley JL, Godfrey WR (2010) Overall survival analysis of a phase II randomized controlled trial of a poxviral-based PSA-targeted immunotherapy in metastatic castration-resistant prostate cancer. J Clin Oncol 28:1099–1105

King C, Tangye SG, Mackay CR (2008) T follicular helper (TFH) cells in normal and dysregulated immune responses. Annu Rev Immunol 26:741–766

Klechevsky E, Morita R, Liu M, Cao Y, Coquery S, Thompson-Snipes L, Briere F, Chaussabel D, Zurawski G, Palucka AK, Reiter Y, Banchereau J, Ueno H (2008) Functional specializations of human epidermal Langerhans cells and CD14+ dermal dendritic cells. Immunity 29:497–510

Klechevsky E, Liu M, Morita R, Banchereau R, Thompson-Snipes L, Palucka AK, Ueno H, Banchereau J (2009) Understanding human myeloid dendritic cell subsets for the rational design of novel vaccines. Hum Immunol 70:281–288

Kukreja A, Hutchinson A, Dhodapkar K, Mazumder A, Vesole D, Angitapalli R, Jagannath S, Dhodapkar MV (2006) Enhancement of clonogenicity of human multiple myeloma by dendritic cells. J Exp Med 203:1859–1865

Lee PP, Yee C, Savage PA, Fong L, Brockstedt D, Weber JS, Johnson D, Swetter S, Thompson J, Greenberg PD, Roederer M, Davis MM (1999) Characterization of circulating T cells specific for tumor-associated antigens in melanoma patients. Nat Med 5:677–685

Li MO, Wan YY, Sanjabi S, Robertson AK, Flavell RA (2005) Transforming growth factor-beta regulation of immune responses. Annu Rev Immunol 24:99–146

Liu YJ (2005) IPC: professional type 1 interferon-producing cells and plasmacytoid dendritic cell precursors. Annu Rev Immunol 23:275–306

Mailliard RB, Wankowicz-Kalinska A, Cai Q, Wesa A, Hilkens CM, Kapsenberg ML, Kirkwood JM, Storkus WJ, Kalinski P (2004) Alpha-type-1 polarized dendritic cells: a novel immunization tool with optimized CTL-inducing activity. Cancer Res 64:5934–5937

Manicassamy S, Ravindran R, Deng J, Oluoch H, Denning TL, Kasturi SP, Rosenthal KM, Evavold BD, Pulendran B (2009) Toll-like receptor 2-dependent induction of vitamin A-metabolizing enzymes in dendritic cells promotes T regulatory responses and inhibits autoimmunity. Nat Med 15:401–409

Matsui T, Connolly JE, Michnevitz M, Chaussabel D, Yu CI, Glaser C, Tindle S, Pypaert M, Freitas H, Piqueras B, Banchereau J, Palucka AK (2009) CD2 distinguishes two subsets of human plasmacytoid dendritic cells with distinct phenotype and functions. J Immunol 182:6815–6823

Maus MV, Thomas AK, Leonard DG, Allman D, Addya K, Schlienger K, Riley JL, June CH (2002) Ex vivo expansion of polyclonal and antigen-specific cytotoxic T lymphocytes by artificial APCs expressing ligands for the T-cell receptor, CD28 and 4-1BB. Nat Biotechnol 20:143–148

Melero I, Hervas-Stubbs S, Glennie M, Pardoll DM, Chen L (2007) Immunostimulatory monoclonal antibodies for cancer therapy. Nat Rev Cancer 7:95–106

Menetrier-Caux C, Gobert M, Caux C (2009) Differences in tumor regulatory T-cell localization and activation status impact patient outcome. Cancer Res 69:7895–7898

Merad M, Ginhoux F, Collin M (2008) Origin, homeostasis and function of langerhans cells and other langerin-expressing dendritic cells. Nat Rev Immunol 8:935–947

Mohamadzadeh M, Berard F, Essert G, Chalouni C, Pulendran B, Davoust J, Bridges G, Palucka AK, Banchereau J (2001) Interleukin 15 skews monocyte differentiation into dendritic cells with features of Langerhans cells. J Exp Med 194:1013–1020

Moore KW, de Waal MR, Coffman RL, O'Garra A (2001) Interleukin-10 and the interleukin-10 receptor. Annu Rev Immunol 19:683–765

Motzer RJ, Rakhit A, Thompson JA, Nemunaitis J, Murphy BA, Ellerhorst J, Schwartz LH, Berg WJ, Bukowski RM (2001) Randomized multicenter phase II trial of subcutaneous recombinant human interleukin-12 versus interferon-alpha 2a for patients with advanced renal cell carcinoma. J Interferon Cytokine Res 21:257–263

Nestle FO, Di Meglio P, Qin JZ, Nickoloff BJ (2009) Skin immune sentinels in health and disease. Nat Rev Immunol 9:679–691

Nossal GJ (1997) Host immunobiology and vaccine development. Lancet 350:1316–1319

Palucka AK, Ueno H, Connolly J, Kerneis-Norvell F, Blanck JP, Johnston DA, Fay J, Banchereau J (2006) Dendritic cells loaded with killed allogeneic melanoma cells can induce objective clinical responses and MART-1 specific CD8+ T-cell immunity. J Immunother 29:545–557

Palucka AK, Ueno H, Fay JW, Banchereau J (2007) Taming cancer by inducing immunity via dendritic cells. Immunol Rev 220:129–150

Panelli MC, Stashower ME, Slade HB, Smith K, Norwood C, Abati A, Fetsch P, Filie A, Walters SA, Astry C, Arico E, Zhao Y, Selleri S, Wang E, Marincola FM (2007) Sequential gene profiling of basal cell carcinomas treated with imiquimod in a placebo-controlled study defines the requirements for tissue rejection. Genome Biol 8:R8

Parmiani G, De Filippo A, Novellino L, Castelli C (2007) Unique human tumor antigens: immunobiology and use in clinical trials. J Immunol 178:1975–1979

Peggs KS, Quezada SA, Korman AJ, Allison JP (2006) Principles and use of anti-CTLA4 antibody in human cancer immunotherapy. Curr Opin Immunol 18(2):206–213

Peggs KS, Quezada SA, Chambers CA, Korman AJ, Allison JP (2009) Blockade of CTLA-4 on both effector and regulatory T cell compartments contributes to the antitumor activity of anti-CTLA-4 antibodies. J Exp Med 206:1717–1725

Pilon-Thomas S, Mackay A, Vohra N, Mule JJ (2010) Blockade of Programmed Death Ligand 1 Enhances the Therapeutic Efficacy of Combination Immunotherapy against Melanoma. J Immunol 184:3442–3449

Polyak K, Hahn WC (2006) Roots and stems: stem cells in cancer. Nat Med 12:296–300

Qi H, Egen JG, Huang AY, Germain RN (2006) Extrafollicular activation of lymph node B cells by antigen-bearing dendritic cells. Science 312:1672–1676

Rabinovich GA, Gabrilovich D, Sotomayor EM (2007) Immunosuppressive strategies that are mediated by Tumor cells. Annu Rev Immunol 25:267–296

Rosin L, DeCamilli P, Butler M, Solimena M, Schmitt HP, Morgenthaler N, Meinck HM (1998) Stiff-man syndrome in a woman with breast cancer: an uncommon central nervous system paraneoplastic syndrome. Neurology 50:94–98

Rossi DJ, Jamieson CH, Weissman IL (2008) Stems cells and the pathways to aging and cancer. Cell 132:681–696

Schmitt N, Morita R, Bourdery L, Bentebibel SE, Zurawski SM, Banchereau J, Ueno H (2009) Human dendritic cells induce the differentiation of interleukin-21-producing T follicular helper-like cells through interleukin-12. Immunity 31:158–169

Seder RA, Darrah PA, Roederer M (2008) T-cell quality in memory and protection: implications for vaccine design. Nat Rev Immunol 8:247–258

Siegal FP, Kadowaki N, Shodell M, Fitzgerald-Bocarsly PA, Shah K, Ho S, Antonenko S, Liu YJ (1999) The nature of the principal type 1 interferon-producing cells in human blood. Science 284:1835–1837

Spisek R, Kukreja A, Chen LC, Matthews P, Mazumder A, Vesole D, Jagannath S, Zebroski HA, Simpson AJ, Ritter G, Durie B, Crowley J, Shaughnessy JD Jr, Scanlan MJ, Gure AO, Barlogie B, Dhodapkar MV (2007) Frequent and specific immunity to the embryonal stem cell associated antigen SOX2 in patients with monoclonal gammopathy. J Exp Med 204:831–840

Stary G, Bangert C, Tauber M, Strohal R, Kopp T, Stingl G (2007) Tumoricidal activity of TLR7/8-activated inflammatory dendritic cells. J Exp Med 204:1441–1451

Steinman RM, Banchereau J (2007) Taking dendritic cells into medicine. Nature 449:419–426

Steinman RM, Hawiger D, Nussenzweig MC (2003) Tolerogenic dendritic cells. Annu Rev Immunol 21:685–711

Tahara H, Sato M, Thurin M, Wang E, Butterfield LH, Disis ML, Fox BA, Lee PP, Khleif SN, Wigginton JM, Ambs S, Akutsu Y, Chaussabel D, Doki Y, Eremin O, Fridman WH, Hirohashi Y, Imai K, Jacobson J, Jinushi M, Kanamoto A, Kashani-Sabet M, Kato K, Kawakami Y, Kirkwood JM, Kleen TO, Lehmann PV, Liotta L, Lotze MT, Maio M, Malyguine A, Masucci G, Matsubara H, Mayrand-Chung S, Nakamura K, Nishikawa H, Palucka AK, Petricoin EF, Pos Z, Ribas A, Rivoltini L, Sato N, Shiku H, Slingluff CA, Streicher H, Stroncek DF, Takeuchi H, Toyota M, Wada H, Wu X, Wulfkuhle J, Yaguchi T, Zeskind B, Zhao Y, Zocca MB, Marincola FM (2009) Emerging concepts in biomarker discovery; The US-Japan workshop on immunological molecular markers in oncology. J Transl Med 7:45

Terabe M, Matsui S, Noben-Trauth N, Chen H, Watson C, Donaldson DD, Carbone DP, Paul WE, Berzofsky JA (2000) NKT cell-mediated repression of tumor immunosurveillance by IL-13 and the IL-4R-STAT6 pathway. Nat Immunol 1:515–520

Terabe M, Ambrosino E, Takaku S, O'Konek JJ, Venzon D, Lonning S, McPherson JM, Berzofsky JA (2009) Synergistic enhancement of CD8+ T cell-mediated tumor vaccine efficacy by an anti-transforming growth factor-beta monoclonal antibody. Clin Cancer Res 15:6560–6569

Townsend AR, Gotch FM, Davey J (1985) Cytotoxic T cells recognize fragments of the influenza nucleoprotein. Cell 42:457–467

Treilleux I, Blay JY, Bendriss-Vermare N, Ray-Coquard I, Bachelot T, Guastalla JP, Bremond A, Goddard S, Pin JJ, Barthelemy-Dubois C, Lebecque S (2004) Dendritic cell infiltration and prognosis of early stage breast cancer. Clin Cancer Res 10:7466–7474

Urosevic M, Dummer R, Conrad C, Beyeler M, Laine E, Burg G, Gilliet M (2005) Disease-independent skin recruitment and activation of plasmacytoid predendritic cells following imiquimod treatment. J Natl Cancer Inst 97:1143–1153 van Herpen CM, van der Voort R, van der Laak JA, Klasen IS, de Graaf AO, van Kempen LC, de Vries IJ, Boer TD, Dolstra H, Torensma R, van Krieken JH, Adema GJ, De Mulder PH (2008) Intratumoral rhIL-12 administration in head and neck squamous cell carcinoma patients induces B cell activation. Int J Cancer 123:2354–2361

Vence L, Palucka AK, Fay JW, Ito T, Liu YJ, Banchereau J, Ueno H (2007) Circulating tumor antigen-specific regulatory T cells in patients with metastatic melanoma. Proc Natl Acad Sci USA 104:20884–20889

Vlad AM, Kettel JC, Alajez NM, Carlos CA, Finn OJ (2004) MUC1 immunobiology: from discovery to clinical applications. Adv Immunol 82:249–293

Volkmann A, Zal T, Stockinger B (1997) Antigen-presenting cells in the thymus that can negatively select MHC class II-restricted T cells recognizing a circulating self antigen. J Immunol 158:693–706

Watts TH (2005) TNF/TNFR family members in costimulation of T cell responses. Annu Rev Immunol 23:23–68

Wei S, Kryczek I, Zou L, Daniel B, Cheng P, Mottram P, Curiel T, Lange A, Zou W (2005) Plasmacytoid dendritic cells induce CD8+ regulatory T cells in human ovarian carcinoma. Cancer Res 65:5020–5026

Wei H, Wang S, Zhang D, Hou S, Qian W, Li B, Guo H, Kou G, He J, Wang H, Guo Y (2009) Targeted delivery of tumor antigens to activated dendritic cells via CD11c molecules induces potent antitumor immunity in mice. Clin Cancer Res 15:4612–4621

Wille-Reece U, Flynn BJ, Lore K, Koup RA, Miles AP, Saul A, Kedl RM, Mattapallil JJ, Weiss WR, Roederer M, Seder RA (2006) Toll-like receptor agonists influence the magnitude and quality of memory T cell responses after prime-boost immunization in nonhuman primates. J Exp Med 203:1249–1258

Wing K, Sakaguchi S (2010) Regulatory T cells exert checks and balances on self tolerance and autoimmunity. Nat Immunol 11:7–13

Wykes M, Pombo A, Jenkins C, MacPherson GG (1998) Dendritic cells interact directly with naive B lymphocytes to transfer antigen and initiate class switching in a primary T-dependent response. J Immunol 161:1313–1319

Yamamura M, Uyemura K, Deans RJ, Weinberg K, Rea TH, Bloom BR, Modlin RL (1991) Defining protective responses to pathogens: cytokine profiles in leprosy lesions. Science 254:277–279

Zaba LC, Fuentes-Duculan J, Steinman RM, Krueger JG, Lowes MA (2007) Normal human dermis contains distinct populations of CD11c+BDCA-1+ dendritic cells and CD163 +FXIIIA+ macrophages. J Clin Invest 117:2517–2525

Zal T, Volkmann A, Stockinger B (1994) Mechanisms of tolerance induction in major histocompatibility complex class II-restricted T cells specific for a blood-borne self-antigen. J Exp Med 180:2089–2099

Zheng Y, Josefowicz S, Chaudhry A, Peng XP, Forbush K, Rudensky AY (2010) Role of conserved non-coding DNA elements in the Foxp3 gene in regulatory T-cell fate. Nature 463:808–812

Zhong G, Reis e, Sousa C, Germain RN (1997) Antigen-unspecific B cells and lymphoid dendritic cells both show extensive surface expression of processed antigen-major histocompatibility class II complexes after soluble protein exposure in vivo or in vitro. J Exp Med 186:673–682

Identification of Human Idiotype-Specific T Cells in Lymphoma and Myeloma

Jinsheng Weng, Sattva S. Neelapu, Alison F. Woo, and Larry W. Kwak

Contents

1 Introduction 194
2 Idiotype Protein as a Tumor Antigen: Discovery Research 194
3 Clinical Investigational New Drug Vaccine Development 195
4 Pivotal Phase III Trials 195
5 Idiotype-Specific T Cell Immunity Elicited by Idiotype Vaccination in Preclinical Models 197
6 Human T Cell Epitopes Identified in Lymphoma-Derived Idiotype Proteins 199
7 Ig Light-Chain as a Source of Idiotype Peptide Recognized by Human T Cells 201
8 Future Directions for Idiotype-Specific T Cell Immunotherapy 204
References 206

Abstract Idiotype protein, among the first identified tumor-specific antigens, has been found to stimulate both humoral and cellular responses in lymphoma and myeloma patients. With the increasing use of B cell depletion treatments such as rituximab in clinic, the cellular response mediated by idiotype-specific T cells has become increasingly important as an adjunct therapy for lymphoma and myeloma. Here, we review the idiotype protein as a tumor antigen and the characteristics of the T cell response elicited idiotype vaccination. We also analyze the T cell epitopes that have been identified in idiotype protein and introduce our new findings of additional T cell epitopes derived from the Ig light chain. Finally, we propose new directions in the generation of idiotype-specific T cells for tumor therapy.

J. Weng (✉), S.S. Neelapu, A.F. Woo, and L.W. Kwak
Department of Lymphoma and Myeloma, The University of Texas M. D. Anderson Cancer Center, Houston, TX 77030, USA
e-mail: jweng@mdanderson.org

G. Dranoff (ed.), *Cancer Immunology and Immunotherapy*,
Current Topics in Microbiology and Immunology 344, DOI 10.1007/82_2010_70

1 Introduction

Vaccination against infectious diseases has been a great success of modern medicine. Since the discovery that many human tumors contain tumor-specific antigens that can stimulate human immune response, there has been much effort to use this knowledge for immunotherapy during the past decades (Hareuveni et al. 1990). The fact that malignant B cell tumors such as lymphoma and myeloma produce a tumor-specific immunoglobulin, known as "idiotype" (Id) protein, has been known for more than 30 years (Sirisinha and Eisen 1971; Lynch et al. 1972). Early studies of idiotype protein immunotherapy were focused on humoral immune responses as anti-idiotype protein antibodies could easily be detected in vaccinated animals or patients (Stevenson and Stevenson 1975). With the development of new techniques in immunology, a cellular response has been frequently observed in idiotype protein-vaccinated patients, particularly with idiotype-specific T cells.

2 Idiotype Protein as a Tumor Antigen: Discovery Research

Idiotype refers to the very tip of the F(ab) region of immunoglobulin that mediates the binding of antibody with specific antigen. Immunoglobulin can either be expressed on the cell surface of lymphoma cell or secreted in the serum by myeloma cells. The cell surface immunoglobulin mediates important cell functions for B cells including antigen recognition, cell growth, and cell survival (Kuppers 2005; Herzog et al. 2009). Under normal conditions, each B cell synthesizes or secretes only one type of immunoglobulin that is unique to the B cell. Since lymphoma and myeloma are clonal B cell tumors, the immunoglobulin produced by lymphoma and myeloma has been considered a tumor-specific antigen (Kwak and Longo 1996). In addition, studies have shown that there are few lymphomas or myelomas that lose the expression of immunoglobulin (Kuppers 2005). Hence, the idiotype proteins of lymphoma or myeloma have several desirable characteristics of an ideal tumor antigen: (1) they are essential to cell function, (2) cell specific, (3) and over expressed in tumors, thus making them ideal candidates as targets for tumor immunotherapy.

The preclinical rationale for idiotype vaccination was first demonstrated by Lynch and Eisen in the 1970s and later confirmed by others in different tumor models (Lynch et al. 1972; Stevenson and Stevenson 1975; Kaminski et al. 1987). Kwak, working in the laboratory of Levy at Stanford University, pioneered the first study translating therapeutic idiotype vaccines to human patients (Kwak et al. 1992). This small pilot study demonstrated that specific antibody responses could be elicited in patients with low-grade lymphoma. Subsequently, the Kwak laboratory at the National Cancer Institute (NCI) discovered that the addition of GM-CSF substantially improved vaccine potency and successfully induced T cell responses in murine lymphoma models (Kwak et al. 1996).

3 Clinical Investigational New Drug Vaccine Development

With dedicated process development support by the Biological Resources Branch at NCI, the first investigational new drug (IND)-supported study of the prototype idiotype vaccine product (patient-specific, hybridoma-generated, idiotype protein chemically linked with keyhole limpet hemocyanin [KLH]) was a phase II clinical trial for previously untreated patients with follicular lymphoma (FL) by the Kwak laboratory (Bendandi et al. 1999). This trial used soluble GM-CSF as an integral part of the vaccine. All patients on this study received treatment with a uniform chemotherapy regimen, which produced a homogeneous group of 20 patients who were all in first complete remission (minimal residual disease state). After a 6-month break following induction therapy (to allow for immune reconstitution after the immunosuppressive effects of chemotherapy), soluble, recombinant GM-CSF was mixed with Id-KLH, and the complete vaccine was injected s.c. in 5 monthly doses. This study was the first to show convincing lymphoma-specific $CD8^+$ T cell responses in the vast majority of patients (85%). In addition, evidence for molecular remissions was obtained in most of the subset of patients whose lymphomas could be detected by this technique. Particularly compelling were the clinical outcomes of this phase II study. After a median follow-up of 9.2 years, the median disease-free survival (DFS) was 8 years and overall survival was 95% (Bendandi et al. 1999). The DFS was superior to that of a historical, ProMACE chemotherapy-treated control group (median DFS, about 2.2 years) (Longo et al. 2000). These results were subsequently confirmed in other, non-IND studies of various vaccine formulations using hybridoma-generated idiotype proteins (Houot and Levy 2009).

4 Pivotal Phase III Trials

Three randomized double-blind placebo controlled multicenter clinical trials were designed to formally determine the clinical efficacy of therapeutic idiotype vaccination in FL. The first phase III trial was initiated by the NCI, and subsequently sponsored by Biovest International, Inc. Patients with previously untreated advanced stage FL were treated with PACE chemotherapy regimen until clinical remission. Patients achieving complete remission were randomized at a ratio of 2:1 to receive Id-KLH (BiovaxID) plus GM-CSF or KLH plus GM-CSF. The primary endpoint for this trial was DFS. About 177 out of 234 enrolled patients achieved complete response and were subsequently randomized to receive either active or control vaccine. Of these, 117 patients maintained remission for the 6-month rest period and received at least one dose of vaccine. This group of patients were treated as intended, and as such constituted the modified intent-to-treat analysis. Seventy-six patients received Id-KLH plus GM-CSF and 41 patients received KLH plus GM-CSF. Both arms were balanced for International Prognostic Index (IPI) and other relevant clinical factors. After a median follow-up of 56.6 months (range 12.6–89.3 months), median time to relapse after randomization for the Id-KLH/GM-CSF arm was 44.2 months vs. 30.6 months for the control arm (P-value = 0.045; HR = 1.6) (Schuster et al. 2009).

The other two phase III trials differed in terms of induction therapy, eligibility of the patients, and method of idiotype production. The Genitope sponsored trial used CVP chemotherapy regimen (cyclophosphamide, vincristine, and prednisone), enrolled complete response and partial response patients, and used recombinant DNA technology for production of idiotype protein. Eligible patients were randomized to receive MyVax (Id-KLH+GM-CSF) or control vaccine (KLH+GM-CSF) in a 2:1 ratio for 6 months after completion of eight cycles of CVP. A series of seven immunizations was administered over 24 weeks. Out of 287 randomized patients 278 received at least 1 vaccination. Forty-one percent of evaluable patients showed specific anti-Id antibody responses. No statistical difference was observed between the two arms in terms of PFS (Levy et al. 2008). The third phase III trial, sponsored by Favrille, investigated the efficacy of recombinant Id-KLH vaccination after treatment with rituximab. Previously untreated and relapsed/refractory FL patients in complete response, partial response or stable disease 2 months after a standard 4-week course of rituximab were randomized 1:1 to receive Id-KLH (Mitumprotimub-t) plus GMCSF or control (Placebo+GM-CSF) vaccine. Patients were immunized six times monthly, and then six times every other month, and then every 3 months until disease progression. The primary efficacy endpoint was time to progression. After a median follow up of 40 months, this trial showed no improvement in time to progression with Mitumprotimub-t plus GM-CSF when compared with control arm (Freedman et al. 2009).

Several differences in the above trials likely account for their disparate results. First, only patients who achieved complete remission were randomized in the BiovaxID clinical trial, whereas the MyVax trial included patients in partial response and the Mitumprotimub-t trial included patients in partial and stable disease. Moreover, the choice of a doxorubicin-containing chemotherapy regimen likely resulted in a higher proportion of patients achieving complete remission in the BiovaxID trial. Results from these trials suggest that a minimal residual disease state may be required for the vaccine-induced immune responses to be effective. Second, BiovaxID was prepared using the heterohybridoma method whereas MyVax and Mitumprotimub-t are recombinant proteins, suggesting that the immunogenicity of the idiotype vaccines may be different between the different formulations. Finally, it is possible that B cell depletion, resulting from the use of rituximab in the Mitumprotimub-t trial, may have had a deleterious effect on subsequent vaccine efficacy. Taken together, we speculate that minimal residual disease status, as exemplified by complete clinical remission, appears to be necessary for the clinical antitumor effect of idiotype vaccines, as demonstrated by the success of BiovaxID in a pivotal phase III trial.

5 Idiotype-Specific T Cell Immunity Elicited by Idiotype Vaccination in Preclinical Models

There are about ten billion different immunoglobulins in humans (Fanning et al. 1996). The acquisition of such huge repertoire of antibodies in one individual is achieved through the mechanism of V(D)J recombination and somatic hypermutation (Butler 1997). The highly variable region of an antibody that mediates the binding of antibody with antigen is composed of multiple domains (Fig. 1) (Berman et al. 1986). Each domain of antibody is encoded by genes that were selected from a large chromosome region. For example, the heavy chain variable region contains at least 55 different variable domain (*V*) genes, plus 27 diversity (*D*) genes, and six joining (*J*) genes that are located together on chromosome 14 (Fanning et al. 1996). The Ig light chain contains 124 IGLV subgroups for lambda light chain on the chromosome 22 and 200 IGKV subgroups for kappa light chain on the chromosome 2 in humans. These *V*, *D*, *J* genes and IGLV and IGLK subgroups are all candidates for the synthesis of heavy and light chain of idiotype protein (Dudley et al. 2005). *V*, *D*, *J* genes and IGLV and IGKV subgroups are selected by cell-type specificity, intra- and inter-locus ordering, and allelic exclusion mechanism and joined together by recombinases, to ensure that every antibody generated is different. After V(D)J recombination, some antibodies undergo further somatic hypermutation in the highly variable region to generate new antibodies for new antigens. Somatic hypermutation only affects the individual B cells and is not transmitted to offspring B cells. Because of V(D)J recombination and somatic hypermutation, it is ensured that there are enough antibodies to recognize and eliminate different types of

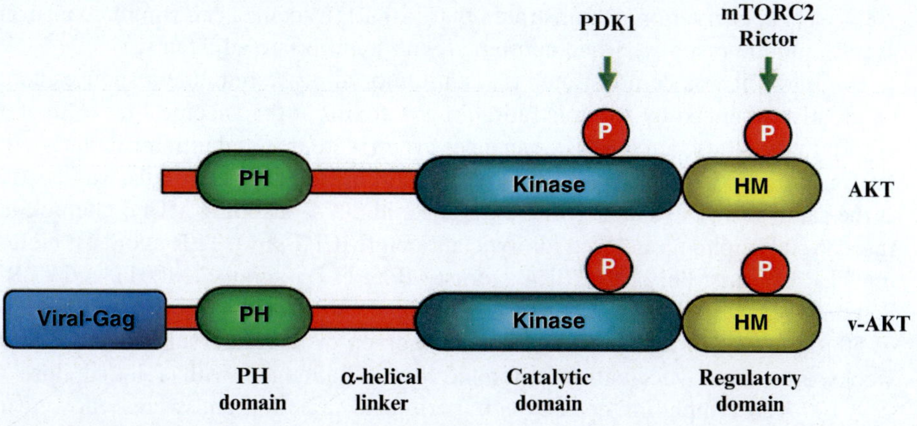

Fig. 1 The term idiotype refers to the unique amino acid sequences within the highly variable regions of the heavy and light chains of the surface immunoglobulin expressed on B cell malignancies. Idiotype includes both three complementarity-determining regions (CDR) and three framework region (FR) of immunoglobulin

antigens in human body. These processes also ensure that each malignant B cell expresses a unique idiotype protein.

Previous studies in mice have shown that idiotype proteins can be engulfed and processed through the exogenous pathway and presented in MHC I and II molecules(Weiss and Bogen 1991). Idiotype protein synthesized in the cytoplasmic compartment can also be processed and presented through the endogenous pathway (Yi et al. 1997). Idiotype-specific T cells can recognize the idiotype epitope derived from idiotype proteins on the cell surface of tumor B cells (Yi et al. 1993). These findings indicate that the idiotype protein can be processed and presented as a target for T cell recognition.

The search for cytokines and experimental adjuvants in preclinical models that could enhance idiotype-specific tumor immunity further suggested a role for T cells. The use of free granulocyte/macrophage colony-stimulating factor (GM-CSF) as an adjuvant drastically enhanced the cellular immune response of Id-KLH vaccination (Kwak et al. 1996). In this study, they investigated that low doses of GM-CSF 10,000 units i.p. or locally s.c. daily for 4 days significantly enhanced protective antitumor immunity induced by s.c. Id-keyhole limpet hemocyanin (KLH) immunization. This effect was critically dependent upon effector CD4 and CD8 T cells and was not associated with any increased anti-idiotypic antibody production. Specifically, 50% of mice immunized with Id-KLH plus GM-CSF on the same day of tumor challenge remained tumor-free at day 80, compared with 17% for Id-KLH alone, when immunization was combined with cyclophosphamide. Depletion of CD4 or CD8 T cells by using anti-CD8 or anti-CD4 antibody drastically decreased the protective role of idiotype vaccine (Kwak et al. 1996). It was likely that the mechanism of GM-CSF in the enhancement of vaccination was related to dendritic cell attraction and activation by GM-CSF (Wadhwa et al. 2003). This observation demonstrated that Id-KLH vaccines can stimulate a strong T cell immune response when combined with appropriate adjuvants.

Similarly, it was demonstrated that antitumor idiotype immune responses could be greatly enhanced by administration of myotoxins at the vaccine sites (Qin et al. 2009). In the study, ten BALB/c mice per group were injected intramuscularly with 6.8 μg cardiotoxin (A) or 0.1 μg crotoxin (B) followed by intramuscular vaccination at the same site 5 days later with 50 μg plasmid DNA encoding MCP3 chemokine-fused A20 lymphoma-derived idiotype antigen (MCP3-sFv). TLR agonists, including TLR3 agonist Poly I:C, TLR4 agonist MPL, TLR7 agonist (M001), and TLR7/8 agonist (M003), respectively, were given on the next day of vaccination at a dose of 50 μg. A total of three vaccinations were given with an interval of 14 days. Two weeks after final vaccination, all mice were challenged with a lethal dose of 2×10^5 A20 lymphoma cells by intraperitoneal injection and were followed for survival for 80 days. The authors found that administration of myotoxins at vaccination sites significantly enhanced idiotype DNA vaccine-induced tumor protection. About 90% mice from myotoxin treated group survived over the 80 days compared to only 10% mice, which survived in the control group. These data were also confirmed with two other chemotactic peptide-fused idiotype DNA vaccines with either defensin2β- or MIP3α-fused antigen. DNA vaccine combinations with Poly I:C (TLR3 agonist), MPL (TLR4 agonist), M001 (TLR7 agonist), and M003 (TLR7/8 agonist), respectively, failed to enhance tumor protection. Both memory and therapeutic antitumor immunity were enhanced by the use of myotoxin, as more than 80% of mice protected by combination DNA vaccine plus cardiotoxin were resistant to tumor rechallenge, compared with less than 40% of mice protected by DNA vaccine alone ($P = 0.01$). Importantly, the authors found that the protective idiotype immunity was mediated by T cells, because depleting $CD8^+$ T cells in vivo after vaccination plus cardiotoxin was clearly associated with reduced tumor protection, and depletion of both $CD4^+$ and $CD8^+$ T cell subsets abrogated protection completely. Of primary revelance, this study was the first to show that humoral immunity, however, was dispensable for antitumor immunity, as DNA vaccine plus cardiotoxin protected both genetically B cell-deficient J_h mice and wild-type mice equally from tumor challenge. More than 80% of tumor-free J_h mice surviving from the primary challenge were surprisingly highly resistant to tumor rechallenge, which suggests that anti-idiotype antibodies did not contribute principally to memory antitumor immunity. The memory antitumor immunity developed in J_h mice was comparable to that found in vaccinated wild-type counterparts.

6 Human T Cell Epitopes Identified in Lymphoma-Derived Idiotype Proteins

Although initial human studies suggest that idiotype-specific T cells can be generated by vaccination, the precise antigenic determinants, or T cell epitopes of idiotype protein, are only partially characterized. The structure and sequence of each idiotype protein is different, and T cell epitopes usually represent a 8–15-amino acid long sequence. These factors make the characterization of idiotype epitope extremely time consuming and expensive. However, characterization of T cell epitopes derived from human idiotype proteins would be highly significant. First, we may be able to identify universal idiotype epitopes shared by patients, thus relieving the effort to prepare idiotype vaccine for each patient. Second, peptide-tetramers can be synthesized and used to monitor T cell immunity in idiotype vaccinated-patients. Third, idiotype peptides could be used to develop novel peptide-vaccine strategies. Finally, idiotype peptides may be used to selectively expand idiotype-specific T cells in vitro for adoptive T cell transfer, as peptides are much more effective antigen for T cell stimulation than the intact idiotype protein (Hansson et al. 2003).

Trojan et al. (2000) combined bioinformatics and in vitro T cell expansion system to identify human immunoglobulin-derived peptides capable of inducing cytotoxic T lymphocyte responses. They cloned 128 heavy chain and 35 light chain sequences from 192 patients and synthesized 794 peptides from 65 patients that were HLA-A2 positive. Among these peptides, 229 (28.8%) were derived from the complementarity-determining regions (CDRs) of the immunoglobulin and the remaining 565 peptides (71.2%) were derived from framework region (FR) motifs. Because of the high homology of amino acid sequences in FR, 29.5% FR-derived peptides were shared by patients. The authors then stimulated purified CD8 T cells from HLA-A2 positive healthy donors with irradiated monocyte-derived peptide-pulsed dendritic cells and restimulated with irradiated, peptide-pulsed, CD40-activated B cells. They found nine FR-derived and one CDR-derived peptide that could stimulate CTLs from healthy donors. Five idiotype peptide-stimulated CTLs could kill both the peptide-pulsed CD40-activated B cells and CLL cells that expressed this peptide. Three peptides could stimulate both allogenic and autologous CTLs (Trojan et al. 2000). This study represents the first large scale and detailed characterization of CD8 T cell epitopes in idiotype protein. Although the percentage of T cell epitopes found in the study was quite low, a framework region (FR3) derived CD8 T cell epitope was found to be shared by patients. This means that one idiotype-peptide specific CTLs may potentially target tumors from several patients. By employing a strategy using heteroclitic peptides, the authors found additional CD8 T cell epitopes from idiotype protein and in their subsequent studies, confirmed that idiotype protein is an immunogenic antigen (Trojan et al. 2000; Harig et al. 2001; Zirlik et al. 2006).

Another important study identifying human T cell epitopes in idiotype protein came from the NCI phase II clinical trial. Instead of using naïve T cells from healthy donors, Baskar et al. (2004) used peripheral blood mononuclear cells (PBMC) from idiotype protein-vaccinated patients. By T cell proliferation and cytokine secretion assays, using that postvaccination patients' PBMC, they demonstrated recognition of multiple CD4 and CD8 T cell epitopes that were exclusively located in the CDRs of idiotype protein. The idiotype-specific CD4 T cells in this study recognized the idiotype protein-pulsed autologous PBMC and HLA-matched EBV B cell lines in an MHC II-dependent manner. Interestingly, the idiotype CD4 T cells recognized the idiotype epitope on multiple HLA class II alleles, including MHC II DR, DQ, and DP, indicating the proximal binding ability of idiotype epitope on the MHC class II molecules. The CD8 T cell line isolated from a post vaccine patient recognized the epitope on the HLA-B08 allele only. Through peptide mapping experiments, they found the minimal determinant of an immunodominant epitope to be composed of critical amino acid residues that may be a product of somatic hypermutation (Baskar et al. 2004). This study confirmed the long-held belief that idiotype vaccination can induce both CD4 and CD8 T cell responses and that there are CD4 and CD8 T cell epitopes in idiotype protein (Bendandi et al. 1999). However, the mapping of most T cell epitopes to the CDR2 and CDR3s of idiotype protein was different from the predominant localization of epitopes to the FR regions by Trojan et al. (2000).

The issue of whether the CDR or FR regions of idiotype protein contribute more T cell epitopes was addressed by another group in Europe, which showed that the CDRs of patients contained more HLA-binding epitopes than the FRs. By using bioinformatics and molecular analysis section (BIMAS) and SYFPEITHI, two online programs, Hansson et al. (2003) found 456 HLA-binding peptides from the CDR but only about 233 HLA-binding epitopes from the FR of the idiotype protein. They also found that most of the predicted peptides were confined to the CDR2-FR3-CDR3 "geographic" region of the Ig-VH region (70%), and that significantly fewer peptides were found within the flanking (FR1-CDR1-FR2 and FR4) regions ($P < 0.01$). Naturally occurring T cells in the myeloma patients' blood recognizing the CDR-derived peptide was found by ELISPOT assay.

Other smaller studies from other groups have tried to characterize the T cell epitopes from the idiotype protein. Wen and Lim (1997) found the CDR3 of the heavy chain of idiotype proteins to contain a strong immunogenic epitope that can stimulate T cell proliferation, cytokine secretion, and cytotoxic activity. Dabadghao et al. (1998) study found that dendritic cells pulsed with idiotype heavy chain are much more immunogenic than dendritic cells pulsed with idiotype light chain, so they hypothesized that idiotype heavy chain may contain more epitopes than the light chain. In the study by Fagerberg et al. (1999), candidate peptides from the heavy chain of idiotype protein responded to the idiotype-specific T cells. In contrast, peptides from idiotype light chain could not be recognized by idiotype-specific T cells, so they concluded that idiotype light chains contain no T cell epitopes.

7 Ig Light-Chain as a Source of Idiotype Peptide Recognized by Human T Cells

The search for T cell epitopes in idiotype proteins will continue to be an area of interest for tumor immunologists, because the identification of immunogenic epitopes can serve as a gateway for developing subsequent immunotherapy, as described earlier. Studies have shown that there is preferential usage of specific variable, diversity, and joining genes at different stages of B cell development and in B cell malignancies (Li et al. 2004a). We propose that there are T cell epitopes in both FR and CDR of idiotype proteins, and the idiotype epitope can stimulate both CD4 and CD8 T cells. One limitation of the studies to date is that they have focused mostly on the heavy chain of idiotype proteins. It is generally believed that the heavy chain contains highly variable diversity-joining parts (VH-D-JH) in the CDR3, which is more immunogenic to T cells (Cohen et al. 2009). However, the idiotype light chains are not well studied to date. Since the highly variable region of idiotype protein contain both heavy chain and light chain and the idiotype light chain are also generated through V(D)J recombination and somatic hypermutation process, it is plausible that the idiotype light chain also contains T cell epitopes.

Recently, we have tried to answer this question with human U266 myeloma cell line and PBMC from healthy donors. The idiotype light chain of U266 was cloned and sequenced with primers published previously (Tiller et al. 2008). Fifteen peptides corresponding to idiotype light chain of U266 idiotype protein were selected based on the binding capacity to HLA-A2 molecules. The peptides were then dissolved in DMSO and used to stimulate PBMC from an HLA-A2-positive healthy donor by using a published protocol (Hida et al. 2002). Briefly, PBMCs (1×10^5/well) obtained from HLA A2 positive healthy donors were incubated with 10 μg/ml (10 μM) peptide in 96-well plate in the presence of 100 U/ml interleukin-2 at day 0 with media that consist of 50% RPMI1640 and 50% AIM-V from Invitrogen. At culture days 4, 7, 10, and 13, half of the cultured media were removed and the cells were restimulated with 10 μg/ml of the peptide. At day 15, the cultured cells were resuspended in fresh medium and mixed with T2 cells loaded with corresponding peptide. T2 cells loaded with HIV peptide were used as a control. After 18 h of coculture, the concentration of IFN-γ in the culture supernatants was collected and measured by ELISA. As shown in Fig. 2, the U266 idiotype light chain-derived peptides P28 (GVTISCSGST) stimulated T cells that secreted a large amount of IFN-γ when cocultured with T2 loaded with P28 peptide, indicating the presence of peptide-specific T cells. The peptide-stimulated T cells were further expanded and analyzed by cytotoxic assay. T2 cells loaded with 40 μM idiotype light chain peptide P28 in the presence of 3 μg/ml β2-microglobulin were labeled with chromium-51 and cocultured with P28 peptide stimulated T cells at different concentrations. As shown in Fig. 3, the P28 peptide stimulated CTLs that can efficiently kill T2 cells loaded with P28 peptide but not T2 cells loaded with HIV peptide, indicating that these T cells are peptide-specific CTLs (Fig. 3). To test

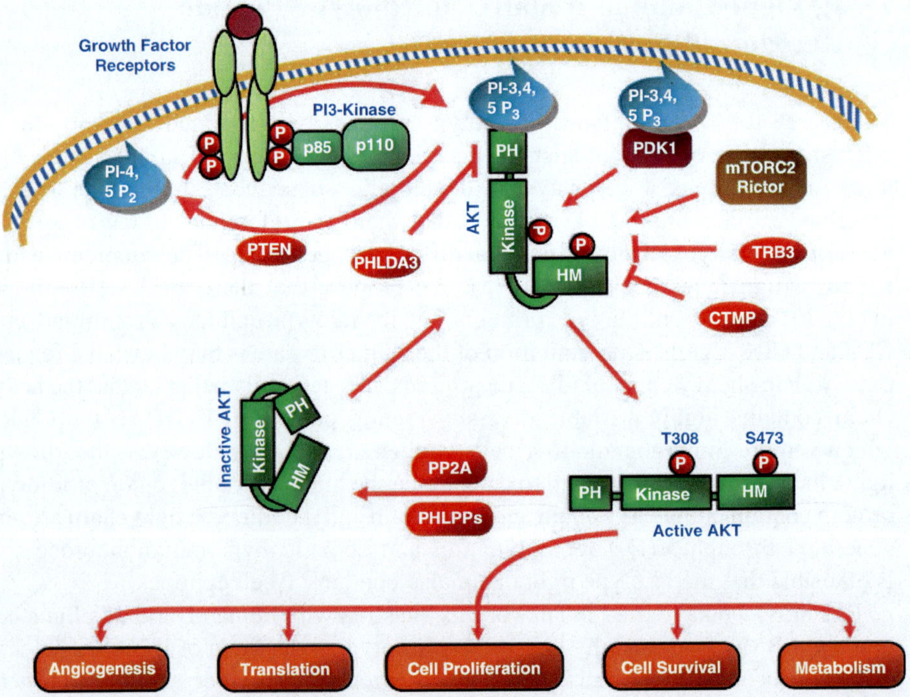

Fig. 2 IFN-γ ELISA. 1×10^5 idiotype light chain peptide-specific T cells secreted a large amount of IFN-γ when cocultured with 1×10^5 T2 cells loaded with 10 μM corresponding peptide (P28) compared with T2 loaded with 10 μM HIV peptide

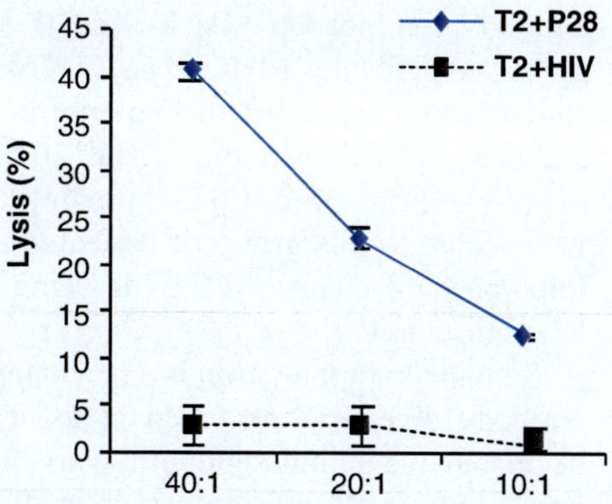

Fig. 3 T2 cell cytotoxic assay. Idiotype light chain peptide (P28)-specific T cells efficiently kill T2 cells loaded with 40 μM corresponding pepetide (P28) compared with T2 loaded with 40 μM HIV peptide

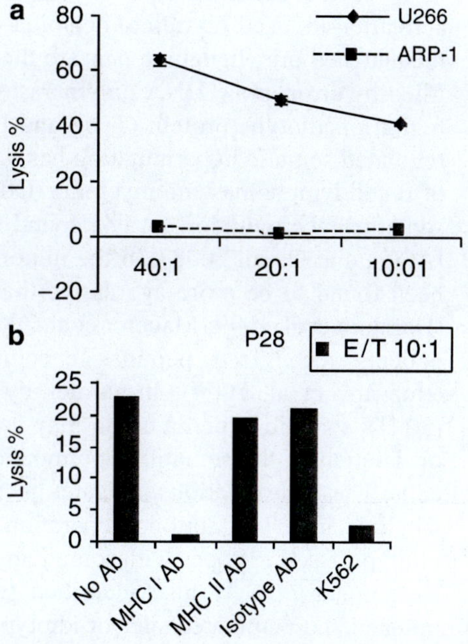

Fig. 4 U266 myeloma cytotoxic assay. (**a**) Idiotype light chain peptide (P28)-specific T cells efficiently kill U266 myeloma cells but not another myeloma (ARP-1 cells), which is HLA-A2 negative. (**b**) The killing of U266 by idiotype light chain peptide (P28)-specific T cells was blocked by MHC class I antibody but not MHC class II antibody, indicating the epitope was presented with MHC class I allele. The idiotype light chain peptide (P28)-specific T cells do not kill K562 cells which are a target of NK cells

whether the peptide was processed and presented by U266 myeloma cells, we cocultured the T cells with U266 myeloma cell at different concentrations. As shown in Fig. 4, idiotype light chain peptide stimulated T cells that can efficiently kill U266 tumor cells but not the control human myeloma ARP-1 cells, indicating that the idiotype light chain peptide was processed and presented on the cell surface of U266 cells. To determine whether the epitope was conjugated with the MHC allele of U266 cells, we performed an MHC antibody blocking assay. U266 myeloma cells were labeled with chromium-51, washed, and incubated with MHC antibodies for 1 h before coculturing with P28 CTLs. As shown in Fig. 4, the killing of U266 by P28 peptide-specific CTLs was blocked by MHC class I antibody but not by MHC class II antibody, indicating that the epitope was presented with the MHC class I allele of U266 cells (Fig. 4). Our preliminary studies have expanded the repertoire of T cell epitopes in idiotype protein. In addition, it is known that about 20% myeloma tumors have lost heavy chain expression; therefore, CTLs targeting the idiotype light chain epitope may be of great value to this group of patients (Cohen et al. 2009). The cytotoxic effect of idiotype light chain of CTLs is being further tested in an *in vivo* system in our laboratory now.

Somatic hypermutation is a mechanism of B cells that is used to further increase antibody diversity and to adapt to new foreign agents. Somatic hypermutation occurs in the immunoglobulin variable region at a rate of 10^{-3} mutations per base pair per cell division, which is 10^{6}-fold higher than the spontaneous mutation rate in somatic cells (Li et al. 2004b). The mechanism of somatic hypermutation involves the deamination of cytosine to uracil in DNA by an enzyme called activation-induced (cytidine) deaminase, or AID (Larson and Maizels 2004). The mismatched uracil:guanine pair are then removed by uracil-DNA glycosylase and filled by error-prone DNA polymerases to create mutations in the highly variable region of idiotype protein (Teng and Papavasiliou 2007). On the one hand, misregulated somatic hypermutation has been found to play a role in the development of B cell lymphomas and myeloma (Odegard and Schatz 2006). On the other hand, somatic hypermutation is also found to contribute to autoimmunity in humans (Atassi and Casali 2008). In the tumor immunity, germline cell lymphomas have been found to be more aggressive than lymphomas with somatic hypermutation (Hamblin et al. 1999; Mauerer et al. 2005). Naturally occurring CTLs isolated from patients recognized peptides encompassing the somatic hypermutation site (Rezvany et al. 2000). In studies by Baskar et al. (2004) and Hansson et al. (2003), somatic hypermutation may have generated T cell epitopes. Replacement or deletion of the somatic hypermuation resulted in the loss of recognition by T cells. These observations indicate that somatic hypermutation may play an important role in T cell epitope generation. In our recent studies, we have identified idiotype T cell epitopes with somatic hypermutations, but epitopes without somatic hypermutation were also identified (data not shown). This indicates that both mutated and unmutated sites of idiotype protein may generate epitopes recognized by CTLs. Since somatic hypermutation affects only individual B cells and the mutations are not transmitted to offspring, the targeting of tumor cells via somatic hypermutation may be a patient-specific strategy.

8 Future Directions for Idiotype-Specific T Cell Immunotherapy

For 30 years, idiotype vaccination has been shown to generate a protective immune response against lymphoma and myeloma tumors, mainly in preclinical models. Future directions will focus on how to improve the effect of the T cell response generated by idiotype vaccination in human patients. As shown by the example of the idiotype-KLH-GMCSF vaccine, an effective vaccine will depend on three factors: tumor antigen, carrier molecules, and vaccine adjuvant. Because KLH has a large molecular weight and is more immunogenic than other molecules, it has become the most widely employed carrier protein for idiotype vaccination. Recently, the alternative conjugation using the maleimide-based method has been reported to significantly enhance the immunogenicity of both human and murine Id-KLH vaccines in preclinical studies (Kafi et al. 2009). The mechanism of GM-CSF in the enhancement of T cell response in idiotype vaccination involved dendritic cell differentiation, migration, and maturation by GM-CSF through the STAT5 signaling pathway (Esashi et al. 2008). Dendritic cells are the most potent antigen presenting cell (APC) to induce antigen-specific T cells in vivo. Recent studies demonstrated that Toll-like receptor signaling pathways also play important roles in the differentiation, maturation, and activation of dendritic cells (Biragyn et al. 2002; Schjetne et al. 2003). Activation of Toll-like receptor signaling by CpG strongly enhances dendritic cell-mediated vaccine efficiency (Speiser et al. 2005). How to incorporate the growing knowledge of Toll-like receptor signaling pathway and dendritic cell activation into our idiotype T cell generation will be important for idiotype vaccination.

The observation that over 50% cancer patients can respond to the adoptive T cell transfer has made the adoptive immunotherapy one of the most attractive strategies (Dudley et al. 2002). A previous study has demonstrated that it is feasible to transfer idiotype-specific T cells from healthy donors to recipients (Kwak et al. 1995). The transferred idiotype-specific T cells protected mice against established tumor in mouse model (Hornung et al. 1995). T cells can also be generated in large number in vitro for adoptive T cell transfer. It has been demonstrated that the success of T cell transfer will depend heavily on the quality of transferred T cells. T cells that belong to central memory (T_{CM}) type but not terminal differentiated type (T_{EM}) can proliferate well and exert a protective role after adoptive transfer (Wherry et al. 2003; Gattinoni et al. 2005). Generating T cells that have a high percentage of T_{CM} cells is essential for the success of adoptive T cell transfer. IL-15 and IL-7 have been reported to increase the percentage of T_{CM} cells in the T cell population (Ku et al. 2000; Schluns et al. 2000; Tan et al. 2002). Recent studies also have demonstrated CD28 and CD27 expression and 4-1BB ligand interaction to increase the pool of T_{CM} cells (Acuto and Michel 2003; Oelke et al. 2003; Topp et al. 2003). Telomeres of T_{CM} cells are characteristically longer than those of T_{EM} cells, which make T_{CM} capable of going through multiple cell divisions (Weng et al. 1997; Rufer et al. 2003). IL-15 is capable of activating telomere synthesis in memory CD8 T cells via Jak3 and PI3K signaling pathways (Li et al. 2005). Further studies of the T cell population will help us to achieve the best culture conditions for preparing idiotype specific T_{CM} cells for adoptive T cell transfer. Moreover, CD4 T cells have proven to be able to improve and expand CD8 T cell function through cytokine- and CD40L-dependent pathways (Bevan 2004). Adoptive transfer of both CD4 and CD8 T cells produced a greater effect than single CD8 T cell transfer

(Ossendorp et al. 1998). Therefore in the future, idiotype-specific adoptive T cell transfer may involve both CD4 and CD8 T cells.

A healthy microenvironment has been demonstrated to be extremely important for the T cell response in vivo. For example, an increase in CD4+CD25+ Treg cell has been observed in lymphoma and myeloma patients (Beyer et al. 2006; Yang et al. 2006). In normal healthy donors, this group of T cells can suppress the autoimmunity mediated by T cells. However, in a tumor environment, this group of T cells can inhibit the immune response of tumor-specific T cells. In both human and mouse studies, it has been shown that the depletion of Treg can drastically increase the antitumor effect of immune system (Sutmuller et al. 2001; Dannull et al. 2005). Moreover CTLs have been reported to express inhibitor molecules, such as PD-1, CTLA4, and B7-1. These molecules can interfere with the cytotoxic function of CTLs, and the inhibition of these molecules has been shown to improve the antitumor immunity by tumor antigen-specific CTLs (Sutmuller et al. 2001; Iwai et al. 2002; Curiel et al. 2003). Taken together, these studies demonstrate that the combination therapy of active immunization and adoptive T cell transfer, together with immune suppressive pathway inhibition, may be the ideal immunotherapy strategy for hematologic malignancies in the future.

References

Acuto O, Michel F (2003) CD28-mediated co-stimulation: a quantitative support for TCR signalling. Nat Rev Immunol 3:939–951

Atassi MZ, Casali P (2008) Molecular mechanisms of autoimmunity. Autoimmunity 41:123–132

Baskar S, Kobrin CB, Kwak LW (2004) Autologous lymphoma vaccines induce human T cell responses against multiple, unique epitopes. J Clin Invest 113:1498–1510

Bendandi M, Gocke CD, Kobrin CB, Benko FA, Sternas LA, Pennington R, Watson TM, Reynolds CW, Gause BL, Duffey PL, Jaffe ES, Creekmore SP, Longo DL, Kwak LW (1999) Complete molecular remissions induced by patient-specific vaccination plus granulocyte-monocyte colony-stimulating factor against lymphoma. Nat Med 5:1171–1177

Berman JE, Malynn BA, Blackwell TK, Alt FW (1986) Regulation of immunoglobulin variable region gene assembly: development of the primary antibody repertoire. Bioessays 5:197–203

Bevan MJ (2004) Helping the CD8(+) T-cell response. Nat Rev Immunol 4:595–602

Beyer M, Kochanek M, Giese T, Endl E, Weihrauch MR, Knolle PA, Classen S, Schultze JL (2006) In vivo peripheral expansion of naive CD4+CD25high FoxP3+ regulatory T cells in patients with multiple myeloma. Blood 107:3940–3949

Biragyn A, Ruffini PA, Leifer CA, Klyushnenkova E, Shakhov A, Chertov O, Shirakawa AK, Farber JM, Segal DM, Oppenheim JJ, Kwak LW (2002) Toll-like receptor 4-dependent activation of dendritic cells by beta-defensin 2. Science 298:1025–1029

Butler JE (1997) Immunoglobulin gene organization and the mechanism of repertoire development. Scand J Immunol 45:455–462

Cohen S, Haimovich J, Hollander N (2009) Dendritic cell-based therapeutic vaccination against myeloma: vaccine formulation determines efficacy against light chain myeloma. J Immunol 182:1667–1673

Curiel TJ, Wei S, Dong H, Alvarez X, Cheng P, Mottram P, Krzysiek R, Knutson KL, Daniel B, Zimmermann MC, David O, Burow M, Gordon A, Dhurandhar N, Myers L, Berggren R,

Hemminki A, Alvarez RD, Emilie D, Curiel DT, Chen L, Zou W (2003) Blockade of B7-H1 improves myeloid dendritic cell-mediated antitumor immunity. Nat Med 9:562–567
Dabadghao S, Bergenbrant S, Anton D, He W, Holm G, Yi Q (1998) Anti-idiotypic T-cell activation in multiple myeloma induced by M-component fragments presented by dendritic cells. Br J Haematol 100:647–654
Dannull J, Su Z, Rizzieri D, Yang BK, Coleman D, Yancey D, Zhang A, Dahm P, Chao N, Gilboa E, Vieweg J (2005) Enhancement of vaccine-mediated antitumor immunity in cancer patients after depletion of regulatory T cells. J Clin Invest 115:3623–3633
Dudley ME, Wunderlich JR, Robbins PF, Yang JC, Hwu P, Schwartzentruber DJ, Topalian SL, Sherry R, Restifo NP, Hubicki AM, Robinson MR, Raffeld M, Duray P, Seipp CA, Rogers-Freezer L, Morton KE, Mavroukakis SA, White DE, Rosenberg SA (2002) Cancer regression and autoimmunity in patients after clonal repopulation with antitumor lymphocytes. Science 298:850–854
Dudley DD, Chaudhuri J, Bassing CH, Alt FW (2005) Mechanism and control of V(D)J recombination versus class switch recombination: similarities and differences. Adv Immunol 86:43–112
Esashi E, Wang YH, Perng O, Qin XF, Liu YJ, Watowich SS (2008) The signal transducer STAT5 inhibits plasmacytoid dendritic cell development by suppressing transcription factor IRF8. Immunity 28:509–520
Fagerberg J, Yi Q, Gigliotti D, Harmenberg U, Ruden U, Persson B, Osterborg A, Mellstedt H (1999) T-cell-epitope mapping of the idiotypic monoclonal IgG heavy and light chains in multiple myeloma. Int J Cancer 80:671–680
Fanning LJ, Connor AM, Wu GE (1996) Development of the immunoglobulin repertoire. Clin Immunol Immunopathol 79:1–14
Freedman A, Neelapu SS, Nichols C, Robertson MJ, Djulbegovic B, Winter JN, Bender JF, Gold DP, Ghalie RG, Stewart ME, Esquibel V, Hamlin P (2009) Placebo-controlled phase III trial of patient-specific immunotherapy with mitumprotimut-T and granulocyte-macrophage colony-stimulating factor after rituximab in patients with follicular lymphoma. J Clin Oncol 27:3036–3043
Gattinoni L, Klebanoff CA, Palmer DC, Wrzesinski C, Kerstann K, Yu Z, Finkelstein SE, Theoret MR, Rosenberg SA, Restifo NP (2005) Acquisition of full effector function in vitro paradoxically impairs the in vivo antitumor efficacy of adoptively transferred CD8+ T cells. J Clin Invest 115:1616–1626
Hamblin TJ, Davis Z, Gardiner A, Oscier DG, Stevenson FK (1999) Unmutated Ig V(H) genes are associated with a more aggressive form of chronic lymphocytic leukemia. Blood 94:1848–1854
Hansson L, Rabbani H, Fagerberg J, Osterborg A, Mellstedt H (2003) T-cell epitopes within the complementarity-determining and framework regions of the tumor-derived immunoglobulin heavy chain in multiple myeloma. Blood 101:4930–4936
Hareuveni M, Gautier C, Kieny MP, Wreschner D, Chambon P, Lathe R (1990) Vaccination against tumor cells expressing breast cancer epithelial tumor antigen. Proc Natl Acad Sci USA 87:9498–9502
Harig S, Witzens M, Krackhardt AM, Trojan A, Barrett P, Broderick R, Zauls AJ, Gribben JG (2001) Induction of cytotoxic T-cell responses against immunoglobulin V region-derived peptides modified at human leukocyte antigen-A2 binding residues. Blood 98:2999–3005
Herzog S, Reth M, Jumaa H (2009) Regulation of B-cell proliferation and differentiation by pre-B-cell receptor signalling. Nat Rev Immunol 9:195–205
Hida N, Maeda Y, Katagiri K, Takasu H, Harada M, Itoh K (2002) A simple culture protocol to detect peptide-specific cytotoxic T lymphocyte precursors in the circulation. Cancer Immunol Immunother 51:219–228
Hornung RL, Longo DL, Bowersox OC, Kwak LW (1995) Tumor antigen-specific immunization of bone marrow transplantation donors as adoptive therapy against established tumor. J Natl Cancer Inst 87:1289–1296

Houot R, Levy R (2009) T-cell modulation combined with intratumoral CpG cures lymphoma in a mouse model without the need for chemotherapy. Blood 113:3546–3552

Iwai Y, Ishida M, Tanaka Y, Okazaki T, Honjo T, Minato N (2002) Involvement of PD-L1 on tumor cells in the escape from host immune system and tumor immunotherapy by PD-L1 blockade. Proc Natl Acad Sci USA 99:12293–12297

Kafi K, Betting DJ, Yamada RE, Bacica M, Steward KK, Timmerman JM (2009) Maleimide conjugation markedly enhances the immunogenicity of both human and murine idiotype-KLH vaccines. Mol Immunol 46:448–456

Kaminski MS, Kitamura K, Maloney DG, Levy R (1987) Idiotype vaccination against murine B cell lymphoma. Inhibition of tumor immunity by free idiotype protein. J Immunol 138:1289–1296

Ku CC, Murakami M, Sakamoto A, Kappler J, Marrack P (2000) Control of homeostasis of CD8+ memory T cells by opposing cytokines. Science 288:675–678

Kuppers R (2005) Mechanisms of B-cell lymphoma pathogenesis. Nat Rev Cancer 5:251–262

Kwak LW, Longo DL (1996) Lymphomas. Cancer Chemother Biol Response Modif 16: 376–440

Kwak LW, Campbell MJ, Czerwinski DK, Hart S, Miller RA, Levy R (1992) Induction of immune responses in patients with B-cell lymphoma against the surface-immunoglobulin idiotype expressed by their tumors. N Engl J Med 327:1209–1215

Kwak LW, Taub DD, Duffey PL, Bensinger WI, Bryant EM, Reynolds CW, Longo DL (1995) Transfer of myeloma idiotype-specific immunity from an actively immunised marrow donor. Lancet 345:1016–1020

Kwak LW, Young HA, Pennington RW, Weeks SD (1996) Vaccination with syngeneic, lymphoma-derived immunoglobulin idiotype combined with granulocyte/macrophage colony-stimulating factor primes mice for a protective T-cell response. Proc Natl Acad Sci USA 93:10972–10977

Larson ED, Maizels N (2004) Transcription-coupled mutagenesis by the DNA deaminase AID. Genome Biol 5:211

Levy R, Robertson M, Ganjoo K, Leonard J, Vose J, Denney D (2008) Results of a Phase 3 trial evaluating safety and efficacy of specific immunotherapy, recombinant idiotype (Id) conjugated to KLH (Id-KLH) with GM-CSF, compared to non-specific immunotherapy, KLH with GM-CSF, in patients with follicular non-Hodgkin's lymphoma (fNHL). AACR Meeting Abstracts 2008, pp LB-204

Li A, Rue M, Zhou J, Wang H, Goldwasser MA, Neuberg D, Dalton V, Zuckerman D, Lyons C, Silverman LB, Sallan SE, Gribben JG (2004a) Utilization of Ig heavy chain variable, diversity, and joining gene segments in children with B-lineage acute lymphoblastic leukemia: implications for the mechanisms of VDJ recombination and for pathogenesis. Blood 103:4602–4609

Li Z, Woo CJ, Iglesias-Ussel MD, Ronai D, Scharff MD (2004b) The generation of antibody diversity through somatic hypermutation and class switch recombination. Genes Dev 18:1–11

Li Y, Zhi W, Wareski P, Weng NP (2005) IL-15 activates telomerase and minimizes telomere loss and may preserve the replicative life span of memory CD8+ T cells in vitro. J Immunol 174:4019–4024

Longo DL, Duffey PL, Gribben JG, Jaffe ES, Curti BD, Gause BL, Janik JE, Braman VM, Esseltine D, Wilson WH, Kaufman D, Wittes RE, Nadler LM, Urba WJ (2000) Combination chemotherapy followed by an immunotoxin (anti-B4-blocked ricin) in patients with indolent lymphoma: results of a phase II study. Cancer J 6:146–150

Lynch RG, Graff RJ, Sirisinha S, Simms ES, Eisen HN (1972) Myeloma proteins as tumor-specific transplantation antigens. Proc Natl Acad Sci USA 69:1540–1544

Mauerer K, Zahrieh D, Gorgun G, Li A, Zhou J, Ansen S, Rassenti LZ, Gribben JG (2005) Immunoglobulin gene segment usage, location and immunogenicity in mutated and unmutated chronic lymphocytic leukaemia. Br J Haematol 129:499–510

Odegard VH, Schatz DG (2006) Targeting of somatic hypermutation. Nat Rev Immunol 6:573–583

Oelke M, Maus MV, Didiano D, June CH, Mackensen A, Schneck JP (2003) Ex vivo induction and expansion of antigen-specific cytotoxic T cells by HLA-Ig-coated artificial antigen-presenting cells. Nat Med 9:619–624

Ossendorp F, Mengede E, Camps M, Filius R, Melief CJ (1998) Specific T helper cell requirement for optimal induction of cytotoxic T lymphocytes against major histocompatibility complex class II negative tumors. J Exp Med 187:693–702

Qin H, Cha SC, Neelapu SS, Lou Y, Wei J, Liu YJ, Kwak LW (2009) Vaccine site inflammation potentiates idiotype DNA vaccine-induced therapeutic T cell-, and not B cell-, dependent antilymphoma immunity. Blood 114:4142–4149

Rezvany MR, Jeddi-Tehrani M, Rabbani H, Ruden U, Hammarstrom L, Osterborg A, Wigzell H, Mellstedt H (2000) Autologous T lymphocytes recognize the tumour-derived immunoglobulin VH-CDR3 region in patients with B-cell chronic lymphocytic leukaemia. Br J Haematol 111:230–238

Rufer N, Zippelius A, Batard P, Pittet MJ, Kurth I, Corthesy P, Cerottini JC, Leyvraz S, Roosnek E, Nabholz M, Romero P (2003) Ex vivo characterization of human CD8+ T subsets with distinct replicative history and partial effector functions. Blood 102:1779–1787

Schjetne KW, Thompson KM, Nilsen N, Flo TH, Fleckenstein B, Iversen JG, Espevik T, Bogen B (2003) Cutting edge: link between innate and adaptive immunity: Toll-like receptor 2 internalizes antigen for presentation to CD4+ T cells and could be an efficient vaccine target. J Immunol 171:32–36

Schluns KS, Kieper WC, Jameson SC, Lefrancois L (2000) Interleukin-7 mediates the homeostasis of naive and memory CD8 T cells in vivo. Nat Immunol 1:426–432

Schuster SJ, Neelapu SS, Gause BL, Muggia FM, Gockerman JP, Sotomayor EM, Winter JN, Flowers CR, Stergiou AM, Kwak LW; for the Biovax IDPIIISI (2009) Idiotype vaccine therapy (BiovaxID) in follicular lymphoma in first complete remission: phase III clinical trial results. J Clin Oncol (Meeting Abstracts) 27:18s

Sirisinha S, Eisen HN (1971) Autoimmune-like antibodies to the ligand-binding sites of myeloma proteins. Proc Natl Acad Sci USA 68:3130–3135

Speiser DE, Lienard D, Rufer N, Rubio-Godoy V, Rimoldi D, Lejeune F, Krieg AM, Cerottini JC, Romero P (2005) Rapid and strong human CD8+ T cell responses to vaccination with peptide, IFA, and CpG oligodeoxynucleotide 7909. J Clin Invest 115:739–746

Stevenson GT, Stevenson FK (1975) Antibody to a molecularly-defined antigen confined to a tumour cell surface. Nature 254:714–716

Sutmuller RP, van Duivenvoorde LM, van Elsas A, Schumacher TN, Wildenberg ME, Allison JP, Toes RE, Offringa R, Melief CJ (2001) Synergism of cytotoxic T lymphocyte-associated antigen 4 blockade and depletion of CD25(+) regulatory T cells in antitumor therapy reveals alternative pathways for suppression of autoreactive cytotoxic T lymphocyte responses. J Exp Med 194:823–832

Tan JT, Ernst B, Kieper WC, LeRoy E, Sprent J, Surh CD (2002) Interleukin (IL)-15 and IL-7 jointly regulate homeostatic proliferation of memory phenotype CD8+ cells but are not required for memory phenotype CD4+ cells. J Exp Med 195:1523–1532

Teng G, Papavasiliou FN (2007) Immunoglobulin somatic hypermutation. Annu Rev Genet 41:107–120

Tiller T, Meffre E, Yurasov S, Tsuiji M, Nussenzweig MC, Wardemann H (2008) Efficient generation of monoclonal antibodies from single human B cells by single cell RT-PCR and expression vector cloning. J Immunol Methods 329:112–124

Topp MS, Riddell SR, Akatsuka Y, Jensen MC, Blattman JN, Greenberg PD (2003) Restoration of CD28 expression in CD28- CD8+ memory effector T cells reconstitutes antigen-induced IL-2 production. J Exp Med 198:947–955

Trojan A, Schultze JL, Witzens M, Vonderheide RH, Ladetto M, Donovan JW, Gribben JG (2000) Immunoglobulin framework-derived peptides function as cytotoxic T-cell epitopes commonly expressed in B-cell malignancies. Nat Med 6:667–672

Wadhwa M, Mellstedt H, Small E, Thorpe R (2003) Immunogenicity of GM-CSF products in cancer patients following immunostimulatory therapy with GM-CSF. Dev Biol (Basel) 112:61–67

Weiss S, Bogen B (1991) MHC class II-restricted presentation of intracellular antigen. Cell 64:767–776

Wen YJ, Lim SH (1997) T cells recognize the VH complementarity-determining region 3 of the idiotypic protein of B cell non-Hodgkin's lymphoma. Eur J Immunol 27:1043–1047

Weng N, Levine BL, June CH, Hodes RJ (1997) Regulation of telomerase RNA template expression in human T lymphocyte development and activation. J Immunol 158:3215–3220

Wherry EJ, Teichgraber V, Becker TC, Masopust D, Kaech SM, Antia R, von Andrian UH, Ahmed R (2003) Lineage relationship and protective immunity of memory CD8 T cell subsets. Nat Immunol 4:225–234

Yang ZZ, Novak AJ, Stenson MJ, Witzig TE, Ansell SM (2006) Intratumoral CD4+CD25+ regulatory T-cell-mediated suppression of infiltrating CD4+ T cells in B-cell non-Hodgkin lymphoma. Blood 107:3639–3646

Yi Q, Bergenbrant S, Osterborg A, Osby E, Ostman R, Bjorkholm M, Holm G, Lefvert AK (1993) T-cell stimulation induced by idiotypes on monoclonal immunoglobulins in patients with monoclonal gammopathies. Scand J Immunol 38:529–534

Yi Q, Dabadghao S, Osterborg A, Bergenbrant S, Holm G (1997) Myeloma bone marrow plasma cells: evidence for their capacity as antigen-presenting cells. Blood 90:1960–1967

Zirlik KM, Zahrieh D, Neuberg D, Gribben JG (2006) Cytotoxic T cells generated against heteroclitic peptides kill primary tumor cells independent of the binding affinity of the native tumor antigen peptide. Blood 108:3865–3870

Modulation of CTLA-4 and GITR for Cancer Immunotherapy

Francesca Avogadri, Jianda Yuan, Arvin Yang, David Schaer, and Jedd D. Wolchok

Contents

1 Introduction 212
2 CTLA-4 Preclinical Data 213
2.1 CTLA-4: A "Brake" on T Cell Activation 214
2.2 Preclinical Studies Using CTLA-4 Blocking Antibodies 217
3 GITR Preclinical 219
3.1 GITR: "Accelerator" of Effector Function 220
3.2 Preclinical Studies Using GITR Agonist Antibody 220
4 Clinical Experiences with CTLA-4 Blockade 222
4.1 CTLA-4 Monotherapy 223
4.2 Postsurgical Adjuvant Therapy 225
4.3 Combinations 226
4.4 Tremelimumab 226
4.5 Immune Related Adverse Effects 227
4.6 Novel Criteria for Antitumor Response to Ipilimumab and Increased Duration of Response 227
4.7 Other Malignancies 228
5 From Clinical Trials, Back to the Bench 229
5.1 Monitoring Antigen-Specific CD4+ and CD8+ T Cell Activity and Polyfunctionality 229

F. Avogadri and D. Schaer
Immunology Program, Sloan-Kettering Institute, New York, NY 10065, USA

J. Yuan
Immunology Program, Sloan-Kettering Institute, New York, NY 10065, USA
Ludwig Center for Cancer Immunotherapy, Immunology Program, Sloan-Kettering Institute, New York, NY 10065, USA

A. Yang and J.D. Wolchok (✉)
Immunology Program, Sloan-Kettering Institute, New York, NY 10065, USA
Melanoma/Sarcoma Service, Department of Medicine, Memorial Sloan-Kettering Cancer Center, New York, NY 10065, USA
Ludwig Center for Cancer Immunotherapy, Immunology Program, Sloan-Kettering Institute, New York, NY 10065, USA
e-mail: wolchokj@mskcc.org

G. Dranoff (ed.), *Cancer Immunology and Immunotherapy*,
Current Topics in Microbiology and Immunology 344, DOI 10.1007/82_2010_49

5.2 Cellular Phenotype Analysis: ICOS, Foxp3, HLA-DR and IDO 230
5.3 ICOS 231
5.4 Foxp3 231
5.5 HLA-DR 231
5.6 IDO 232
5.7 Antibody Responses 232
5.8 The "Immunogram": A Tool to Synthesize Immune Monitoring 233
6 Future Directions 233
References 236

Abstract The rational manipulation of antigen-specific T cells to reignite a tumor-specific immune response in cancer patients is a challenge for cancer immunotherapy. Targeting coinhibitory and costimulatory T cell receptors with specific antibodies in cancer patients is an emerging approach to T cell manipulation, namely "immune modulation." Cytotoxic T-lymphocyte antigen-4 (CTLA-4) and glucocorticoid-induced tumor necrosis factor family receptor (GITR) are potential targets for immune modulation through anti-CTLA-4 blocking antibodies and anti-GITR agonistic antibodies, respectively. In this review, we first discuss preclinical findings key to the understanding of the mechanisms of action of these immunomodulatory antibodies and the preclinical evidence of antitumor activity which preceded translation into the clinic. We next describe the outcomes and immune related adverse effects associated with anti-CTLA-4 based clinical trials with particular emphasis on specific biomarkers used to elucidate the mechanisms of tumor immunity in patients. The experience with anti-CTLA-4 therapy and the durable clinical benefit observed provide proof of principle to effective antitumor immune modulation and the promise of future clinical immune modulatory antibodies.

1 Introduction

In the late nineteenth century, the antitumor effects of Coley's toxin provided the first suggestive evidence that the immune system could be harnessed to combat cancer. Over 100 years later, we now possess a better understanding of mechanisms of T cell activation and the technology to manipulate these findings in the clinical setting. Current clinical, immunotherapeutic treatments, although not exclusively effective in one disease, have been most successful in melanoma. FDA approved treatments for melanoma include the adjuvant use of high-dose interferon alpha and high-dose IL-2 in the metastastic setting. The complete list of approved therapies for melanoma only requires the addition of dacarbazine (DTIC), the only FDA approved chemotherapeutic agent for melanoma. The modest response rates for both IL-2 and DTIC coupled with recent epidemiological data demonstrating an increasing incidence of melanoma provide incentive for alternative strategies. Recent advances in immunology have led to a more profound insight regarding the function of costimulatory and coinhibitory receptors expressed by different T cell subsets, providing a novel approach to optimize immunotherapies through immune modulation.

During the primary activation of naïve T lymphocytes, the immune system utilizes various checks and balances to maintain tolerance to self while assuring appropriate activation against foreign and self antigens. Although primary antigen recognition occurs through the interactions of the T cell receptor (TCR) and peptide-MHC complexes, without costimulation through CD28 binding to either B7-1 (CD80) or B7-2 (CD86), cognate antigen recognition will result only in T cell anergy induction (Linsley and Ledbetter 1993). This first check is followed by additional signals mediated by coinhibitory/costimulatory receptors, such as cytotoxic T-lymphocyte antigen-4 (CTLA-4) and glucocorticoid-induced tumor necrosis factor family receptor (GITR), which further shape the resulting effector function and dictate its efficacy and duration. Since their discovery, much effort has been put into understanding the immunomodulatory properties of CTLA-4 and GITR in mice. The development of antibodies specifically targeting these receptors and modulating their functions has provided a new perspective for immunotherapeutic approaches.

Under physiological stimulus, TCR binding causes activation of a complex signaling cascade culminating in downstream activation of the NF-κB, NFAT pathways and target gene transcription (Chan et al. 1995; Zhang et al. 1998; van Leeuwen and Samelson 1999; Tybulewicz et al. 2003). However, naive T cells require CD28 costimulation to maintain this cascade. When CD28 is activated, it potentiates the cascade through activation of PI3K and Sos resulting in stabilization of mRNA for NF-κB, NFAT (Pages et al. 1994). The importance of costimulation in T cell physiology is highlighted by CD28−/− mice which have dramatic reduction in the ability to maintain T cell activation (Lucas et al. 1995). Thus, CD28 provides the first checkpoint in T cell activation, sensing the expression of CD80/CD86 on an activated antigen presenting cell (APC). If the APC has not experienced the proper "danger signals" (e.g., cytokines, TLR, Fc Receptor stimulus), it will not optimally upregulate the expression of CD80/CD86. This need for CD28 costimulation is thought to reduce inadvertent activation of possibly self-reactive T cell clones in the periphery, which have escaped thymic deletion. Reinforcing this checkpoint is CTLA-4, which acts as a coinhibitory molecule. Antagonizing CD28 T cell costimulation, CTLA-4 binds with much greater affinity to CD80/CD86 and effectively shuts off TCR signaling (van der Merwe et al. 1997).

2 CTLA-4 Preclinical Data

CTLA-4 is a member of the CD28:B7 immunoglobulin superfamily. In contrast to CD28, CTLA-4 is normally expressed at low levels on the surface of naive effector T cells (Teff) and mainly exists in prepackaged vesicles inside the cytosol (Alegre et al. 1996). When the TCR stimulus to the naive T cell is too strong or lasts too long, CTLA-4 is recruited to the cell surface in a polar manner with release at the site of the immunological synapse (IS) (Linsley et al. 1996). Once at the IS, CTLA-4 can now compete with CD28 for CD80/CD86 (Chuang et al. 1999; Carreno et al. 2000; Cinek et al. 2000), effectively shutting off TCR signaling (van der Merwe et al. 1997). While CTLA-4 translocation to the cell membrane has been shown to depend on many events downstream of TCR signaling (reviewed in (Rudd et al. 2009)), it is not yet entirely clear how CTLA-4 mediates TCR signaling shut down upon binding to CD80/CD86. CTLA-4 does not have traditional immune tyrosine inhibitory motif (ITIM) domains, which are known to recruit regulatory proteins through binding of SH2 domains to phosphorylated tyrosine residues in the (I/V/L/S)xYxx(L/V) motif (Blank et al. 2009). However, CTLA-4 does have other tyrosine motifs which have been shown to recruit phosphatases SHP-2, and PP2A, yet the functional significance of these interactions remain unclear. For instance, SHP-2 also associates with CD28 and has been shown to potentiate the TCR cascade (Gadina et al. 1998). Although PP2A may act as a negative regulator of the TCR cascade, whether or not it does this through its interactions with CTLA-4 is also not fully established (Chuang et al. 2000). Besides directing downstream signaling events, it is thought that CTLA-4 may function simply to sequester CD80/CD86 away from CD28 because of its higher affinity for these molecules. In fact, mutant CTLA-4 molecules with levels of surface expression that lack tyrosines or prolines in their cytoplasmic tail are still able to suppress CD80-mediated CD28 activation signals (Carreno et al. 2000; Cinek et al. 2000).

Once it has been triggered, CTLA-4 may destabilize components of the super molecular activation complex (SMAC) in the IS. In fact, CTLA-4 was shown to alter lipid raft formation, resulting in reduced phosphorylation of linker for the activation of T cells (LAT) after TCR and CD28 stimulation (Martin et al. 2001). This block in IS formation applies also to ZAP-70 microclusters which are needed to maintain calcium flux and downstream events in TCR signaling (Bunnell et al. 2002; Schneider et al. 2008). Thus, CTLA-4 requires initial TCR signaling for its membrane targeting, and subsequently shuts off these early activation events.

2.1 CTLA-4: A "Brake" on T Cell Activation

The importance of CTLA-4 control of T cell activation was originally demonstrated by studies showing that blockade of CTLA-4:B7 interactions enhanced T cell responses in vitro (Walunas et al. 1994). In vivo adoptive transfer experiments confirmed that anti-CTLA-4 antibodies or Fab fragments greatly enhanced the accumulation of OVA-specific CD4+ T cells following peptide immunization (Kearney et al. 1995). Further proof of the major role for CTLA-4 in inhibiting T cell expansion came from the phenotype of CTLA-4−/− mice, which die within 3–4 weeks of birth because of lymphoproliferation and fatal tissue destruction in multiple organs (Waterhouse et al. 1995; Tivol et al. 1995). Administration of recombinant CTLA-4-Ig protected CTLA-4−/− mice from lethal lymphoproliferation (Tivol et al. 1997), corroborating the concept that CTLA-4 is a negative regulator of CD28-dependent T cell responses in vivo, which is further supported by evidence that CTLA-4/B7-1/B7-2 triple KO mice lack lymphoproliferative disease (Mandelbrot et al. 1999).

2.1.1 Cell Intrinsic Suppression

Both CD4+ and CD8+ T cells show higher proliferative potential and an activated phenotype when lacking CTLA-4 in vitro and in vivo (Chambers et al. 1997, 1998, 1999; Greenwald et al. 2001, 2002; McCoy et al. 1999). Interestingly, lack of CTLA-4 had a more dramatic effect on the proliferation of CD4+ T cells in vivo, resulting in a skewing of the CD4/CD8 ratio toward CD4+ T cells. In addition, CD4+ T cells were necessary and sufficient for the massive infiltration of peripheral organs, and CD8+ T cell activation was entirely CD4+ T cell dependent (Chambers et al. 1997). The function of CTLA-4 in CD4+ T cells was then more closely investigated using TCR transgenic mice. Lack of CTLA-4 enhanced both primary and secondary peptide-specific responses of CD4+ and TCR tg and DO11 TCR tg CD4+ T cells (Chambers et al. 1999; Greenwald et al. 2001). CTLA-4−/− DO11 TCR tg T cells were also resistant to tolerance induction. Additionally, experiments with anti-CTLA-4 blocking antibodies consistently showed that CTLA-4 engagement induced peripheral CD4+ T cell tolerance (Perez et al. 1997) and regulated CD4+ T cell activation in a cell intrinsic manner by modulating cell cycle progression (Greenwald et al. 2001, 2002). To investigate the role of CTLA-4 in CD8+ T cells, adoptive transfer experiments were performed with pmel-1 TCR tg mice, specific for the self antigen gp100, which showed that lack of CTLA-4 did not have evident cell intrinsic effects on CD8+ T cells. In fact, pmel-1 CTLA-4−/− mice developed autoimmune hypopigmentation in a CD4+ T cell dependent manner (Gattinoni et al. 2006). However, experiments with 2CT TCR tg T cells indicated that secondary CD8+ responses significantly increased in the absence of CTLA-4 (Chambers et al. 1998). Similarly, in response to a dendritic cell based vaccine, 318 TCR tg T cells proliferated more in the presence of anti-CTLA-4 neutralizing antibodies in a CD4-independent fashion (McCoy et al. 1999). Consistent with CTLA-4−/− mice, TCR transgenic mice lacking CTLA-4 developed lymphoproliferative disease, although with a delayed onset, which was abrogated in a RAG−/− background. This indicated that T cells specific for an endogenous self-antigen are likely required to trigger tissue destruction in the absence of CTLA-4.

2.1.2 Cell Extrinsic Suppression

Reconstitution of RAG1/2−/− animals with wild type (WT) and/or CTLA-4−/− bone marrow cells or T cells demonstrated that tissue damage induced by transferred CTLA-4−/− cells could be inhibited in a dose-dependent manner by concomitant transfer of WT cells (Bachmann et al. 1999; Tivol and Gorski 2002; Friedline et al. 2009). These experiments suggested that CTLA-4 dependent inhibition is not only cell autonomous. In fact, CD25+CD4+ T cells and not CD8+ T cells or NKT cells were required to mediate the CTLA-4-dependent extrinsic immune-suppression, in an IL-10 independent fashion (Friedline et al. 2009). This *trans*-regulation depended on the persistent presence of WT suppressor cells and was reversible. Tolerized CTLA-4−/− Teff cells in WT:KO chimeras became pathogenic when transferred into a new Rag1−/− recipient without WT cells. Overall, these experiments showed that regulatory T cells (Tregs) expressing CTLA-4 maintain self tolerance and immune homeostasis in a dominant fashion. This was confirmed by the phenotype of conditional knockout mice lacking CTLA-4 in the CD4+Foxp3+ Treg cell compartment (CKO) (Wing et al. 2008), which developed systemic lymphoproliferation, indicating that CTLA-4 deficiency in Foxp3+ T cells is sufficient to destabilize immune homeostasis. Of note, the onset of disease in CKO mice is delayed as compared to CTLA-4, indicating that CTLA-4 expression on effector cells contributes to control disease progression. These findings indicate that the extrinsic suppressive mechanism of CTLA-4 has a more pronounced role in immune homeostasis and self tolerance as compared to the intrinsic suppression.

The relative contribution of CTLA-4 blockade on Tregs versus Teffs can be different in different disease models. For instance, blocking CTLA-4 on Tregs alone is not sufficient to promote T cell mediated tumor rejection in a mouse melanoma model that is responsive to anti-CTLA-4 treatment in combination with vaccine (Peggs et al. 2009; Quezada et al. 2006). In this case, blocking CTLA-4 on Teffs is necessary to induce tumor immunity, although additional CTLA-4 blockade on Tregs has added effects that lead to maximal tumor immunity. By contrast, in a T cell-mediated colitis model (Read et al. 2000), anti-CTLA-4 mAb induced colitis by primarily affecting Tregs and not colitogenic Teffs (Read et al. 2006). The nature of the target antigen and the inflammatory stimulus that trigger the response may explain the different outcomes. In addition, a CTLA-4 splice variant (liCTLA-4) has recently been identified which is expressed at high levels on resting T cells (Vijayakrishnan et al. 2004). As liCTLA-4 lacks the B7 binding domain, its suppressive function is absent in CTLA-4−/− mice, but is not abrogated by anti-CTLA-4 blocking antibodies, perhaps explaining some of the discrepancies observed. Similarly, the fact that CTLA-4 deficient Tregs express more IL-10 and TGF-β as compared to WT Tregs (Tang et al. 2004) might also account for some of the differences.

The mechanism(s) underlying the extrinsic inhibitory effect of CTLA-4 is/are still largely unknown. It is possible that CTLA-4 expressing Tregs directly inhibit Teffs through the release of immunosuppressive cytokines. Another possible scenario is that CTLA-4 expressing Tregs "condition" other cells, which in turn inhibit Teffs. It has been shown, for example, that CTLA-4 positive TCR tg T cells failed to form long-term interactions with APCs in the presence of antigen in vitro and in vivo (Schneider et al. 2006), suggesting that dendritic cells may be important to induce/maintain CTLA-4-dependent Treg-mediated immune suppression. Indeed, CD4 + CD25+ cells can induce dendritic cells to express enzyme indoleamine 2,3-dioxygenase (IDO) in vitro (Fallarino et al. 2003), possibly via a CTLA-4 dependent mechanism. Similarly, CTLA-4 expression on Foxp3+ Tregs mediates downregulation of CD80 and CD86 on splenic dendritic cells in vitro (Wing et al. 2008).

The CTLA-4 dependent suppressive activity of T regs in vivo may therefore be mediated, at least in part, by APCs such as dendritic cells.

2.2 *Preclinical Studies Using CTLA-4 Blocking Antibodies*

As an immunosuppressive role of CTLA-4 was becoming apparent, the possibility that inhibiting CTLA-4:B7 interaction could have beneficial antitumor effects, by enhancing tumor-specific T cell responses, was hypothesized.

2.2.1 Monotherapy

The initial evidence that blocking CTLA-4 with anti-CTLA-4 antibody could treat established tumors came from studies done in transplantable tumor models of colon carcinoma (51BLim10), fibrosarcoma (Sa1N and CSA1M), ovarian carcinoma (OV-HM), and prostate cancer (TRAMPC1) (Leach et al. 1996; Kwon et al. 1997; Yang et al. 1997). Not only did these models demonstrate that blocking CTLA-4 caused tumor regression as a single agent, but they also showed that the immunity generated provided protection to subsequent challenge with the same tumor. While the use of anti-CTLA-4 as a single agent to treat established tumors showed very promising results in immunogenic cell lines, the beneficial effect was only marginal in the case of established poorly immunogenic tumors (immunogenicity being defined in general as the ability of an irradiated cell line to induce rejection of a subsequent challenge with the same cell line).

2.2.2 CTLA-4 and Active/Passive Immunization

Combination of anti-CTLA-4 with GM-CSF-expressing tumor vaccines resulted in the regression of the poorly immunogenic SM1 mammary tumor (Hurwitz et al. 1998) and B16 melanoma (van Elsas et al. 1999). The same approach showed promising effects in the transgenic adenocarcinoma of the mouse prostate (TRAMP) mouse model, decreasing tumor incidence and grade (Hurwitz et al. 2000). In these preclinical models, treatment with anti-CTLA-4 or the GM-CSF expressing vaccine alone was not sufficient to mediate tumor regression, but the combination of the two treatments had a synergistic effect. The nature of the immune response required for tumor rejection varied depending on the tumor model. In fact, both CD4+ and CD8+ T cell responses could mediate rejection of the SM1 mammary tumor; by contrast, rejection of B16 was mediated by CD8+ T cells and natural killer (NK) cells as well as required perforin and Fas/FasL interactions, but not CD4+ T cells and TNFα (van Elsas et al. 2001).

CTLA-4 blockade has also shown synergistic effects with other vaccination strategies, such as TRP-2 peptide in CpG-ODN adjuvant (Davila et al. 2003) or TRP-2, gp100, and PSMA xenogeneic DNA vaccines (Gregor et al. 2004) for melanoma and prostate cancer. Interestingly, CTLA-4 blockade did not provide additional benefit when combined with an idiotypic vaccine that induced dormancy in mice with BCL1 lymphoma, suggesting that anti-CTLA-4 might not enhance antigen-specific antitumor effects that are B cell mediated (Pop et al. 2005).

The possibility that CTLA-4 blockade could enhance the antitumor potency of adoptive T cell transfer has also been investigated in mice. Although the transfer of OVA-specific CD8+ T cells along with anti-CTLA-4 showed synergistic CD4-dependent effects against the OVA-expressing thymoma E.G7 (Shrikant et al. 1999), lack of CTLA-4 expression did not enhance antitumor efficacy of adoptively transferred gp100-specific CD8+ T cells in conjunction with rFPhgp100 vaccine and rhIL2 (Gattinoni et al. 2006). This could possibly be due to differences in the antigen and/or the adjuvant used to activate the transferred T cells. Further experiments would be important to address these discrepancies.

2.2.3 CTLA-4 and Chemotherapy/Radiotherapy/Tumor Ablation

Synergy between ionizing radiation therapy and anti-CTLA-4 has been reported in the 4T1 and TSA mammary tumor and MCA38 colon carcinoma models (Demaria et al. 2005). Combination of the two treatments showed a systemic antitumor effect that inhibited the growth of a distant tumor outside the radiation field, suggesting that the combination of CTLA-4 blockade and local radiation enhanced a tumor-specific immune response. It is possible that while radiation provided a source of antigen or increased MHC I expression/peptide processing on tumor cells and stroma (Reits et al. 2006; Zhang et al. 2007), anti-CTLA-4 treatment synergistically empowered the effects of cross-presentation. Anti-CTLA-4 also enhanced antitumor immunity when combined with in situ tumor destructive cryoablation or radiofrequency ablation in a transplantable melanoma model expressing the nonself model antigen OVA (den Brok et al. 2006). It will be interesting to see whether such synergy occurs in nonmanipulated tumors and if tolerance against self antigens can be averted by this means.

Furthermore, CTLA-4 blockade has shown significant therapeutic benefits in mice bearing the MOPC-315 transplantable plasmacytoma tumor, when combined with a subtherapeutic dose of the chemotherapeutic agent melphalan, perhaps reflecting a synergy provided by targeting multiple immunoregulatory pathways (Mokyr et al. 1998a, b). The combination between chemotherapy and CTLA-4 blockade in animal models warrants further investigation. It will be interesting to dissect whether possible synergies require an effect of the chemotherapeutic agents on immune cells or tumors.

2.2.4 CTLA-4 and Other Immunostimulatory Strategies

CTLA-4 blocking antibody dramatically enhanced the antitumor efficacy of a recombinant oncolytic virus developed to preferentially target breast cancer cells

(Gao et al. 2009). Targeting tumor cells with viruses may therefore represent a valuable approach to enhance inflammation at the tumor site and to increase tumor immunogenicity locally, thus providing a window of opportunity for treatment with anti-CTLA-4.

Another way to increase the efficacy of anti-CTLA-4 blockade could be to combine it with other monoclonal antibodies that target immune receptors. It has been recently shown that combining anti-CTLA-4 with the agonistic anti-OX40 mAb (OX86) potentiates the systemic effects of intratumoral CpG treatments in a mouse lymphoma model (Houot and Levy 2009). Several other immunomodulatory mAbs have shown potent anticancer effects in mouse models including the anti-GITR agonistic mAb DTA-1, described later in this chapter, and might be future candidates to combine with anti-CTLA-4.

3 GITR Preclinical

GITR was originally described by Nocentini et al. after being cloned from dexamethasone-treated murine T cell hybridomas (Nocentini et al. 1997). Unlike CD28 and CTLA-4, GITR has a very low basal expression on naive CD4+ and CD8+ T cells (Ronchetti et al. 2004). This is in contrast to Treg cells which express both CTLA-4 and GITR at high levels constitutively. After activation, both naive and Treg cells upregulate expression of GITR which lasts several days and is highest in tumor infiltrating lymphocytes (Tone et al. 2003; Cohen unpublished results).

GITR ligand (GITR-L) is expressed at low levels by APCs such as macrophages, dendritic cells, and B cells. Like CD80/CD86, GITR-L is upregulated upon activation with stimuli such as TLR ligands (Tone et al. 2003; Suvas et al. 2005). Similar to other members of the TNF superfamily, GITR contains TNF receptor associate factor (TRAF) binding domains in its cytoplasmic tail; however, it does not contain so called death domains which directly mediate apoptosis found on Fas and Trail (reviewed in Nocentini and Riccardi (2005)). Through yeast two hybrid screening, GITR was shown to interact specifically with TRAF 1, 2, and 3 which mediate downstream signaling from the receptor. Stimulation of GITR can cause activation of NF-κB (Nocentini et al. 1997; Ronchetti et al. 2004). In addition, GITR has been shown to activate members of the MAPK pathway, including p38, JNK, and ERK (Esparza and Arch 2005). By activating these pathways and their downstream events, GITR ligation is in turn believed to enhance T cell survival by upregulating IL-2Rα, IL-2, and IFNγ, along with rescuing T cells from anti-CD3 mediated apoptosis (Ronchetti et al. 2004). While GITR does not have canonical death domains in its cytoplasmic tail, GITR has been shown to bind to the death domain containing protein, Siva (Spinicelli et al. 2002). As a result of its interaction with Siva, Spinicelli et al. demonstrated that GITR ligation can induce apoptosis in Cos7 cells. However, how this interaction modulates GITR function in primary T cells has yet to be established.

3.1 GITR: "Accelerator" of Effector Function

Triggering or blocking GITR signaling on immune cells has provided most of the evidence that GITR may be a T cell costimulatory receptor. GITR ligation by GITR-L enhances both CD4+ and CD8+ T cell proliferation and effector functions, particularly in the setting of suboptimal TCR stimulation (Tone et al. 2003; Kanamaru et al. 2004; Kohm et al. 2004; Ronchetti et al. 2004). In contrast, blocking GITR-GITR-L signaling with anti-GITR-L antibodies inhibited lymphocyte proliferation (Stephens et al. 2004). Consistent with this idea, injection of anti-GITR agonistic antibody in neonatal mice induced overt autoimmune disease (Shimizu et al. 2002).

Similar to the differential roles that CTLA-4 plays on various T cell subsets, GITR stimulation may affect Tregs differently from Teffs. Treatment of Tregs with anti-GITR polyclonal sera (McHugh et al. 2002) or with the rat monoclonal anti-GITR antibody DTA-1 (Shimizu et al. 2002) inhibited the suppression induced in vitro by CD4+ CD25+ T cells when cocultured with CD4+ CD25− or CD8+ T cells with anti-CD3 stimulation and irradiated APCs. Addition of recombinant GITRL or cells transfected with GITRL to Treg/Teff cocultures had similar outcomes (Tone et al. 2003).

These experiments raised the question regarding the relative contribution of GITR signaling to Tregs and Teffs. Experiments done in vitro have shown that GITR stimulation induced direct proliferation of Tregs (McHugh et al. 2002; Ronchetti et al. 2002) and of effector cells (Ronchetti et al. 2002; Tone et al. 2003; Kanamaru et al. 2004). In addition to the direct proliferative effects, GITR ligation on Teffs may allow these cells to overcome Treg-mediated suppression (Stephens et al. 2004; Zhou et al. 2007). Other data showed that GITR ligation on Tregs could also indirectly contribute to immunostimulation by inhibiting their suppressive activity (Shimizu et al. 2002; Ronchetti et al. 2004).

Interestingly, studies done with GITR KO mice showed that GITR-deficient lymphocytes proliferate more and are more sensitive to activation induced cell death (AICD) as compared to lymphocytes expressing GITR (Ronchetti et al. 2002), supporting a role for this pathway in lymphocyte proliferation/survival. CD4+CD25+ T cells lacking GITR, instead, were equally able to suppress when compared to WT CD4+CD25+ T cells, suggesting that GITR signaling may be more relevant on Teffs rather than Tregs.

3.2 Preclinical Studies Using GITR Agonist Antibody

The observation that GITR stimulation has immunostimulatory effects in vitro and induced autoimmunity in vivo prompted the investigation of the antitumor potency of triggering this pathway.

3.2.1 Monotherapy

Injection of the anti-GITR agonistic antibody DTA-1 eradicated established Meth A fibrosarcoma and CT26 carcinoma in an IFN-γ dependent manner and induced tumor specific CD4+ and CD8+ T cell responses (Ko et al. 2005). This immunomodulatory antibody was most effective eight days after tumor inoculation, possibly implying a requirement for tumor-dependent T cell priming and/or the establishment of a structured tumor microenvironment. DTA-1 treatment could also induce concomitant tumor immunity that resulted in rejection of a distal poorly immunogenic B16 melanoma (Turk et al. 2004). The growth of the primary B16 melanoma was transiently slowed by a single DTA-1 dose and the tumor was rejected by multiple DTA-1 doses (at day 1, 4, and 9 after tumor inoculation) in a T cell (both CD4+ and CD8+) and NK cell dependent fashion. In this model, DTA-1's mechanism of action required IFN-γ and FasL, but not perforin while inducing tumor immunity through endogenous T cell response against B16 (Ramirez-Montagut et al. 2006). Furthermore, as observed in vitro, DTA-1 treatment also expanded Foxp3+ Tregs in vivo. Interestingly, the expanded Tregs retained their suppressive capabilities, as assessed by ex vivo suppression assays, but their expansion did not impact negatively on tumor growth. While Tregs are still suppressive in the periphery, we have recently demonstrated, using the B16 melanoma model, that GITR modulation has a profound effect on intra-tumor Tregs. Treatment with DTA-1 causes a significant impairment of intra-tumor Treg accumulation and loss of FoxP3 expression (Cohen et al. 2010). This results in a much more favorable intra-tumor Teff:Treg ratio and enhanced tumor-specific CD8+ T-cell activity. Impairment of Treg infiltration was lost if Tregs were GITR−/−, and the protective effect of DTA-1 was reduced in reconstituted RAG1−/− mice if either the Treg or Teff subset were GITR-negative and absent if both were negative. Our recent data further corroborates the concept that DTA-1 administration has effects on both Teffs and Tregs in vivo, both of which may be important to the generation of tumor immunity.

3.2.2 GITR and Active Immunization

Consistent with the hypothesis that DTA-1 has a direct role on Teff cell expansion and activation, administration of DTA-1 enhanced effector and memory CD8+ T cell responses to self antigens improved tumor protection when combined with a xenogenic DNA vaccine for gp100 or TRP-2 (Cohen et al. 2006). Importantly, DTA-1 was most effective when boosting vaccine-induced CD8+ T cells before the second immunization. By contrast, DTA-1 administration before the first immunization failed to enhance tumor rejection, possibly by enhancing AICD rather than T cell expansion. This indicated that triggering GITR signaling with DTA-1 in vivo has different outcomes on T cell activation depending on the timing with respect to the antigenic stimulation. The exact reason for this is unknown, but it may reflect differences in the signaling pathways activated at different stages of priming.

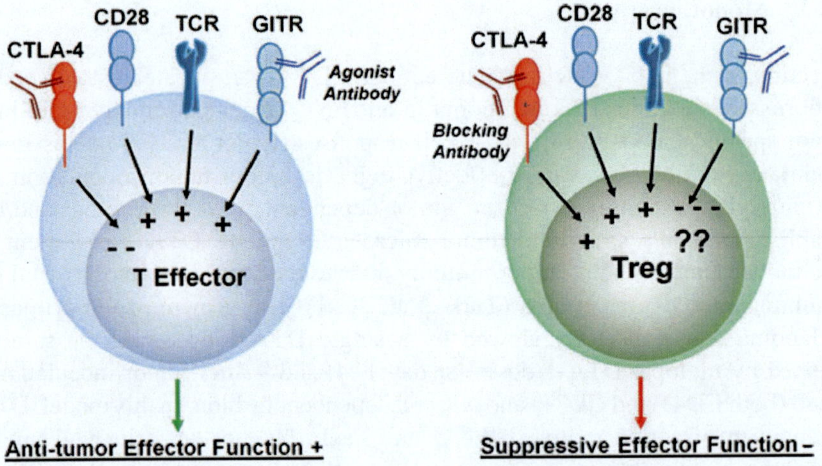

Fig. 1 Differential outcomes of CTLA-4 and GITR monoclonal antibody therapy on different T cell lineages. Although CTLA-4 and GITR are present on both Teffs and Tregs, it has become apparent that each lineage incorporates signals from these receptors differently. In Teffs, CTLA-4 provides a strong negative signal which blocks positive stimuli from the TCR and CD28 during priming. GITR on the other hand, provides additional positive stimuli that may overcome CTLA-4's negative effect. Unlike Teffs, Tregs express CTLA-4 and GITR constitutively, an initial clue to a variation in their roles. In fact, Tregs have been shown to be nonfunctional without CTLA-4 expression. This suggests that Tregs may see signals from CTLA-4 as a "positive stimulus" as part of their "suppressive effector functions." Likewise, evidence has shown that under certain conditions, GITR ligation on Tregs may negatively modulate their suppressive ability. The divergent incorporation of signals from these receptors is why the effects of antibody therapy to these receptors may have different effects on each lineage. Blocking CTLA-4 antibodies prevents negative signals to Teffs while at the same time stopping Tregs from receiving positive stimuli. Agonist GITR antibodies work in reverse, providing costimulatory signals to Teffs whereas Tregs may see this stimulus in a negative manner. Thus, while these antibodies enhance desired Teff antitumor activity, they may have the added benefit of negating the suppressive functions of Tregs

This consideration will be extremely important when designing combination cancer immunotherapies based on the use of DTA-1.

Overall, immune modulation of CTLA-4 and GITR with blocking and agonistic monoclonal antibodies, respectively, has proven effective in a variety of preclinical tumor models. Although the mechanism of action differs for the two antibodies, they share the complexity of affecting distinct T cell populations with opposing outcomes, as illustrated in Fig. 1.

4 Clinical Experiences with CTLA-4 Blockade

Clinical application of immunomodulatory antibodies has presented a new approach to systemic anticancer therapy. These agents are designed to activate the patient's immune system to eliminate cancer as opposed to administration of cytotoxic agents directed at the tumor itself (treating the patient versus treating the cancer).

Given these fundamental differences from cytotoxic chemotherapy, it was not unexpected to observe differences in the kinetics of the antitumor response, duration of response, and immune related adverse effects. In fact, the efficacy of ipilimumab, an anti-CTLA-4 antibody, appears to be independent of currently accepted negative clinical prognostic factors (Wolchok et al. 2009a).

Currently, there are two available CTLA-4 blocking monoclonal antibodies, ipilimumab (MDX-010) and tremelimumab (CP-675,206) (Phan et al. 2003; Ribas et al. 2005, 2008; Weber 2008). Both antibodies were developed in mice transgenic for human immunoglobulin genes, thereby producing fully human antibodies against CTLA-4. These agents have been most extensively studied in melanoma; however, there have also been durable responses noted in prostate, ovarian, breast, and renal cell cancer (Table 1). For metastatic melanoma in particular, anti-CTLA-4 blockade opens up a new avenue of treatment for patients that have very few options and have only a historical 6–9 month median survival without therapy.

4.1 CTLA-4 Monotherapy

In an initial trial of 17 patients with unresectable melanoma treated with ipilimumab, there were two partial responses (PRs) at the starting dose of 3 mg/kg administered as a single dose. These responses were durable and treatment was well tolerated but for a mild rash (Tchekmedyian et al. 2002). A second pilot trial was conducted with patients that had been prior participants in tumor vaccine studies for metastatic disease. Nine patients who were previously treated with a GM-CSF secreting tumor cell vaccine, including seven with metastatic melanoma and two with ovarian carcinoma, were treated with a single dose of ipilimumab at 3 mg/kg. Here, there was some evidence of efficacy with tumor biopsies of five melanoma patients revealing necrosis, and in the ovarian cancer patients there was a decrease or stabilization of CA-125, an ovarian cancer tumor marker (Hodi et al. 2003). Ipilimumab was then combined with a gp100 peptide vaccine in a phase I clinical trial, where 14 stage IV melanoma patients were treated with 3 mg/kg ipilimumab followed by a gp100 peptide vaccine. While three objective responses were noted including two complete responses (CRs), accrual was discontinued when >3 individuals developed grade III and IV immune related adverse events (irAEs) including dermatitis, enterocolitis, hypophysitis, and hepatitis (Phan et al. 2003). Following this, 56 patients with stage IV melanoma previously vaccinated with gp100 peptide received ipilimumab with an overall response rate (ORR) of 13% (7/56) with two CRs and five PRs. Interestingly, 36% of patients with irAEs experienced tumor regression compared with 5% of patients without irAEs (Attia et al. 2005).

Several dose escalation trials followed; in one trial, 88 patients with either unresectable stage III or IV melanoma received ipilimumab with a dose escalation from 2.8 mg/kg up to 20 mg/kg. Four patients obtained objective responses with one CR and three PRs, and an additional 14 patients had prolonged stable disease (SD)

Table 1 Select anti-CTLA-4 antibody clinical trials

Reference	# Pts	Drug – schedule mg/kg	Response rate	Immune related adverse effects	Median OS
Wolchok et al. (2009c)	217	Ipilimumab Melanoma Dose escalation: 0.3 mg/kg versus 3 mg/kg versus 10 mg/kg q3weeks ×4 cycles, then q3months	10 mg/kg BORR 11.1% Disease control rate 29.2% 2 CR, 6 PR, 13 SD	70% (50/71) Grade 3 or 4 – (18/71)	11.4 months 1 year survival 48.6%
			3 mg/kg BORR 4.2% Disease control rate 26.4% 0 CR, 3 PR, 16 SD	65% (46/7 1) Grade 3 or 4 – 7% (5/71)	8.7 months 1 year survival 39.3%
			0.3 mg/kg BORR 9% Disease control rate 13.7% 0 CR, 0 PR, 10 SD	26% (19/72) Grade 3 or 4 – 0% (0/72)	8.6 months 1 year survival 39.6%
Weber et al. (2009)	115	Ipilimumab with or without budesonide Melanoma 10 mg/kg q3weeks ×4 cycles followed by q3months	Budesonide + Ipilimumab BORR 12.1% Disease control rate 31% 1 CR, 6 PR, 11 SD	32.7%	17.7 months 1 year survival 62.4%
			Ipilimumab BORR 15.8% Disease control rate 35% 0 CR, 9 PR, 11 SD	35%	19.3 months 1 year survival 62.4%
Camacho et al. (2009)	117	Tremelimumab Melanoma 3, 6, 10 mg/kg (28 pts) Phase II 10 mg/kg versus 15 mg/kg (89)	10 mg/kg (41 pts) BORR 21% 1 CR, 3 PR, 12 SD	84% (37/44) Grade 3 or 4 – 27% (7/44)	10.0 months 1 year survival 32%
			15 mg/kg (43 pts) BORR 42% 1 CR, 3 PR, 14 SD	73% (33/45) Grade 3 or 4 – 13% (6/45)	11.5 months 1 year survival 46%

with a median time of 194 days. The objective responders also maintained a long duration of response of greater than 638 days (Weber et al. 2008). Another phase II trial of 139 patients treated at doses from 3–9 mg/kg of ipilimumab with or without peptide vaccine resulted in a 17% ORR with 3 CRs and 20 PRs. Sixty two percent of the patients had some form of irAEs which in this study was statistically associated with a higher likelihood of antitumor response (Downey et al. 2007).

Subsequently, there was a dose–response relationship demonstrated in a double-blind phase II trial of ipilimumab with three dose levels administered as a monotherapy to 217 unresectable stage III/IV patients. These patients received 0.3, 3, or 10 mg/kg of antibody every 3 weeks for four doses, followed by a maintenance dose once every 12 weeks starting at week 24 in the setting of SD or better without grade III/IV toxicity. The 10 mg/kg cohort had the greatest response rate at 11% with a median overall survival of 14 months. Consequently, the 10 mg/kg dosage is considered the optimal dosing to achieve clinical benefit although associated with the greatest rate of irAEs (Wolchok et al. 2009c). It is important to note that most irAEs can be easily medically managed with corticosteroids using simple algorithms. In fact, use of immunosuppressive drugs does not interfere with antitumor effects, for unclear reasons at this time. In an additional phase II trial of ipilimumab in advanced stage melanoma patients progressing on prior therapies, 150 patients were treated with 10 mg/kg of ipilimumab and the best overall response rate (BORR) was shown to be 5.8% (O'Day et al. 2008). A phase III registration trial which began in 2006 is currently ongoing comparing combined DTIC and ipilimumab with DTIC alone as front-line therapy. A separate phase III registration trial with 676 enrolled patients for second-line therapy with ipilimumab has just been completed, assessing the safety and efficacy of ipilimumab in combination with gp100 peptide vaccines, or single agents.

4.2 Postsurgical Adjuvant Therapy

Ipilimumab has also been tested in the adjuvant setting for high risk patients that had been rendered free of disease by surgery. In this trial, anti-CTLA-4 therapy was given at 0.3, 1 or 3 mg/kg every 4 weeks combined with a gp100, MART-1, and tyrosinase peptide vaccine to 19 stage III and IV resected melanoma patients. Eight patients experienced evidence of irAEs with three patients experiencing grade III gastrointestinal toxicity. Interestingly, 3 of 8 patients with irAEs experienced relapse while 9 out of 11 patients without irAEs experienced relapse (Sanderson et al. 2005). Similar results were seen in a subsequent phase II trial of ipilimumab at 3 mg/kg with a multipeptide vaccine in 25 patients who had resected stage IIIC/IV melanoma with no evidence of disease, which resulted in ten relapses at 22 months (Weber et al. 2006). Finally, the efficacy of ipilimumab in the adjuvant setting will soon be determined by an ongoing phase III double blinded placebo controlled clinical trial for stage III melanoma patients with no evidence of disease, with an estimated enrollment of 950 patients.

4.3 Combinations

Ipilimumab has also been combined with standard therapies. In a phase I/II clinical trial, 36 patients were treated with 0.1–3 mg/kg of ipilimumab every 3 weeks combined with IL-2. However, the ORR of 22% with three CRs and five PRs suggested no synergistic effect in combining IL-2 compared to ipilimumab alone (Maker et al. 2005b). Chemotherapy has also been rationally combined with ipilimumab on the basis of the potential for tumor antigen release, or depletion of Tregs. In a phase II randomized trial, 72 patients were treated with 3 mg/kg of ipilimumab, with or without DTIC. From this trial, it appeared that DTIC augmented the efficacy of ipilimumab with a 21.6% disease control rate in the ipilimumab alone arm and 31.4% in the combination arm (Hersh et al. 2008). In a follow up report, the investigators demonstrated an overall 57% 1 year survival rate with the combined DTIC and ipilimumab arm having a superior survival rate (Hersh et al. 2009). Currently ongoing is another three arm trial with 60 patients, where ipilimumab is being administered alone or in combination with carboplatin and paclitaxel, or with DTIC (NCT00796991).

4.4 Tremelimumab

A dose escalation study with tremelimumab ranging from 0.03 to 15 mg/kg in 34 patients demonstrated durable responses with eight objective responses, including two CRs, two PRs and four patients with SD (Ribas et al. 2005). A follow up phase II study of 20 patients receiving tremelimumab at 10 mg/kg monthly and ten patients receiving 15 mg/kg every 3 months resulted in five total responders with four occurring in individuals who developed irAEs (Reuben et al. 2006). In a third phase II study, 84 patients received tremelimumab at 10 mg/kg or 15 mg/kg with an ORR of 10% and medium survival of 10.2 months at the 10 mg/kg dose, and with a 7% ORR and 11.5 month median survival at the 15 mg/kg dose (Camacho et al. 2009). A further phase II trial at 15 mg/kg for stage IV malignant melanoma patients who had progressed on prior chemotherapy was conducted with an endpoint of achieving at least a 15% ORR. Reported at the American Society of Clinical Oncology (ASCO) 2008 Meeting, this trial of 258 patients treated with tremelimumab showed an ORR of 8.3% with a median survival of 10.0 months (Kirkwood et al. 2008). A large randomized phase III trial has been completed with tremelimumab 15 mg/kg compared to either DTIC or temozolomide in 550 patients. Unfortunately this trial was halted in its second interim analysis with a median overall survival of 10.7 months for the chemotherapy arm and 11.7 months for the tremelimumab arm. The hazard ratio was 1.05 with survival curves overlapping and thus it did not meet its primary endpoint (Ribas 2008).

4.5 *Immune Related Adverse Effects*

Since the initial studies with ipilimumab, there has been evidence of irAEs, most of which included diarrhea, colitis, rash, hypophysitis, and rare incidences of uveitis and adrenal insufficiency (Blansfield et al. 2005). To determine if the incidence of diarrhea could be decreased, 115 stage IV melanoma patients participated in a randomized phase II trial with ipilimumab with or without budesonide, a nonabsorbed oral steroid. These patients were treated with or without budesonide and received ipilimumab at 10 mg/kg every 3 weeks for four doses. Overall, ipilimumab was well tolerated with the best ORR of 12.1% in the budesonide arm and 15.8% in the placebo controlled arm, with no effect of budesonide on the rate of grade III or greater diarrhea (Weber et al. 2009). As noted above, most irAEs are easily managed with corticosteroids and those few patients with steroid-refractory disease respond to TNF-blocking agents or mycophenolate. Intriguingly, despite the rapid resolution of symptoms from irAEs using immunosuppressive medications, such drugs do not seem to temper antitumor effects.

4.6 *Novel Criteria for Antitumor Response to Ipilimumab and Increased Duration of Response*

Traditional standards for evaluation of antitumor response have been based on the Response Evaluation Criteria in Solid Tumors (RECIST) or WHO criteria, which may not adequately reflect the patterns of response for immunotherapies. A set of novel immune related response criteria (irRC) was recently proposed to more accurately describe the clinical activity of immunotherapies. It has not been uncommon to see late responses, sometimes happening 5–6 months after initiating treatment, even occurring after progression of index and/or new lesions. This may be related to the time needed for specific activation of the immune system to recognize antigens expressed by individual tumors, or a function of the kinetics regarding immune mediated tumor destruction. This should be contrasted with relatively short periods of time expected for observation of direct cytotoxic effects from chemotherapy. In addition, radiological evidence of progression of disease at early time points may reflect a heterogenous mixture of inflammation, edema, and lymphocytic infiltration as opposed to true increase in tumor volume.

To develop irRC, phase II clinical trial data from the ipilimumab program were utilized to define four patterns of response: (1) decrease in baseline lesions without evidence of new lesions, (2) durable SD with possible slow, steady decline in tumor burden, (3) response of tumor volume after initial increase in total tumor burden, and (4) response in the presence of new lesions. All of these response patterns were associated with increased overall survival (Wolchok et al. 2009b). Duration of response also appears to be increased in comparison to standard therapies. In fact, a recent ASCO abstract provided updated survival data from three phase II clinical trials of pretreated advanced stage melanoma patients. Here, they showed that the

18 month overall survival ranged from 34.5 to 39.4% for the 288 previously treated melanoma patients (O'Day et al. 2009).

4.7 Other Malignancies

While the vast clinical experience of CTLA-4 blockade has been with melanoma, there is increasing evidence of efficacy in other malignancies. In prostate cancer, ipilimumab was studied in a phase II trial of comparing ipilimumab with or without docetaxel in chemotherapy-naive hormone refractory prostate cancer patients. Six of 43 patients with three in each arm had decreases of PSA >50%. Three patients had durable PSA responses greater than 79, 169, and 280 days. Immune related adverse effects were similar to those noted in melanoma, including adrenal insufficiency and colitis (Small et al. 2006). Other combinatorial treatment strategies include a phase I/II clinical trial in 45 metastatic castrate resistant prostate cancer patients treated with ipilimumab and radiation therapy. Here, ten patients had decreases of PSA greater than 50% while radiation therapy did not appear to impact the effects of ipilimumab (Slovin et al. 2009). A combinatorial approach using a PSA-TRICOM vaccine, a pox based viral vector expressing PSA and three costimulatory molecules including ICAM-I, LFA-3, and B7.1 and GM-CSF, has been tested in combination with ipilimumab in 30 metastatic castrate resistant prostate cancer patients as well. Twenty-four chemotherapy naive patients had an increased PSA doubling time from 2.5 to 6 months. In addition, 14 of 30 patients had PSA decreases from baseline or peak PSA on study. The therapy was well tolerated with no dose limiting toxicity, although again there was a correlation with increasing dose and incidence of irAE (Mohebtash et al. 2009). While most trials have been performed in solid malignancies, a phase I trial of ipilimumab has been performed in 18 non-Hodgkin's lymphoma patients. The therapy was safely tolerated and two patients had a clinical response, with one CR and one durable PR (Ansell et al. 2009). Ipilimumab has also been tested in relapsed allogeneic transplant patients, based on the hypothesis that CTLA-4 blockade could augment the graft versus tumor effect. Interestingly, in the 29 patients receiving a single infusion of ipilimumab at either 0.1 mg/kg or 3 mg/kg, there was no exacerbation of graft versus host disease, although four patients experienced organ specific immune related adverse effects including grade 3 arthritis, grade 2 hyperthyroidism, and recurrent grade 4 pneumonitis. In that trial, there were three overall responders with two CRs and one PR (Bashey et al. 2009). Tremelimumab has been evaluated in 25 advanced breast cancer patients. A phase I open label trial of tremelimumab combined with exemestane resulted in a best response of eight patients with SD lasting a median of 8 months. The expected dose limiting toxicities included transient grade 3 transaminitis, diarrhea, and thyroiditis (Vonderheide et al. 2009). A phase II trial of tremelimumab versus best supportive care in 87 patients with nonsmall cell lung cancer has also been reported. Two of 44 (4.8%) patients treated with tremelimumab experienced an objective response, compared with zero in the best supportive care group (Zatloukal et al. 2009). Ipilimumab is also being tested in lung cancer in a phase II trial comparing carboplatin and paclitaxel with or without ipilimumab (NCT00527735). For renal cell carcinoma, anti-CTLA-4 antibodies have been tested alone and with sunitinib. In a phase II trial of ipilimumab, 61 patients were treated in sequential cohorts of increased doses. Twenty-one patients were treated at 3 mg/kg followed by 1 mg/kg q3weeks with one PR. Five of the 40 patients at 3 mg/kg every 3 weeks had PRs (Yang et al. 2007). Finally, tremelimumab has been combined with sunitinib, a multitargeted tyrosine kinase inhibitor, in a phase I clinical trial. The combination with sunitinib was chosen on the basis of evidence of sunitinib inhibiting myeloid-derived suppressor cells. There were five PRs noted in the 21 patients treated. There were multiple adverse effects noted including a ruptured diverticula, grade 3 mucositis, sudden death, and acute renal failure (Gordon et al. 2009).

There are other clinical trials with either ipilimumab or tremelimumab that are still ongoing and have not yet been reported. These include ipilimumab in unresectable pancreatic cancer and advanced hepatocellular carcinoma (NCT00836407) (NCT01008358) along with neoadjuvant ipilimumab being assessed in urothelial carcinoma undergoing surgical resection (NCT00362713). The later trial will provide an ideal trial design to assess the impact of immune modulation on the local tumor microenvironment. Adoptive T cell therapy is also being combined with ipilimumab in treatment of metastatic melanoma patients. NY-ESO-1 specific CD8+ T cells are currently being studied in cyclophosphamide treated metastatic melanoma patients with or without CTLA-4 blockade (NCT00871481). If successful, this strategy would support anti-CTLA-4 therapy preventing possible local tumor microenvironment inhibition of Teffs. (NCT00871481).

5 From Clinical Trials, Back to the Bench

As described above, anti-CTLA-4 therapy has shown clinical activity as an immune modulator, inducing durable objective responses as a monotherapy, and demonstrating efficacy with combination therapies that direct the immune response to the cancer. However, we have yet to fully investigate the heterogeneity of responses that have been observed with anti-CTLA-4 therapy. Detailed analysis of anti-CTLA-4 treated patients may assist us in discovering mechanisms that are critical to the antitumor response. This section outlines several current directions in the field of immune monitoring i.e., the study of individual responses to anti-CTLA-4 therapy.

5.1 Monitoring Antigen-Specific CD4+ and CD8+ T Cell Activity and Polyfunctionality

Antigen-specific T cell activity can be evaluated using in vitro stimulation assays, or by staining peripheral T cells with antigen-specific MHC tetramers. Such analyses were recently conducted on selected melanoma patients receiving ipilimumab (Yuan et al. 2008). Of eight clinical responders, five demonstrated antibody, $CD4^+$, and $CD8^+$

responses to NY-ESO-1, a prototypical cancer testis antigen. In contrast, only 1/7 nonresponders mounted a $CD4^+$ response, but no $CD8^+$ or antibody response (Yuan et al. 2008). These data imply that antigen-specific immunity may be associated with clinical benefit, and suggest a rationale for future trials combining vaccination to NY-ESO-1 or other antigens with anti-CTLA-4 therapy.

Using the same techniques, specificity to other antigens has also been investigated. In a phase I trial of 24 prostate cancer patients treated with ipilimumab +GM-CSF, no antigen-specific T cell responses were detected against PSA or other known prostate differentiation antigens, including PAP, PSMA, EphA2, or survivin (Fong et al. 2009). However, in an analysis of a melanoma patient experiencing CR from treatment with ipilimumab, both Melan-A-specific peripheral T cells and tumor-infiltrating T cells were identified (Klein et al. 2009). These Melan-A/MART1 specific $CD8^+$ cells were expanded in culture, and were demonstrated to exhibit potent killing activity in vitro against SK-Mel-14, a Melan-A-expressing cell line. This case report calls for further studies examining Melan-A-specific immunity as a possible marker for positive therapeutic response (Klein et al. 2009). In some cases, peripheral T cell specificity may not capture intratumoral immune events as analysis of patients receiving tremelimumab showed no trend of increased gp100, Melan-A/MART1, or tyrosinase-specific peripheral $CD8^+$ cells (Comin-Anduix et al. 2008). Still, analysis of tumor infiltrate in regressing lesions demonstrated marked enrichment of gp100-specific $CD8^+$ cells, which suggests that peripheral specificity may not always correlate with intratumoral T cell specificity (Comin-Anduix et al. 2008).

Polyfunctional T cell subsets – T cell subsets that generate multiple cytokines – can be measured by multiparametric flow cytometry, and are markers of robust immune activity. Polyfunctional T cells have been associated with nonprogression of HIV2 infection (Makedonas and Betts 2006; Duvall et al. 2008) and vaccine responses to Hepatitis B virus (De Rosa et al. 2004) and vaccinia (Precopio et al. 2007). Recently, polyfunctional $CD8^+$ T cells were also demonstrated in a melanoma patient receiving adjuvant therapy with GM-CSF DNA and gp100/tyrosinase peptide vaccines with polyfunctionality coinciding at the time point of maximal IFN-γ production (Perales et al. 2008). An analysis of polyfunctionality in ipilimumab patients found that patients experiencing clinical benefit demonstrated $CD4^+$, $CD8^+$, and/or antibody responses to NY-ESO-1. In fact, T cells from clinical benefiters were found to be polyfunctional, producing IFN-γ, MIP-1β, and/or TNFα in response to NY-ESO-1 peptide stimulation, while none of the nine nonresponders demonstrated a polyfunctional T cell response. These results suggest that antigen-specific polyfunctionality could be a possible marker of anti-CTLA-4 activity (Yuan et al. 2008).

5.2 *Cellular Phenotype Analysis: ICOS, Foxp3, HLA-DR and IDO*

Another immune monitoring strategy is to utilize flow cytometric analysis and other techniques to examine changes in cellular phenotype, with the hope of identifying biomarkers for clinical response.

5.3 *ICOS*

ICOS is a T cell specific surface protein structurally related to CD28 and CTLA-4, which becomes expressed on the cell surface following T cell activation (Hutloff et al. 1999; Liakou et al. 2008). T cells expressing intermediate levels of ICOS are associated with synthesis of the T_H2 cytokines IL-4, IL-5, and IL-13, whereas T cells expressing high levels of ICOS ($ICOS^{high}$) correlate with the production of IL-10, an immunosuppressive cytokine, in some studies (Lohning et al. 2003). Studies showing a relationship between ICOS expression with increased Teff cell survival (Burmeister et al. 2008) serve to highlight the significance of ICOS as a possible marker of anti-CTLA-4 activity. This has been recently investigated in a series of six bladder cancer patients receiving anti-CTLA-4 therapy preoperatively. In these patients, an increase in the number of $CD4^{+}ICOS^{high}$ cells was observed in peripheral blood mononuclear cells and in tumor infiltrates. These cells exhibited increased IFN-γ production, and in 3/3 of these patients who had NY-ESO-1 expressing tumors, IFN-γ was produced in response to stimulation with NY-ESO-1 peptides (Liakou et al. 2008). These data imply that ICOS expression could be correlated with clinical activity; however, this must be further investigated.

5.4 *Foxp3*

Foxp3, a member of the forkhead box family of transcription factors, is necessary for Treg function. The overall frequency of Foxp3+ Treg cells in untreated cancer patients tends to be higher than in normal healthy donors, which implies that Foxp3 levels may correlate with tumor immune evasion (Liakou et al. 2008). The role of Foxp3 as a biomarker of anti-CTLA-4 induced Treg modulation is being investigated. In the series of bladder patients above, Foxp3 expression was not consistently altered by CTLA-4 blockade (Liakou et al. 2008). In an analysis of eight patients receiving tremelimumab, no statistical change was seen in predosing and postdosing levels of peripheral Foxp3 mRNA production. However, a recent analysis of tumor biopsies taken at week 0 and week 4 in ipilimumab patients showed a statistical correlation of clinical benefit with changes from pretreatment Foxp3 expression (Hamid et al. 2009).

5.5 *HLA-DR*

Several markers of T cell activation have been screened as possible biomarkers for anti-CTLA-4 activity. HLA-DR is a cell surface molecule which appears on both $CD25^{+}$ and $CD25^{-}$ T cells late after activation. In a recent analysis of 30 patients treated with ipilimumab, posttreatment increases in the percentage of HLA-DR expression were seen in both $CD4^{+}CD25^{-}$ and $CD4^{+}CD25^{+}$ cells. (Maker et al.

2005a) A separate analysis demonstrated that HLA-DR expression on $CD8^+$ cells after two doses of tremelimumab could differentiate responders from nonresponders (comin-Anduix et al. 2008). Further work must be performed to validate HLA-DR expression as a biomarker.

5.6 *IDO*

Treg cells from tumor-draining lymph nodes in mouse models have been shown to become highly activated by exposure to the immunoregulatory enzyme indoleamine 2,3-dioxygenase (IDO), an enzyme expressed in specific subsets of plasmacytoid dendritic cells (Sharma et al. 2009). Additionally, blockade of IDO expression has been shown to convert Tregs into a nonsuppressive, proinflammatory phenotype similar to T_H17 cells. As such, IDO has been implicated as a "switch" for Treg mediated immune regulation, and thus levels of IDO expression could be used as a biomarker. To date, this has yet to be validated. Analysis of pre and postdosing tumor biopsies in four patients receiving tremelimumab failed to show an association of IDO^+ T cell staining with tumor response (Ribas et al. 2009). Analysis of tumor biopsies in ipilimumab patients showed a statistical correlation of clinical benefit with week 0 IDO expression (Hamid et al. 2009). Further studies are pending.

5.7 *Antibody Responses*

Differentiation antigens (for example, PSA, Melan-A/MART1, and gp100), cancer testis antigens (for example, NY-ESO-1 and MAGE), and products of DNA damage (for example, Bcr/Abl or mutated p53) have all been associated with antigen-specific humoral and/or T cell responses (Houghton et al. 1982; Chen et al. 1997; Perales et al. 2002; Nakada et al. 2003). CTLA-4 blockade may indirectly activate the humoral response by stimulating CD4-mediated priming of B cells, thereby inducing antibody production against tumor antigens.

In a recent serologic analysis of melanoma patients treated with ipilimumab, 22% of patients (9/41) produced antibodies against NY-ESO-1, an antigen expressed in a significant fraction of melanoma, lung, and bladder cancer specimens (Gnjatic et al. 2008). The majority (66%) of these patients experienced clinical benefit, and of the three nonresponders, one had a transient mixed response and another had a PR prior to requiring steroids for treatment-related colitis (Gnjatic et al. 2008). Anti-CTLA-4 induced NY-ESO-1 antibody responses have also been demonstrated in prostate cancer patients (Fong et al. 2009). Further investigation must be conducted to determine whether such antibodies are protective, or are simply surrogates for another protective immune process.

Antibodies against products secreted from tumors have also been observed with CTLA-4 blockade. Some patients who have responded clinically to anti-CTLA-4 therapy developed high titers of antibodies against MHC class I chain-related protein A (MICA) (Fong and Small 2008). MICA and related proteins including ULBP normally stimulate NK or $CD8^+$ T cell mediated cytotoxicity by binding to NK cell receptor NKG2D. However, tumor metastases may evolve to shed soluble MICA or ULBP, thereby suppressing cytolytic activity (Paschen et al. 2009). It is possible that part of the clinical benefit from anti-CTLA-4-induced anti-MICA antibody production may be the reduced soluble MICA enabling better NK-mediated tumor killing (Jinushi et al. 2006; Fong and Small 2008).

5.8 *The "Immunogram": A Tool to Synthesize Immune Monitoring*

The ever expanding and evolving data from correlative immunologic studies of patients undergoing immune modulation may in fact become overwhelming. To mitigate this, we introduced the concept of the "immunogram," which synthesizes current immune monitoring data and allows us to distill important lessons from individual patients. The immunogram is simply a modular, chronological illustration of treatment history, dissected radiographic response, blood counts, serologic measurements of immune response, cellular phenotype markers, and measurements of antigen-specific response. With changes in technology and data collection, the immunogram can evolve to include different types of information.

The immunogram of patient IMF-16 (Fig. 2) anecdotally validates a wealth of data regarding the mechanism of anti-CTLA-4 therapy (Yuan et al. 2010). For example, the immunogram illustrates that steroid treatment in this patient did not clearly affect therapy and that early lymphocyte expansion, along with ICOS increases, may predict clinical outcome. In addition, responses seen may also be correlated with NY-ESO-1 specific T cell and B cell activity. This immunogram prompted a follow-up study analyzing the tumor-antigen and tumor-infiltrating lymphocyte profile of the resected "escape" lesion. Here, we learned that NY-ESO-1-specific T cells were engaging the tumor, which was still expressing NY-ESO-1 antigen, but that Tregs were heavily abundant in the tumor. This suggests that, in IMF-16, tumor escape was mediated by Treg suppression of antigen-specific Teff activity. The immunogram – a newly-described graphical synthesis of treatment data and immune correlates in individual patients – may help us to confirm, reject, or formulate hypotheses of the mechanism of anti-CTLA-4 activity.

6 Future Directions

Immunomodulation with monoclonal antibodies targeting immune receptors, such as CTLA-4 and GITR, has shown efficacy as an anticancer therapeutic approach both as a single agent and in combination with other drugs in different pre-clinical tumor models. Experiments done in mice indicate that anti-CTLA-4 is effective on

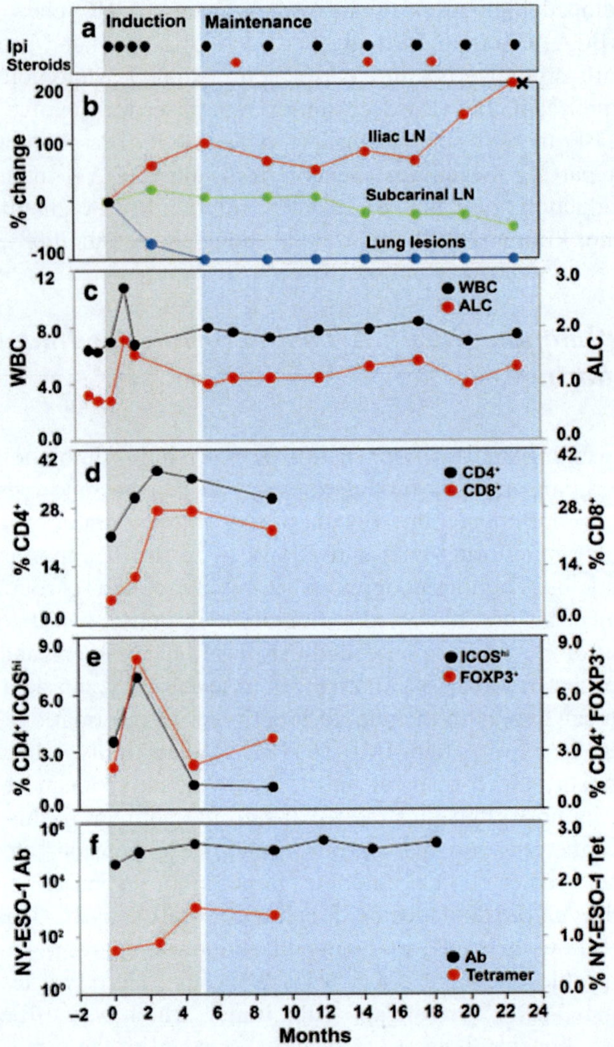

Fig. 2 Immunogram of patient IMF-16. (**a**) Patient IMF-16 received ipilimumab therapy as part of protocol CA183-008, and received four induction doses at 10 mg/kg every 3 weeks followed by maintenance doses every 3 months. The patient received intermittent low-dose oral steroids to treat grade 2 rash and pruritis; (**b**) Response of target lesions is illustrated as percent change of maximal tumor diameter from baseline. The patient underwent resection of progressive iliac lymph nodes ("x"); (**c**) WBC and ALC are graphed in $\times 10^3/\text{mm}^3$ units; (**d**) Peripheral $CD4^+$ and $CD8^+$ lines expanded with therapy, measured by flow cytometry; (**e**) Peripheral expressions of phenotype markers ICOS and Foxp3 were both transiently expanded with therapy; (**f**) NY-ESO-1 titers are graphed in $\log_{10}$ as an inverse titer. $CD8^+$ NY-ESO-1 specific function was measured by flow cytometry using HLA-A*0201/NY-ESO-$1_{157-165}$ tetramer stain. (Reproduced with permission from Yuan et al. 2010). *Ipi* ipilimumab, *LN* lymph node, *Tet* tetramer, *ALC* absolute lymphocyte count

tumor bearing hosts if a certain threshold of "tumor-immunogenicity" is reached. For example, the tumor itself can be intrinsically immunogenic or rendered immunogenic by other means such as transfection, vaccination, or immunomodulation. Conventional chemotherapeutic agents or radiotherapy have also shown efficacy in combination with anti-CTLA-4. This might depend on effects of the chemo/radiotherapy on "tumor-immunogenicity" either by directly affecting immune cell populations (e.g., Inducing lymphopenia and promoting activation of adaptive immune responses during recovery from lymphopenia) or by favoring antigen release, increasing MHC I expression and/or inducing local inflammation. Further dissecting the effects of conventional therapies on tumor immunogenicity when combined with CTLA-4 blockade will be important to provide more rationale for clinical studies.

Although the amount of preclinical work done with anti-GITR agonist antibody is not yet as thorough as what has been done with anti-CTLA-4, it is very clear that DTA-1 has striking antitumor properties in mouse models both as a monotherapy and in combination with vaccines. The mechanisms of action of DTA-1 are still under investigation and its relative effect on Tregs versus Teffs or perhaps other cells, such as endothelial cells, is not yet entirely clear. Anti-GITR is therefore an interesting new drug to test in patients and to consider for combinations with other immunomodulatory antibodies and vaccines.

Conceptually, optimal tumor vaccination would involve production of increased amounts of tumor antigen in order to drive a tumor specific response. There are currently promising small molecule inhibitors targeting melanoma harboring genetic mutations including BRAF, the presence of which appears to confer sensitivity to BRAF inhibitors. Preliminary phase I and II clinical trials have reported high rates of response, however, with a median duration of response reported to be only 6 months. We hypothesize that the antigenic release with these small molecule inhibitors coupled with immune modulating antibodies to lower the immune threshold for antitumor response may be synergistic in providing long-lasting tumor immunity.

Finally, durable responses induced by anti-CTLA-4 therapy correlate with markers of immune activity such as antigen-specific $CD4^+$ or $CD8^+$ cytokine release, antitumor antibody formation, or cellular phenotype differentiation. Some patients exhibit atypical responses to anti-CTLA-4 therapy, demonstrating transient/delayed responses or heterogeneity by lesion site. Such atypical responses may offer insight into the mechanism of anti-CTLA-4 therapy. Immune monitoring of individual patients enables us to hypothesize regarding the mechanism of anti-CTLA-4 therapy. When analyzed in a compendium, such analyses might assist us in determining which immune processes are key, which combination therapies to pursue, and which immune parameters can be used to guide treatment fine-tuning of the immune system to achieve an optimal clinical result.

Acknowledgments The authors would like to thank Dr. Stephanie Terzulli and Brian Ginsberg for reviewing the manuscript and Drs. Lloyd Old and David Page for their scientific guidance and assistance in generating the immunogram.

References

Alegre ML, Noel PJ, Eisfelder BJ, Chuang E, Clark MR, Reiner SL, Thompson CB (1996) Regulation of surface and intracellular expression of CTLA4 on mouse T cells. J Immunol 157:4762–4770

Ansell SM, Hurvitz SA, Koenig PA, LaPlant BR, Kabat BF, Fernando D, Habermann TM, Inwards DJ, Verma M, Yamada R, Erlichman C, Lowy I, Timmerman JM (2009) Phase I study of ipilimumab, an anti-CTLA-4 monoclonal antibody, in patients with relapsed and refractory B-cell non-Hodgkin lymphoma. Clin Cancer Res 15:6446–6453

Attia P, Phan GQ, Maker AV, Robinson MR, Quezado MM, Yang JC, Sherry RM, Topalian SL, Kammula US, Royal RE, Restifo NP, Haworth LR, Levy C, Mavroukakis SA, Nichol G, Yellin MJ, Rosenberg SA (2005) Autoimmunity correlates with tumor regression in patients with metastatic melanoma treated with anti-cytotoxic T-lymphocyte antigen-4. J Clin Oncol 23:6043–6053

Bachmann MF, Kohler G, Ecabert B, Mak TW, Kopf M (1999) Cutting edge: lymphoproliferative disease in the absence of CTLA-4 is not T cell autonomous. J Immunol 163:1128–1131

Bashey A, Medina B, Corringham S, Pasek M, Carrier E, Vrooman L, Lowy I, Solomon SR, Morris LE, Holland HK, Mason JR, Alyea EP, Soiffer RJ, Ball ED (2009) CTLA4 blockade with ipilimumab to treat relapse of malignancy after allogeneic hematopoietic cell transplantation. Blood 113:1581–1588

Blank U, Launay P, Benhamou M, Monteiro RC (2009) Inhibitory ITAMs as novel regulators of immunity. Immunol Rev 232:59–71

Blansfield JA, Beck KE, Tran K, Yang JC, Hughes MS, Kammula US, Royal RE, Topalian SL, Haworth LR, Levy C, Rosenberg SA, Sherry RM (2005) Cytotoxic T-lymphocyte-associated antigen-4 blockage can induce autoimmune hypophysitis in patients with metastatic melanoma and renal cancer. J Immunother 28:593–598

Bunnell SC, Hong DI, Kardon JR, Yamazaki T, McGlade CJ, Barr VA, Samelson LE (2002) T cell receptor ligation induces the formation of dynamically regulated signaling assemblies. J Cell Biol 158:1263–1275

Burmeister Y, Lischke T, Dahler AC, Mages HW, Lam KP, Coyle AJ, Kroczek RA, Hutloff A (2008) ICOS controls the pool size of effector-memory and regulatory T cells. J Immunol 180:774–782

Camacho LH, Antonia S, Sosman J, Kirkwood JM, Gajewski TF, Redman B, Pavlov D, Bulanhagui C, Bozon VA, Gomez-Navarro J, Ribas A (2009) Phase I/II trial of tremelimumab in patients with metastatic melanoma. J Clin Oncol 27:1075–1081

Carreno BM, Bennett F, Chau TA, Ling V, Luxenberg D, Jussif J, Baroja ML, Madrenas J (2000) CTLA-4 (CD152) can inhibit T cell activation by two different mechanisms depending on its level of cell surface expression. J Immunol 165:1352–1356

Chambers CA, Sullivan TJ, Allison JP (1997) Lymphoproliferation in CTLA-4-deficient mice is mediated by costimulation-dependent activation of CD4+ T cells. Immunity 7:885–895

Chambers CA, Sullivan TJ, Truong T, Allison JP (1998) Secondary but not primary T cell responses are enhanced in CTLA-4-deficient CD8+ T cells. Eur J Immunol 28:3137–3143

Chambers CA, Kuhns MS, Allison JP (1999) Cytotoxic T lymphocyte antigen-4 (CTLA-4) regulates primary and secondary peptide-specific CD4(+) T cell responses. Proc Natl Acad Sci USA 96:8603–8608

Chan AC, Dalton M, Johnson R, Kong GH, Wang T, Thoma R, Kurosaki T (1995) Activation of ZAP-70 kinase activity by phosphorylation of tyrosine 493 is required for lymphocyte antigen receptor function. EMBO J 14:2499–2508

Chen YT, Scanlan MJ, Sahin U, Tureci O, Gure AO, Tsang S, Williamson B, Stockert E, Pfreundschuh M, Old LJ (1997) A testicular antigen aberrantly expressed in human cancers detected by autologous antibody screening. Proc Natl Acad Sci USA 94:1914–1918

Chuang E, Lee KM, Robbins MD, Duerr JM, Alegre ML, Hambor JE, Neveu MJ, Bluestone JA, Thompson CB (1999) Regulation of cytotoxic T lymphocyte-associated molecule-4 by Src kinases. J Immun 162:1270–1277

Chuang E, Fisher TS, Morgan RW, Robbins MD, Duerr JM, Vander Heiden MG, Gardner JP, Hambor JE, Neveu MJ, Thompson CB (2000) The CD28 and CTLA-4 receptors associate with the serine/threonine phosphatase PP2A. Immunity 13:313–322

Cinek T, Sadra A, Imboden JB (2000) Cutting edge: tyrosine-independent transmission of inhibitory signals by CTLA-4. J Immunol 164:5–8

Cohen AD, Diab A, Perales MA, Wolchok JD, Rizzuto G, Merghoub T, Huggins D, Liu C, Turk MJ, Restifo NP, Sakaguchi S, Houghton AN (2006) Agonist anti-GITR antibody enhances vaccine-induced CD8(+) T-cell responses and tumor immunity. Cancer Res 66: 4904–4912

Cohen AD, Schaer DA, Liu C, Li Y, Hirschhorn-Cymmerman D, Kim SC, Diab A, Rizzuto G, Duan F, Perales MA, Merghoub T, Houghton AN, Wolchok JD (2010) Agonist anti-GITR monoclonal antibody induces melanoma tumor immunity in mice by altering regulatory T cell stability and intra-tumor accumulation. In Press

Comin-Anduix B, Lee Y, Jalil J, Algazi A, de la Rocha P, Camacho LH, Bozon VA, Bulanhagui CA, Seja E, Villanueva A, Straatsma BR, Gualberto A, Economou JS, Glaspy JA, Gomez-Navarro J, Ribas A (2008) Detailed analysis of immunologic effects of the cytotoxic T lymphocyte-associated antigen 4-blocking monoclonal antibody tremelimumab in peripheral blood of patients with melanoma. J Transl Med 6:22

Davila E, Kennedy R, Celis E (2003) Generation of antitumor immunity by cytotoxic T lymphocyte epitope peptide vaccination, CpG-oligodeoxynucleotide adjuvant, and CTLA-4 blockade. Cancer Res 63:3281–3288

De Rosa SC, Lu FX, Yu J, Perfetto SP, Falloon J, Moser S, Evans TG, Koup R, Miller CJ, Roederer M (2004) Vaccination in humans generates broad T cell cytokine responses. J Immunol 173:5372–5380

Demaria S, Bhardwaj N, McBride WH, Formenti SC (2005) Combining radiotherapy and immunotherapy: a revived partnership. Int J Radiat Oncol Biol Phys 63:655–666

den Brok MH, Sutmuller RP, Nierkens S, Bennink EJ, Frielink C, Toonen LW, Boerman OC, Figdor CG, Ruers TJ, Adema GJ (2006) Efficient loading of dendritic cells following cryo and radiofrequency ablation in combination with immune modulation induces anti-tumour immunity. Br J Cancer 95:896–905

Downey SG, Klapper JA, Smith FO, Yang JC, Sherry RM, Royal RE, Kammula US, Hughes MS, Allen TE, Levy CL, Yellin M, Nichol G, White DE, Steinberg SM, Rosenberg SA (2007) Prognostic factors related to clinical response in patients with metastatic melanoma treated by CTL-associated antigen-4 blockade. Clin Cancer Res 13:6681–6688

Duvall MG, Precopio ML, Ambrozak DA, Jaye A, McMichael AJ, Whittle HC, Roederer M, Rowland-Jones SL, Koup RA (2008) Polyfunctional T cell responses are a hallmark of HIV-2 infection. Eur J Immunol 38:350–363

Esparza EM, Arch RH (2005) Glucocorticoid-induced TNF receptor functions as a costimulatory receptor that promotes survival in early phases of T cell activation. J Immunol 174: 7869–7874

Fallarino F, Grohmann U, Hwang KW, Orabona C, Vacca C, Bianchi R, Belladonna ML, Fioretti MC, Alegre ML, Puccetti P (2003) Modulation of tryptophan catabolism by regulatory T cells. Nat Immunol 4:1206–1212

Fong L, Small EJ (2008) Anti-cytotoxic T-lymphocyte antigen-4 antibody: the first in an emerging class of immunomodulatory antibodies for cancer treatment. J Clin Oncol 26:5275–5283

Fong L, Kwek SS, O'Brien S, Kavanagh B, McNeel DG, Weinberg V, Lin AM, Rosenberg J, Ryan CJ, Rini BI, Small EJ (2009) Potentiating endogenous antitumor immunity to prostate cancer through combination immunotherapy with CTLA4 blockade and GM-CSF. Cancer Res 69:609–615

Friedline RH, Brown DS, Nguyen H, Kornfeld H, Lee J, Zhang Y, Appleby M, Der SD, Kang J, Chambers CA (2009) CD4+ regulatory T cells require CTLA-4 for the maintenance of systemic tolerance. J Exp Med 206:421–434

Gadina M, Stancato LM, Bacon CM, Larner AC, O'Shea JJ (1998) Involvement of SHP-2 in multiple aspects of IL-2 signaling: evidence for a positive regulatory role. J Immunol 160:4657–4661

Gao Y, Whitaker-Dowling P, Griffin JA, Barmada MA, Bergman I (2009) Recombinant vesicular stomatitis virus targeted to Her2/neu combined with anti-CTLA4 antibody eliminates implanted mammary tumors. Cancer Gene Ther 16:44–52

Gattinoni L, Ranganathan A, Surman DR, Palmer DC, Antony PA, Theoret MR, Heimann DM, Rosenberg SA, Restifo NP (2006) CTLA-4 dysregulation of self/tumor-reactive CD8+ T-cell function is CD4+ T-cell dependent. Blood 108:3818–3823

Gnjatic S, Yuan J, Ritter E, Jungbluth AA, Gallardo H, Terzulli S, Ritter G, Houghton A, Old LJ, Allison JP, Wolchok JD (2008) Serum antibodies as predictive markers of clinical response to anti-CTLA-4 (Ipimilumab) treatment in advanced melanoma patients. In: ASCO 2008 Annual Meeting

Gordon MS, Stein M, Shannon P, Eddy S, Tyler A, Catlett L, Hsyu P, Huang B, Healey D, Rini BI (2009) Phase I dose escalation trial of tremelimumab plus sunitinib in patients (pts) with metastatic renal cell carcinoma (mRCC). J Clin Oncol (Meeting Abstracts) 27 Abstract no: 5115

Greenwald RJ, Boussiotis VA, Lorsbach RB, Abbas AK, Sharpe AH (2001) CTLA-4 regulates induction of anergy in vivo. Immunity 14:145–155

Greenwald RJ, Oosterwegel MA, van der Woude D, Kubal A, Mandelbrot DA, Boussiotis VA, Sharpe AH (2002) CTLA-4 regulates cell cycle progression during a primary immune response. Eur J Immunol 32:366–373

Gregor PD, Wolchok JD, Ferrone CR, Buchinshky H, Guevara-Patino JA, Perales MA, Mortazavi F, Bacich D, Heston W, Latouche JB, Sadelain M, Allison JP, Scher HI, Houghton AN (2004) CTLA-4 blockade in combination with xenogeneic DNA vaccines enhances T-cell responses, tumor immunity and autoimmunity to self antigens in animal and cellular model systems. Vaccine 22:1700–1708

Hamid O, Tsuchihasi Z, Alaparthy S, Galbraith S, Berman D (2009) Association of baseline and on-study tumor biopsy markers with clinical activity in patients (pts) with advanced melanoma treated with ipilimumab. In: 2009 ASCO annual meeting, Orlando, FL

Hersh EM, Weber JS, Powderly JD, Khan K, Pavlick AC, Samlowski WE, O'Day SJ, Nichol G, Yellin MJ, Cramner L (2008) Disease control and long-term survival in chemotherapy-naive patients with advanced melanoma treated with ipilimumab (MDX-010) with or without dacarbazine. J Clin Oncol (Meeting Abstracts) 26 Abstract no: 9022

Hersh E, Weber J, Powderly J, Pavlik A, Nichol G, Yellin M, Cranmer L, Urba W, O'Day S (2009) Long-term survival of patients (pts) with advanced melanoma treated with ipilimumab with or without dacarbazine. J Clin Oncol (Meeting Abstracts) 27 Abstract no: 9038

Hodi FS, Mihm MC, Soiffer RJ, Haluska FG, Butler M, Seiden MV, Davis T, Henry-Spires R, MacRae S, Willman A, Padera R, Jaklitsch MT, Shankar S, Chen TC, Korman A, Allison JP, Dranoff G (2003) Biologic activity of cytotoxic T lymphocyte-associated antigen 4 antibody blockade in previously vaccinated metastatic melanoma and ovarian carcinoma patients. Proc Natl Acad Sci USA 100:4712–4717

Houghton AN, Eisinger M, Albino AP, Cairncross JG, Old LJ (1982) Surface antigens of melanocytes and melanomas. Markers of melanocyte differentiation and melanoma subsets. J Exp Med 156:1755–1766

Houot R, Levy R (2009) T-cell modulation combined with intratumoral CpG cures lymphoma in a mouse model without the need for chemotherapy. Blood 113:3546–3552

Hurwitz AA, Yu TF, Leach DR, Allison JP (1998) CTLA-4 blockade synergizes with tumor-derived granulocyte-macrophage colony-stimulating factor for treatment of an experimental mammary carcinoma. Proc Natl Acad Sci USA 95:10067–10071

Hurwitz AA, Foster BA, Kwon ED, Truong T, Choi EM, Greenberg NM, Burg MB, Allison JP (2000) Combination immunotherapy of primary prostate cancer in a transgenic mouse model using CTLA-4 blockade. Cancer Res 60:2444–2448

Hutloff A, Dittrich AM, Beier KC, Eljaschewitsch B, Kraft R, Anagnostopoulos I, Kroczek RA (1999) ICOS is an inducible T-cell co-stimulator structurally and functionally related to CD28. Nature 397:263–266

Jinushi M, Hodi FS, Dranoff G (2006) Therapy-induced antibodies to MHC class I chain-related protein A antagonize immune suppression and stimulate antitumor cytotoxicity. Proc Natl Acad Sci USA 103:9190–9195

Kanamaru F, Youngnak P, Hashiguchi M, Nishioka T, Takahashi T, Sakaguchi S, Ishikawa I, Azuma M (2004) Costimulation via glucocorticoid-induced TNF receptor in both conventional and CD25+ regulatory CD4+ T cells. J Immunol 172:7306–7314

Kearney ER, Walunas TL, Karr RW, Morton PA, Loh DY, Bluestone JA, Jenkins MK (1995) Antigen-dependent clonal expansion of a trace population of antigen-specific CD4+ T cells in vivo is dependent on CD28 costimulation and inhibited by CTLA-4. J Immunol 155:1032–1036

Kirkwood JM, Lorigan P, Hersey P, Hauschild A, Robert C, McDermott DF, Gomez-Navarro J, Liang JQ, Bulanhagui CA (2008) A phase II trial of tremelimumab (CP-675,206) in patients with advanced refractory or relapsed melanoma. J Clin Oncol (Meeting Abstracts) 26 Abstract no: 9023

Klein O, Ebert LM, Nicholaou T, Browning J, Russell SE, Zuber M, Jackson HM, Dimopoulos N, Tan BS, Hoos A, Luescher IF, Davis ID, Chen W, Cebon J (2009) Melan-A-specific cytotoxic T cells are associated with tumor regression and autoimmunity following treatment with anti-CTLA-4. Clin Cancer Res 15:2507–2513

Ko K, Yamazaki S, Nakamura K, Nishioka T, Hirota K, Yamaguchi T, Shimizu J, Nomura T, Chiba T, Sakaguchi S (2005) Treatment of advanced tumors with agonistic anti-GITR mAb and its effects on tumor-infiltrating Foxp3 + CD25 + CD4+ regulatory T cells. J Exp Med 202:885–891

Kohm AP, Williams JS, Miller SD (2004) Cutting edge: ligation of the glucocorticoid-induced TNF receptor enhances autoreactive CD4+ T cell activation and experimental autoimmune encephalomyelitis. J Immunol 172:4686–4690

Kwon ED, Hurwitz AA, Foster BA, Madias C, Feldhaus AL, Greenberg NM, Burg MB, Allison JP (1997) Manipulation of T cell costimulatory and inhibitory signals for immunotherapy of prostate cancer. Proc Natl Acad Sci USA 94:8099–8103

Leach DR, Krummel MF, Allison JP (1996) Enhancement of antitumor immunity by CTLA-4 blockade. Science 271:1734–1736

Liakou CI, Kamat A, Tang DN, Chen H, Sun J, Troncoso P, Logothetis C, Sharma P (2008) CTLA-4 blockade increases IFNgamma-producing CD4 + ICOShi cells to shift the ratio of effector to regulatory T cells in cancer patients. Proc Natl Acad Sci USA 105:14987–14992

Linsley PS, Ledbetter JA (1993) The role of the CD28 receptor during T cell responses to antigen. Annu Rev Immunol 11:191–212

Linsley PS, Bradshaw J, Greene J, Peach R, Bennett KL, Mittler RS (1996) Intracellular trafficking of CTLA-4 and focal localization towards sites of TCR engagement. Immunity 4:535–543

Lohning M, Hutloff A, Kallinich T, Mages HW, Bonhagen K, Radbruch A, Hamelmann E, Kroczek RA (2003) Expression of ICOS in vivo defines CD4+ effector T cells with high inflammatory potential and a strong bias for secretion of interleukin 10. J Exp Med 197:181–193

Lucas PJ, Negishi I, Nakayama K, Fields LE, Loh DY (1995) Naive CD28-deficient T cells can initiate but not sustain an in vitro antigen-specific immune response. J Immunol 154:5757–5768

Makedonas G, Betts MR (2006) Polyfunctional analysis of human t cell responses: importance in vaccine immunogenicity and natural infection. Springer Semin Immunopathol 28:209–219

Maker AV, Attia P, Rosenberg SA (2005a) Analysis of the cellular mechanism of anti-tumor responses and autoimmunity in patients treated with CTLA-4 blockade. J Immunol 175:7746–7754

Maker AV, Phan GQ, Attia P, Yang JC, Sherry RM, Topalian SL, Kammula US, Royal RE, Haworth LR, Levy C, Kleiner D, Mavroukakis SA, Yellin M, Rosenberg SA (2005b) Tumor regression and autoimmunity in patients treated with cytotoxic T lymphocyte-associated antigen 4 blockade and interleukin 2: a phase I/II study. Ann Surg Oncol 12:1005–1016

Mandelbrot DA, McAdam AJ, Sharpe AH (1999) B7-1 or B7-2 is required to produce the lymphoproliferative phenotype in mice lacking cytotoxic T lymphocyte-associated antigen 4 (CTLA-4). J Exp Med 189:435–440

Martin M, Schneider H, Azouz A, Rudd CE (2001) Cytotoxic T lymphocyte antigen 4 and CD28 modulate cell surface raft expression in their regulation of T cell function. J Exp Med 194: 1675–1681

McCoy KD, Hermans IF, Fraser JH, Le Gros G, Ronchese F (1999) Cytotoxic T lymphocyte-associated antigen 4 (CTLA-4) can regulate dendritic cell-induced activation and cytotoxicity of CD8(+) T cells independently of CD4(+) T cell help. J Exp Med 189:1157–1162

McHugh RS, Whitters MJ, Piccirillo CA, Young DA, Shevach EM, Collins M, Byrne MC (2002) CD4(+)CD25(+) immunoregulatory T cells: gene expression analysis reveals a functional role for the glucocorticoid-induced TNF receptor. Immunity 16:311–323

Mohebtash M, Madan RA, Arlen PM, Rauckhorst M, Tsang KY, Cereda V, Vergati M, Poole DJ, Dahut WL, Schlom J, Gulley JL (2009) Phase I trial of targeted therapy with PSA-TRICOM vaccine (V) and ipilimumab (ipi) in patients (pts) with metastatic castration-resistant prostate cancer (mCRPC). J Clin Oncol (Meeting Abstracts) 27 Abstract no: 5144

Mokyr MB, Kalinichenko T, Gorelik L, Bluestone JA (1998a) Realization of the therapeutic potential of CTLA-4 blockade in low-dose chemotherapy-treated tumor-bearing mice. Cancer Res 58:5301–5304

Mokyr MB, Kalinichenko TV, Gorelik L, Bluestone JA (1998b) Importance of the B7-2 molecule for low dose melphalan-induced acquisition of tumor-eradicating immunity by mice bearing a large MOPC-315 tumor. J Immunol 160:1866–1874

Nakada T, Noguchi Y, Satoh S, Ono T, Saika T, Kurashige T, Gnjatic S, Ritter G, Chen YT, Stockert E, Nasu Y, Tsushima T, Kumon H, Old LJ, Nakayama E (2003) NY-ESO-1 mRNA expression and immunogenicity in advanced prostate cancer. Cancer Immun 3:10

Nocentini G, Riccardi C (2005) GITR: a multifaceted regulator of immunity belonging to the tumor necrosis factor receptor superfamily. Eur J Immunol 35:1016–1022

Nocentini G, Giunchi L, Ronchetti S, Krausz LT, Bartoli A, Moraca R, Migliorati G, Riccardi C (1997) A new member of the tumor necrosis factor/nerve growth factor receptor family inhibits T cell receptor-induced apoptosis. Proc Natl Acad Sci USA 94:6216–6221

O'Day SJ, Ibrahim R, DePril V, Maio M, Chiarion-Sileni V, Gajewski TF, Pehamberger H, Hoos A, Humphrey R, Wolchock J (2008) Efficacy and safety of ipilimumab induction and maintenance dosing in patients with advanced melanoma who progressed on one or more prior therapies. J Clin Oncol (Meeting Abstracts) 26: 9021

O'Day S, Weber J, Lebbe C, Maio M, Pehamberger H, Harmankaya K, Siegel J, Hoos A, Humphrey R, Wolchok J (2009) Effect of ipilimumab treatment on 18-month survival: update of patients (pts) with advanced melanoma treated with 10 mg/kg ipilimumab in three phase II clinical trials. J Clin Oncol (Meeting Abstracts) 27 Abstract no: 9033

Pages F, Ragueneau M, Rottapel R, Truneh A, Nunes J, Imbert J, Olive D (1994) Binding of phosphatidylinositol-3-OH kinase to CD28 is required for T-cell signalling. Nature 369: 327–329

Paschen A, Sucker A, Hill B, Moll I, Zapatka M, Nguyen XD, Sim GC, Gutmann I, Hassel J, Becker JC, Steinle A, Schadendorf D, Ugurel S (2009) Differential clinical significance of individual NKG2D ligands in melanoma: soluble ULBP2 as an indicator of poor prognosis superior to S100B. Clin Cancer Res 15:5208–5215

Peggs KS, Quezada SA, Chambers CA, Korman AJ, Allison JP (2009) Blockade of CTLA-4 on both effector and regulatory T cell compartments contributes to the antitumor activity of anti-CTLA-4 antibodies. J Exp Med 206:1717–1725

Perales MA, Blachere NE, Engelhorn ME, Ferrone CR, Gold JS, Gregor PD, Noffz G, Wolchok JD, Houghton AN (2002) Strategies to overcome immune ignorance and tolerance. Semin Cancer Biol 12:63–71

Perales MA, Yuan J, Powel S, Gallardo HF, Rasalan TS, Gonzalez C, Manukian G, Wang J, Zhang Y, Chapman PB, Krown SE, Livingston PO, Ejadi S, Panageas KS, Engelhorn ME, Terzulli SL, Houghton AN, Wolchok JD (2008) Phase I/II study of GM-CSF DNA as an adjuvant for a multipeptide cancer vaccine in patients with advanced melanoma. Mol Ther 16:2022–2029

Perez VL, Van Parijs L, Biuckians A, Zheng XX, Strom TB, Abbas AK (1997) Induction of peripheral T cell tolerance in vivo requires CTLA-4 engagement. Immunity 6:411–417

Phan GQ, Yang JC, Sherry RM, Hwu P, Topalian SL, Schwartzentruber DJ, Restifo NP, Haworth LR, Seipp CA, Freezer LJ, Morton KE, Mavroukakis SA, Duray PH, Steinberg SM, Allison JP, Davis TA, Rosenberg SA (2003) Cancer regression and autoimmunity induced by cytotoxic T lymphocyte-associated antigen 4 blockade in patients with metastatic melanoma. Proc Natl Acad Sci USA 100:8372–8377

Pop LM, Smallshaw JE, Tucker TF, Stevenson FK, Vitetta ES (2005) Failure of vaccination with idiotypic protein or DNA, (+/-IL-2), the depletion of regulatory T cells, or the blockade of CTLA-4 to prolong dormancy in mice with BCL1 lymphoma. J Immunother 28:525–534

Precopio ML, Betts MR, Parrino J, Price DA, Gostick E, Ambrozak DR, Asher TE, Douek DC, Harari A, Pantaleo G, Bailer R, Graham BS, Roederer M, Koup RA (2007) Immunization with vaccinia virus induces polyfunctional and phenotypically distinctive CD8(+) T cell responses. J Exp Med 204:1405–1416

Quezada SA, Peggs KS, Curran MA, Allison JP (2006) CTLA4 blockade and GM-CSF combination immunotherapy alters the intratumor balance of effector and regulatory T cells. J Clin Invest 116:1935–1945

Ramirez-Montagut T, Chow A, Hirschhorn-Cymerman D, Terwey TH, Kochman AA, Lu S, Miles RC, Sakaguchi S, Houghton AN, van den Brink MR (2006) Glucocorticoid-induced TNF receptor family related gene activation overcomes tolerance/ignorance to melanoma differentiation antigens and enhances antitumor immunity. J Immunol 176:6434–6442

Read S, Malmstrom V, Powrie F (2000) Cytotoxic T lymphocyte-associated antigen 4 plays an essential role in the function of CD25(+)CD4(+) regulatory cells that control intestinal inflammation. J Exp Med 192:295–302

Read S, Greenwald R, Izcue A, Robinson N, Mandelbrot D, Francisco L, Sharpe AH, Powrie F (2006) Blockade of CTLA-4 on CD4 + CD25+ regulatory T cells abrogates their function in vivo. J Immunol 177:4376–4383

Reits EA, Hodge JW, Herberts CA, Groothuis TA, Chakraborty M, Wansley EK, Camphausen K, Luiten RM, de Ru AH, Neijssen J, Griekspoor A, Mesman E, Verreck FA, Spits H, Schlom J, van Veelen P, Neefjes JJ (2006) Radiation modulates the peptide repertoire, enhances MHC class I expression, and induces successful antitumor immunotherapy. J Exp Med 203:1259–1271

Reuben JM, Lee BN, Li C, Gomez-Navarro J, Bozon VA, Parker CA, Hernandez IM, Gutierrez C, Lopez-Berestein G, Camacho LH (2006) Biologic and immunomodulatory events after CTLA-4 blockade with ticilimumab in patients with advanced malignant melanoma. Cancer 106:2437–2444

Ribas A (2008) Overcoming immunologic tolerance to melanoma: targeting CTLA-4 with tremelimumab (CP-675, 206). Oncologist 13(Suppl 4):10–15

Ribas A, Camacho LH, Lopez-Berestein G, Pavlov D, Bulanhagui CA, Millham R, Comin-Anduix B, Reuben JM, Seja E, Parker CA, Sharma A, Glaspy JA, Gomez-Navarro J (2005) Antitumor activity in melanoma and anti-self responses in a phase I trial with the anti-cytotoxic T lymphocyte-associated antigen 4 monoclonal antibody CP-675, 206. J Clin Oncol 23:8968–8977

Ribas A, Hauschild A, Kefford R, Gomez-Navarro J, Pavlov D, Marshall MA (2008) Phase III, open-label, randomized, comparative study of tremelimumab (CP-675,206) and chemotherapy (temozolomide [TMZ] or dacarbazine [DTIC]) in patients with advanced melanoma. J Clin Oncol (Meeting Abstracts) 26 Abstract no: LBA9011

Ribas A, Comin-Anduix B, Economou JS, Donahue TR, de la Rocha P, Morris LF, Jalil J, Dissette VB, Shintaku IP, Glaspy JA, Gomez-Navarro J, Cochran AJ (2009) Intratumoral immune cell infiltrates, FoxP3, and indoleamine 2, 3-dioxygenase in patients with melanoma undergoing CTLA4 blockade. Clin Cancer Res 15:390–399

Ronchetti S, Nocentini G, Riccardi C, Pandolfi PP (2002) Role of GITR in activation response of T lymphocytes. Blood 100:350–352

Ronchetti S, Zollo O, Bruscoli S, Agostini M, Bianchini R, Nocentini G, Ayroldi E, Riccardi C (2004) GITR, a member of the TNF receptor superfamily, is costimulatory to mouse T lymphocyte subpopulations. Eur J Immunol 34:613–622

Rudd CE, Taylor A, Schneider H (2009) CD28 and CTLA-4 coreceptor expression and signal transduction. Immunol Rev 229:12–26

Sanderson K, Scotland R, Lee P, Liu D, Groshen S, Snively J, Sian S, Nichol G, Davis T, Keler T, Yellin M, Weber J (2005) Autoimmunity in a phase I trial of a fully human anti-cytotoxic T-lymphocyte antigen-4 monoclonal antibody with multiple melanoma peptides and Montanide ISA 51 for patients with resected stages III and IV melanoma. J Clin Oncol 23:741–750

Schneider H, Downey J, Smith A, Zinselmeyer BH, Rush C, Brewer JM, Wei B, Hogg N, Garside P, Rudd CE (2006) Reversal of the TCR stop signal by CTLA-4. Science 313:1972–1975

Schneider H, Smith X, Liu H, Bismuth G, Rudd CE (2008) CTLA-4 disrupts ZAP70 microcluster formation with reduced T cell/APC dwell times and calcium mobilization. Eur J Immunol 38:40–47

Sharma MD, Hou DY, Liu Y, Koni PA, Metz R, Chandler P, Mellor AL, He Y, Munn DH (2009) Indoleamine 2, 3-dioxygenase controls conversion of Foxp3+ Tregs to TH17-like cells in tumor-draining lymph nodes. Blood 113:6102–6111

Shimizu J, Yamazaki S, Takahashi T, Ishida Y, Sakaguchi S (2002) Stimulation of CD25(+)CD4(+) regulatory T cells through GITR breaks immunological self-tolerance. Nat Immunol 3:135–142

Shrikant P, Khoruts A, Mescher MF (1999) CTLA-4 blockade reverses CD8+ T cell tolerance to tumor by a CD4+ T cell- and IL-2-dependent mechanism. Immunity 11:483–493

Slovin SF, Beer TM, Higano CS, Tejwani S, Hamid O, Picus J, Harzstark A, Scher HI, Lan Z, Lowy I, Prostate Cancer Clinical Trials Consortium (2009) Initial phase II experience of ipilimumab (IPI) alone and in combination with radiotherapy (XRT) in patients with metastatic castration-resistant prostate cancer (mCRPC). J Clin Oncol (Meeting Abstracts) 27 Abstract no: 5138

Small E, Higano C, Tchekmedyian N, Sartor O, Stein B, Young R, Vestal J, Moseley W, Fischkoff S, Lowy I (2006) Randomized phase II study comparing 4 monthly doses of ipilimumab (MDX-010) as a single agent or in combination with a single dose of docetaxel in patients with hormone-refractory prostate cancer. J Clin Oncol (Meeting Abstracts) 24 Abstract no: 4609

Spinicelli S, Nocentini G, Ronchetti S, Krausz LT, Bianchini R, Riccardi C (2002) GITR interacts with the pro-apoptotic protein Siva and induces apoptosis. Cell Death Differ 9:1382–1384

Stephens GL, McHugh RS, Whitters MJ, Young DA, Luxenberg D, Carreno BM, Collins M, Shevach EM (2004) Engagement of glucocorticoid-induced TNFR family-related receptor on effector T cells by its ligand mediates resistance to suppression by CD4 + CD25+ T cells. J Immunol 173:5008–5020

Suvas S, Kim B, Sarangi PP, Tone M, Waldmann H, Rouse BT (2005) In vivo kinetics of GITR and GITR ligand expression and their functional significance in regulating viral immunopathology. J Virol 79:11935–11942

Tang Q, Boden EK, Henriksen KJ, Bour-Jordan H, Bi M, Bluestone JA (2004) Distinct roles of CTLA-4 and TGF-beta in CD4 + CD25+ regulatory T cell function. Eur J Immunol 34:2996–3005

Tchekmedyian S, Glaspy J, Korman A, Keler T, Deo Y, Davis TA (2002) MDX-010 (human anti-CTLA4): a phase I trial in malignant melanoma. Proc Am Soc Clin Oncol 21 Abstract no: 56

Tivol EA, Gorski J (2002) Re-establishing peripheral tolerance in the absence of CTLA-4: complementation by wild-type T cells points to an indirect role for CTLA-4. J Immunol 169:1852–1858

Tivol EA, Borriello F, Schweitzer AN, Lynch WP, Bluestone JA, Sharpe AH (1995) Loss of CTLA-4 leads to massive lymphoproliferation and fatal multiorgan tissue destruction, revealing a critical negative regulatory role of CTLA-4. Immunity 3:541–547

Tivol EA, Boyd SD, McKeon S, Borriello F, Nickerson P, Strom TB, Sharpe AH (1997) CTLA4Ig prevents lymphoproliferation and fatal multiorgan tissue destruction in CTLA-4-deficient mice. J Immunol 158:5091–5094

Tone M, Tone Y, Adams E, Yates SF, Frewin MR, Cobbold SP, Waldmann H (2003) Mouse glucocorticoid-induced tumor necrosis factor receptor ligand is costimulatory for T cells. Proc Natl Acad Sci USA 100:15059–15064

Turk MJ, Guevara-Patino JA, Rizzuto GA, Engelhorn ME, Sakaguchi S, Houghton AN (2004) Concomitant tumor immunity to a poorly immunogenic melanoma is prevented by regulatory T cells. J Exp Med 200:771–782

Tybulewicz VL, Ardouin L, Prisco A, Reynolds LF (2003) Vav1: a key signal transducer downstream of the TCR. Immunol Rev 192:42–52

van der Merwe PA, Bodian DL, Daenke S, Linsley P, Davis SJ (1997) CD80 (B7-1) binds both CD28 and CTLA-4 with a low affinity and very fast kinetics. J Exp Med 185:393–403

van Elsas A, Hurwitz AA, Allison JP (1999) Combination immunotherapy of B16 melanoma using anti-cytotoxic T lymphocyte-associated antigen 4 (CTLA-4) and granulocyte/macrophage colony-stimulating factor (GM-CSF)-producing vaccines induces rejection of subcutaneous and metastatic tumors accompanied by autoimmune depigmentation. J Exp Med 190: 355–366

van Elsas A, Sutmuller RP, Hurwitz AA, Ziskin J, Villasenor J, Medema JP, Overwijk WW, Restifo NP, Melief CJ, Offringa R, Allison JP (2001) Elucidating the autoimmune and antitumor effector mechanisms of a treatment based on cytotoxic T lymphocyte antigen-4 blockade in combination with a B16 melanoma vaccine: comparison of prophylaxis and therapy. J Exp Med 194:481–489

van Leeuwen JE, Samelson LE (1999) T cell antigen-receptor signal transduction. Curr Opin Immunol 11:242–248

Vijayakrishnan L, Slavik JM, Illes Z, Greenwald RJ, Rainbow D, Greve B, Peterson LB, Hafler DA, Freeman GJ, Sharpe AH, Wicker LS, Kuchroo VK (2004) An autoimmune disease-associated CTLA-4 splice variant lacking the B7 binding domain signals negatively in T cells. Immunity 20:563–575

Vonderheide RH, LoRusso PM, Khalil M, Heath E, Khaira D, Soulieres D, Dorazio P, Mariani GL, Usari T, Domchek SM (2009) Tremelimumab in combination with exemestane as novel immunotherapy for patients with advanced breast cancer. J Clin Oncol (Meeting Abstracts) 27 Abstract no: 3034

Walunas TL, Lenschow DJ, Bakker CY, Linsley PS, Freeman GJ, Green JM, Thompson CB, Bluestone JA (1994) CTLA-4 can function as a negative regulator of T cell activation. Immunity 1:405–413

Waterhouse P, Penninger JM, Timms E, Wakeham A, Shahinian A, Lee KP, Thompson CB, Griesser H, Mak TW (1995) Lymphoproliferative disorders with early lethality in mice deficient in Ctla-4. Science 270:985–988

Weber J (2008) Overcoming immunologic tolerance to melanoma: targeting CTLA-4 with ipilimumab (MDX-010). Oncologist 13(Suppl 4):16–25

Weber JS, Targan S, Scotland R, Snively J, Garcia M, Yellin M, Fischkoff S, Nichol G (2006) Phase II trial of extended dose anti-CTLA-4 antibody ipilimumab (formerly MDX-010) with a multi-peptide vaccine for resected stages IIIC and IV melanoma. J Clin Oncol (Meeting Abstracts) 24 Abstract no: 2510

Weber JS, O'Day S, Urba W, Powderly J, Nichol G, Yellin M, Snively J, Hersh E (2008) Phase I/II study of ipilimumab for patients with metastatic melanoma. J Clin Oncol 26:5950–5956

Weber J, Thompson JA, Hamid O, Minor D, Amin A, Ron I, Ridolfi R, Assi H, Maraveyas A, Berman D, Siegel J, O'Day SJ (2009) A randomized, double-blind, placebo-controlled, phase II study comparing the tolerability and efficacy of ipilimumab administered with or without prophylactic budesonide in patients with unresectable stage III or IV melanoma. Clin Cancer Res 15:5591–5598

Wing K, Onishi Y, Prieto-Martin P, Yamaguchi T, Miyara M, Fehervari Z, Nomura T, Sakaguchi S (2008) CTLA-4 control over Foxp3+ regulatory T cell function. Science 322:271–275

Wolchok JD, de Pril V, Linette G, Waterfield W, Gajewski T, Chiarion-Sileni V, Ibrahim R, Chin K, Hoos A, Hamid O (2009a) Efficacy of ipilimumab 10 mg/kg in advanced melanoma patients (pts) with good and poor prognostic factors. J Clin Oncol (Meeting Abstracts) 27 Abstract no: 9036

Wolchok JD, Hoos A, O'Day S, Weber JS, Hamid O, Lebbe C, Maio M, Binder M, Bohnsack O, Nichol G, Humphrey R, Hodi FS (2009b) Guidelines for the evaluation of immune therapy activity in solid tumors: immune-related response criteria. Clin Cancer Res 15:7412–7420

Wolchok JD, Neyns B, Linette G, Negrier S, Lutzky J, Thomas L, Waterfield W, Schadendorf D, Smylie M, Guthrie T Jr, Grob JJ, Chesney J, Chin K, Chen K, Hoos A, O'Day SJ, Lebbe C (2009c) Ipilimumab monotherapy in patients with pretreated advanced melanoma: a randomised, double-blind, multicentre, phase 2, dose-ranging study. Lancet Oncol 11:155–164

Yang YF, Zou JP, Mu J, Wijesuriya R, Ono S, Walunas T, Bluestone J, Fujiwara H, Hamaoka T (1997) Enhanced induction of antitumor T-cell responses by cytotoxic T lymphocyte-associated molecule-4 blockade: the effect is manifested only at the restricted tumor-bearing stages. Cancer Res 57:4036–4041

Yang JC, Hughes M, Kammula U, Royal R, Sherry RM, Topalian SL, Suri KB, Levy C, Allen T, Mavroukakis S, Lowy I, White DE, Rosenberg SA (2007) Ipilimumab (anti-CTLA4 antibody) causes regression of metastatic renal cell cancer associated with enteritis and hypophysitis. J Immunother 30:825–830

Yuan J, Gnjatic S, Li H, Powel S, Gallardo HF, Ritter E, Ku GY, Jungbluth AA, Segal NH, Rasalan TS, Manukian G, Xu Y, Roman RA, Terzulli SL, Heywood M, Pogoriler E, Ritter G, Old LJ, Allison JP, Wolchok JD (2008) CTLA-4 blockade enhances polyfunctional NY-ESO-1 specific T cell responses in metastatic melanoma patients with clinical benefit. Proc Natl Acad Sci USA 105:20410–20415

Yuan J, Page DB, Ku GY, Li Y, Mu Z, Ariyan C, Gallardo HF, Roman RA, Heine AI, Terzulli SL, Gnjatic S, Ritter G, Jungbluth AA, Allison JP, Old LJ, Wolchok JD (2010) Correlation of clinical and immunological data in a metastatic melanoma patient with heterogeneous tumor responses to ipilimumab therapy. Cancer Immun 10:1

Zatloukal P, Heo DS, Park K, Kang J, Butts C, Bradford D, Graziano S, Huang B, Healey D (2009) Randomized phase II clinical trial comparing tremelimumab (CP-675,206) with best supportive care (BSC) following first-line platinum-based therapy in patients (pts) with advanced non-small cell lung cancer (NSCLC). J Clin Oncol (Meeting Abstracts) 27 Abstract no: 8071

Zhang W, Sloan-Lancaster J, Kitchen J, Trible RP, Samelson LE (1998) LAT: the ZAP-70 tyrosine kinase substrate that links T cell receptor to cellular activation. Cell 92:83–92

Zhang B, Bowerman NA, Salama JK, Schmidt H, Spiotto MT, Schietinger A, Yu P, Fu YX, Weichselbaum RR, Rowley DA, Kranz DM, Schreiber H (2007) Induced sensitization of tumor stroma leads to eradication of established cancer by T cells. J Exp Med 204:49–55

Zhou P, L'Italien L, Hodges D, Schebye XM (2007) Pivotal roles of CD4+ effector T cells in mediating agonistic anti-GITR mAb-induced-immune activation and tumor immunity in CT26 tumors. J Immunol 179:7365–7375

Immunobiology of Cancer Therapies Targeting CD137 and B7-H1/PD-1 Cosignal Pathways

Shengdian Wang and Lieping Chen

Contents

1 Introduction 246
2 The Costimulatory CD137 Signaling Pathway 248
2.1 The Expression of CD137L and CD137 248
2.2 Role of CD137 Cosignaling in Effector/Memory T Cells 249
3 Strategies to Augment Tumor Immunity by Stimulating CD137 250
3.1 Tumor Therapy with Agonist Anti-CD137 Antibody 250
3.2 Whole Cell Vaccines with Capacity to Stimulate CD137 252
3.3 Adoptive Transfer of T Cells with CD137 Costimulation 253
4 The Coinhibitory B7-H1/PD-1 Signaling Pathway 254
4.1 Expression of B7-H1, B7-DC and PD-1 254
4.2 Complex Interactions Among B7-H1, B7-DC, B7-1, PD-1, and Possible Additional Binding Partners 255
4.3 B7-H1/PD-1 Interaction in the Suppression of Immune Responses 256
5 Manipulation of B7-H1/PD-1 Pathway in Tumor Immunotherapy 257
5.1 B7-H1/PD-1 Pathway in the Evasion of Tumor Immunity 257
5.2 Blocking B7-H1/PD-1 Pathway in Cancer Therapy 259
References 260

Abstract Cancer immunotherapy is finally entering a new era with manipulation of cosignaling pathways as a therapeutic approach, for which the principle was proved nearly two decades ago. In addition to CTLA-4, CD137 and B7-H1/PD-1 pathways are two new targets in the stage. CD137 pathway is costimulatory and its agonistic antibody delivers potent signal to drive T cell growth and activation. On the other hand, blockade of B7-H1/PD-1 pathway with antagonistic antibody has shown to

---

S.Wang
Center for Infection and Immunity, Institute for Biophysics, Chinese Academy of Sciences, Beijing, China
L. Chen (✉)
Sidney Kimmel Comprehensive Cancer Center and Department of Oncology, Johns Hopkins University School of Medicine, Baltimore, MD, USA
e-mail: lchen42@jhmi.edu

G. Dranoff (ed.), *Cancer Immunology and Immunotherapy*,
Current Topics in Microbiology and Immunology 344, DOI 10.1007/82_2010_81

protect ongoing T cell responses from impairment by immune evasion mechanism in cancer microenvironment. With these tools in hand, a mechanism-based design of combined immunotherapy with high efficacy is becoming a reality.

Abbreviations

APCs	Antigen presenting cells
DCs	Dendritic cells
HSV	Herpes simplex virus
IDO	Indoleamine-2,3-dioxygenase
LCMV	Lymphocytic choriomeningitis virus
mAb	Monoclonal antibody
MDCs	Myeloid DCs
MHC	Major histocompatibility complex
NK	Natural killer
OVA	Ovalbumin
TCR	T cell receptor
TDLN	Tumor-draining lymph node
TIL	Tumor infiltrating T lymphocytes
TNF	Tumor necrosis factor

1 Introduction

T-lymphocytes play a pivotal role in the control of cancer progression. The inherent genetic instability in tumor cells results in the expression of aberrant antigenic epitopes or the overexpression of normally repressed genes that could be recognized by T cells of the host immune system (Pardoll 2003). However, the engagement of T-cell receptors (TCRs) on T cells by the antigenic peptide/major histocompatibility complex (MHC) on the surface of antigen-presenting cells is often not sufficient to drive the activation of naive T cells leading to optimal immune responses (Lenschow et al. 1996; Chen et al. 1994). Productive T-cell activation requires a second antigen-independent cosignal, the "costimulatory signal" provided by the interaction of accessory surface molecules between T cells and antigen presenting cells (APCs). In the absence of costimulation, TCR-mediated activation of T cells resulted in antigen-specific unresponsiveness (termed T-cell anergy), rendering the T cells unable to respond to subsequent exposure to antigen (Schwartz 2003; Harding et al. 1992). On the other hand, activated T cells are under tight control by different sets of cell surface molecules through "co-inhibitory signal" to attenuate T cell responses. These co-inhibitory signals are inducible or strengthen in responding to activation and has been shown to be a very powerful mechanism in negative regulation of T cell-mediated immune responses (Chen 2004).

CD28 is the first identified costimulatory receptor constitutively expressed on naïve T cells. Upon binding to its ligands, B7-1 (CD80) and B7-2 (CD86) on APCs, CD28 provides a potent costimulatory signal to T cells activated through their TCRs, which enhances T-cell proliferation by induction of IL-2 transcription, expression of IL-2 receptor CD25 and also confers critical survival signals to T cells through the Bcl-XL pathway. Once T cells are activated, a closely related molecule, cytotoxic T-lymphocyte antigen-4 (CTLA-4) (CD152), is induced to express on the surface of activated T cells. CTLA-4 has higher affinity than CD28 for the same ligands but appears to inhibit IL-2 production, IL-2 receptor expression, and cell cycle progression, which attenuate the immune responses and prevent autoimmune diseases (Carreno and Collins 2002; Sharpe and Freeman 2002). At present, a broad array of proteins has been identified to be involved in T-cell costimulation. The specific binding between the paired costimulatory ligands and receptors enhance or inhibit T cell responses by costimulatory signaling or coinhibitory signaling through TCRs. These cosignaling interactions form a delicate network to regulate and control initiation, expansion, development of effector and memory T cell responses as well as T cell homeostasis at multiple stages of the immune responses (Chen 2004; Wang and Chen 2004).

In the last two decades, the identification of tumor-associated antigens led to development of a variety of vaccine strategies for tumor immunotherapy, including peptides, proteins, whole cells, recombinant viral vectors, and antigen-pulsed dendritic cells, aiming to parallel the successes achieved in developing vaccines for infectious diseases. However, the attempts to target human cancers have been significantly less successful than was initially envisaged possible. In some instances, failure of consistent clinical responses including tumor regression has occurred despite impressive immunologic responses, particularly those elicited using anchor-modified epitopes as immunogens. The adoptive transfer of antigen-specific T-cells has also showed limited success in patients with melanoma and renal cell carcinoma (Morgan et al. 2006). These results offer evidences that generation of a large *in vivo* population of tumor-reactive $CD8^+$ T cells is not singularly sufficient to mediate clinically significant tumor regression. This conclusion is not so surprised because the challenges of delivering effective vaccines or immunotherapies for tumor are aligned much more closely with those associated with therapy of chronic or even ongoing infections than more acute infections, in which the majority of the successes have come with prophylactic vaccination strategies. Once the antigen-specific T cells are fully activated to become effector cells, most of them are dead of apoptosis and less develop into functional memory T cells compared to acute viral infection. Persistent antigen stimulation result in corruption of effector T cell functions such as in chronic viral infections or tumor-bearing state. Ex vivo analysis of tumor infiltrating lymphocytes (TILs) has generally demonstrated a dysfunctional state (Lee et al. 1999), which can be reversed upon culture *in vitro* (Radoja et al. 2001). It is obvious that the long-term maintenance of potent T-cells represents a significant challenge in patients with established or recurrent tumors. Fortunately, the positive and negative costimulatory pathways have been showed to play critical roles in regulating the survival and functional corruptions (including anergy, tolerance, exhaustion, and dysfunction) of effector T cell in the settings of persistent antigen stimulation, such as chronic viral infections and the tumor-bearing state. In this context, CD137 and B7-H1/PD-1 cosignaling pathways are most promising candidates for manipulation to achieve long-term potent anti-tumor T cell responses in patients.

2 The Costimulatory CD137 Signaling Pathway

2.1 The Expression of CD137L and CD137

CD137 (4-1BB, ILA, TNFRFS9) belongs to the tumor necrosis factor (TNF) receptor superfamily and is inducibly expressed on T cells following stimulation through the TCR complex (Pollok et al. 1993). With soluble antigens, such as superantigens or ovalbumin (OVA) delivered with lipopolysaccharide (LPS), CD137 is expressed only transiently on the T cells *in vivo* (Takahashi et al. 1999). However, CD137 expression can be prolonged with persistent antigen stimulation, such as cardiac allograft rejection, adenovirus delivered antigen, persistent herpes simplex virus (HSV)-1 infection, or severe influenza infection (Tan et al. 2000; Seo et al. 2003; Lin et al. 2009). Thus, the effects of CD137 on activated T cells may depend in part on its expression pattern in the particular model studied. In addition to antigen stimulation, the cytokines of interleukin 2 (IL-2) and IL-15 can induce expression of CD137 on memory but not naive $CD8^+$ T cells *in vitro*, which may contribute to memory T cell survival after antigen clearance (Pulle et al. 2006; Sabbagh et al. 2007). Both $CD8^+$ and $CD4^+$ T cells, including Th1 and Th2 cells, can be induced to express CD137; however, at least in some circumstances, $CD8^+$ T cells can upregulate CD137 more rapidly and to higher levels than $CD4^+$ T cells (Wen et al. 2002; Futagawa et al. 2002). In addition to its well-established role as an inducible costimulatory receptor on T cells, CD137 was also expressed on activated natural killer (NK), dendritic cells (DCs), hepatoma cells and blood vessels from individuals with malignant tumors (Futagawa et al. 2002; Broll et al. 2001; Melero et al. 1998a; Schwarz et al. 1995).

CD137L, a member of TNF superfamily, was found to be expressed following stimulation on professional APCs including DCs and macrophages as well as activated B cells (Alderson et al. 1994; Pollok et al. 1994), and is also expressed on myeloid progenitors and hematopoietic stem cells (Lee et al. 2008; Jiang et al. 2008). CD137L expression appears to be tightly regulated *in vivo*, such that its expression during an ongoing immune response *in vivo* is difficult to be detected at the protein level (Lin et al. 2009). However, during chronic and inflammatory conditions CD137L is more readily detectable at the mRNA or protein level (Tan et al. 2000; Lin et al. 2009; Mack et al. 2008). The low and transient level of

CD137L expression has made it difficult to study the immediate effects of CD137L binding to CD137 *in vivo*.

When coupled with a strong signal through the TCR, engagement of CD137 can induce IL-2 production of T cells independent of CD28 ligation. Early studies demonstrated that ligation of CD137 by either cell surface CD137L or specific antibodies provide a costimulatory signal to T cells, including both $CD4^+$ and $CD8^+$ T cells, enhancing proliferation, cytokine production, and particularly survival (Takahashi et al. 1999; Schwarz et al. 1995; Alderson et al. 1994; Shuford et al. 1997; Hurtado et al. 1997). The costimulatory signal has been shown to be more potent for $CD8^+$ T cells than $CD4^+$ T cells (Shuford et al. 1997). Later studies point to the role of CD137 engagement in augmenting rather than initiating T-cell response and in sustaining their effector functions.

CD137 engagement on DCs using antibodies or transfected ligand enhances their production of inflammatory cytokines, including IL-12 (p40/70) and IL-6, and enhances their ability to activate T cells (Futagawa et al. 2002; Wilcox et al. 2002). However, the relative importance of CD137 signaling in APCs versus T cells during an ongoing immune response is unknown. Since anti-CD137 induced enhancement of T-cell expansion *in vivo* appears to act primarily through CD137 on the T cells rather than on the APCs (Sabbagh et al. 2008). Similarly, anti-CD137-induced expansion of adoptively-transferred memory T cells required CD137 on the T cells but not in the host (Zhu et al. 2007), arguing for direct effects of CD137 in the T cells.

2.2 Role of CD137 Cosignaling in Effector/Memory T Cells

The up-regulation of CD137 on antigen-experienced T cells suggests that CD137 cosignaling may target these primed T cells differentially, influencing those T cells preferentially with highest avidity receptors. When wild-type or CD137L-deficient mice were infected intraperitoneally with influenza A/X31, the primary expansion and contraction of $CD8^+$ T cells was indistinguishable over the first 2 weeks of the response. However, there was a two- to threefold defect in the number of $CD8^+$ T cells persisting at 3–5 weeks after infection, and a two- to threefold decrease in the recall response to influenza A/PR8 in the CD137L-deficient mice (Bertram et al. 2002). This observation revealed a role for CD137L in controlling influenza specific effector-memory T-cell numbers late in the primary response. In an adoptive transfer experiment, TCR-transgenic T cells were cultured with OVA antigen peptide followed by human IL-15 to produce the cells with the surface phenotype of central-memory T cells ($CD62L^{high}$ $CD44^{high}$ $IL\text{-}7R^+$ $CCR7^+$ $CD69^+$) (Manjunath et al. 2001). Transfer of these *in vitro*-derived "memory phenotype" cells into otherwise unmanipulated naive-wild-type or CD137L-deficient mice showed that the absence of CD137L in the host resulted in a two- to threefold decrease in the number of adoptively transferred T cells recovered in the spleen and bone marrow compared with wild-type mice by 3 weeks post transfer under conditions where the rate of cell division (about one or two divisions in 3 weeks) was indistinguishable in the mice (Pulle et al. 2006). Taken together, the CD137/CD137L interaction may play a role in survival of effector-memory CD8$^+$ T cell after antigen has been cleared.

Our recent study found that systemic administration of anti-CD137 antibodies induced expansion of CD4$^+$ and CD8$^+$ T cells with memory but not naïve phenotype in mice (Zhu et al. 2007). The T cell activation and proliferation is antigen independent. CD137 is required on the T cells and is dispensable in the host for anti-CD137 to expand memory T cells. With systemic antibody treatment, both CD4$^+$ and CD8$^+$ memory T cells were expanded, and this expansion was due to increased division as measured by bromodeoxyuridine incorporation. In contrast, CD137L deficiency influenced the CD8$^+$ but not the CD4$^+$ memory T-cell pool largely through effects on survival rather than on cell division (Pulle et al. 2006). It is possible that the supraphysiological anti-CD137 or overexpressed CD137L signal is sufficient to drive T-cell proliferation, whereas the endogenous level of CD137L in the host may not be sufficient for this effect. In summary, data from both knockout mice as well as from systemic treatment of unimmunized mice with stimulatory anti-CD137 antibodies support a role for CD137 on memory T cells receiving signals from CD137L in the host to maintain CD8$^+$ T-cell memory.

3 Strategies to Augment Tumor Immunity by Stimulating CD137

Ligation of costimulatory receptor CD137 by either its ligand or agonistic antibodies has been shown to provide a potent costimulatory signal, which is more potent for CD8$^+$ T cells than for CD4$^+$ T cells. Particularly, CD137 is specifically expressed on antigen-activated T cells and provides a potent costimulatory signal for enhancing the functions of effector/memory T cells and for maintaining the T cells survival. These results raise great interest in manipulation of the CD137 pathway as a therapeutic target for cancer therapy.

3.1 Tumor Therapy with Agonist Anti-CD137 Antibody

In an early study, agonist anti-CD137 mAb was shown to induce regression of established tumors including the poor immunogenic Ag104A sarcoma and the highly tumorigenic p815 mastocytoma in mouse models (Melero et al. 1997). The anti-tumor effect required both CD4$^+$ and CD8$^+$ T cells and was accompanied by marked augmentation of tumor-specific CTL activity. Subsequent studies showed that agonist anti-CD137 mAbs induced the complete regression of many types of established tumors induced by transplantable syngeneic mouse tumor lines (May et al. 2002; Kim et al. 2001; Lynch 2008).

The mechanisms of CD137 mAb-mediated tumor regression are yet to be elucidated. Several possible mechanisms include the breaking of immunological ignorance, prevention of T cell tolerance/anergy and deletion, and are largely dependent on the models employed. In an established C3 tumor model, CTLs against a model tumor antigen, human papillomavirus E7 oncoprotein, are not anergic or deleted, but remain naïve. Immunological ignorance of specific CTLs appears to prevent anti–CD137 mAb from activating tumor immunity, since anti–CD137 mAb itself neither activates tumor-specific CTLs nor induces the regression of established C3 tumors. Similar observations were made in the TC-1 lung carcinoma and B16-F10 melanoma models. Immunization with E7 tumor peptide in the presence of adjuvant stimulated E7-specific $CD8^+$ CTL, leading to elimination of T cell ignorance, albeit is still insufficient to regress the established C3 tumor. In combination with anti-CD137 mAb, a high level of E7-specific CTLs was elicited, leading to the complete regression of established C3 tumors *in vivo*. These studies indicate that cancer cells may not be able to initiate antigen-specific CTL response and initial trigger of such responses is critical. Similarly, treatment of tumor-bearing mice with Flt3L (a cytokine that promotes the generation of large numbers of DCs *in vivo*) resulted in the generation of effective $CD8^+$ T-cell-mediated immune responses by enhancing the efficiency of antigen presentation to T cells. There was a clear cooperative effect when Flt3L and anti-CD137 treatments were combined in tumor-bearing mice (Miller et al. 2002). Treatment of mice that have been immunized with either GM-CSF-secreting tumor cells or a DC-based vaccine with CD137 mAb also results in augmentation of the anti-tumor immune responses (Li et al. 2007; Ito et al. 2004). Collectively, these results suggest that selective stimulation of antigen-specific T cells is prerequisite for CD137 agonists to operate. Interestingly, several reports in rodent models have also shown synergistic effects of agonistic anti-CD137 mAb in combination with anti-tumor necrosis factor-related apoptosis-inducing ligand (TRAIL) and CD40 mAbs (Uno et al. 2006), with intratumoral introduction of the IL-12 gene (Xu et al. 2005), or with chemotherapy or radiotherapy (McMillin et al. 2006; Shi and Siemann 2006). These observations provide important information for developing combination studies in the clinic.

A somewhat unusual feature accompanied with anti-CD137 mAb therapy is diminished pathology in autoimmune disease models. Sun and colleagues showed that the same agonist anti-CD137 antibody used to promote anti-tumor immunity resulted in ameliorating both the incidence and severity of experimental autoimmune encephalomyelitis (EAE) (Sun et al. 2002a). Many other studies have confirmed the beneficial effects of anti-CD137 mAb in various autoimmune disease models including rheumatoid arthritis (Seo et al. 2004), and systemic lupus erythematosis (Vinay et al. 2006). In a transplantation model, anti-CD137 was also shown to inhibit rejection of intestinal allografts in mice (Wang et al. 2003a). Although a complete understanding of these differential effects is lacking, the promotion of regulatory T cell development and activity is believed to play a role. Additional potential explanations for immune suppression in some settings include the apparent ability to delete $CD4^+$ T cells, retard B-cell function, and upregulation of indoleamine-2,3-dioxygenase (IDO) and IFN-γ (Sun et al. 2002a, 2002b; Seo et al. 2004; Vinay et al. 2006). Therefore, anti-CD137 mAb represents a unique immunotherapeutic agent that could be applied to both immune potentiating for tumor immunity and immune suppressive for certain autoimmune diseases.

3.2 Whole Cell Vaccines with Capacity to Stimulate CD137

Introduction of costimulatory molecules into tumor cells to improve its ability as better APCs has become a common therapeutic vaccine in tumor immunotherapy. Transfection of tumor cells to express CD137L showed to enhance immunogenicity of murine P815 mastocytoma or AG104A sarcoma lines by developing a strong CTL response, which rejected these tumors (Melero et al. 1998b). Although CD137 is an independent costimulator, optimal effect of CD137L in CTL stimulation may require B7-CD28 interaction since blockade of this interaction by antibodies down-regulated the expression of CD137 on T cells and decreased CTL activity. Furthermore, co-expression of CD137L and B7-1 in the poorly immunogenic AG104A sarcoma enhanced the induction of effector CTL and the rejection of the wild-type tumor while neither CD137L nor B7-1 single transfectants were effective (Melero et al. 1998b). In a later study using the A20, a B-cell lymphoma cell line, a similar result was obtained (Guinn et al. 1999). These results suggest that a synergistic effect between the CD137 and the CD28 co-stimulatory pathways in the anti-tumor immune responses. Although CD137 can function independently of CD28 to deliver a co-mitogenic signal for T cell proliferation and IL-2 production (DeBenedette et al. 1997), B7-CD28 costimulatory signaling is required for the optimal expression of CD137 on T cells, which in return further promote the anti-tumor functions of the activated T cells.

In order to deliver CD137L to tumor for tumor therapy, a replication-defective adenovirus expressing CD137L gene was constructed. In a syngeneic mouse model of liver tumor metastasis induced by intrahepatic injection of the poorly immunogenic MCA26 colon cancer cells, various combinations of replication-defective adenoviruses expressing IL-12 and CD137L cDNA were injected into the established liver tumor. The long-term survival rate of mice treated with the combination of IL-12 and CD137L were significantly improved over that of animals in the control groups. *In vivo* depletion of NK cells or $CD8^+$ T cells completely abolished the long-term survival advantage of the IL-12 plus CD137L-treated animals (Martinet et al. 2000). When combined with IL-12 gene transfer, systemic administration of the Ig-CD137L fusion protein can generate a better antitumor response than local gene delivery. In this combination therapy, the Ig-CD137L is as potent as the agonistic anti-CD137 antibody for the treatment of hepatic MCA26 colon carcinoma, resulting in 50% complete tumor regression and long-term survival. In long-term surviving mice, both treatment modalities induced persistent tumor-specific CTL activity (Xu et al. 2005).

It would appear that the transfection of CD137L cDNA into tumor cells as a whole cell tumor vaccine may not be as effective as anti-CD137 mAb. In the murine sarcoma line Ag104, the tumor cells which express CD137L had no therapeutic activity unless they were also transfected with B7-1 (Melero et al. 1998b). However, the injection of anti-CD137 mAb into mice with the same tumor (Ag104) caused tumor destruction (Melero et al. 1997). In order to create a vaccine that stimulate the immune system as a monoclonal antibody does, Ye and colleagues constructed a vector encoding cell-bound single-chain Fv fragments from a hybridoma secreting CD137 mAb, and transfected to express this gene into K1735 melanoma cells which expressed low levels of MHC class I molecules and were poorly immunogenicity. Mice vaccinated with modified tumor cells rejected established wild-type K1735 tumors growing as subcutaneous nodules or in the lung (Ye et al. 2002).

3.3 *Adoptive Transfer of T Cells with CD137 Costimulation*

Adoptive transfer of tumor-reactive T cells represents an effective immunotherapeutic strategy for cancer treatment. Clinical trials have demonstrated beneficial effects of adoptive immunotherapy in malignant melanoma (Dudley et al. 2002; Yee et al. 2002), renal cell carcinoma (Kawai et al. 2003), EBV-associated nasopharyngeal carcinoma (Straathof et al. 2005), Hodgkin's Disease (Bollard et al. 2004) and glioma (Tsuboi et al. 2003) with ex vivo expanded CTLs. Efficacy of T-cell adoptive transfer may be improved through optimization of *in vitro* expansion, characterization of effector populations, and/or by enhancing the function and survival of transferred CTLs to facilitate establishment of immunologic memory.

Several studies have examined the possibility of using CD137 costimulation for the generation of tumor-reactive T cells for adoptive immunotherapy. Addition of an agonistic anti-CD137 mAb to *in vitro* cultures of tumor-draining lymph node (TDLN) cells with anti-CD3/anti-CD28 antibodies enhanced expansion, type 1 cytokine production, and survival of T cells. When anti-CD3/anti-CD28/anti-CD137-expanded TDLN cells were adoptively transferred into MCA 205 tumor-bearing mice, significantly fewer metastatic lesions and prolonged survival of mice were observed compared with TDLN cells stimulated without anti-CD137 (Li et al. 2003). Strome et al. (2000) isolated T cells from the TDLN of mice bearing disseminated micrometastasis of a poorly immunogenic, MHC class I-negative A9P squamous cell carcinoma. The T cells expended with combination of anti-CD3/anti-CD28/anti-CD137 were more effective than those activated by anti-CD3 alone or anti-CD3/anti-CD28 in mediating antitumor reactivity.

Currently, a majority of investigators generated T cells for clinical trials of adoptive immunotherapy by repetitive TCR-based stimulation of peripheral blood lymphocytes using various APCs. The CD28 costimulation is a commonly used approach for expanding T cells since B7/CD28 pathway is widely considered an important costimulatory pathway for TCR activation. However, bead-based anti-CD3/CD28 artificial APCs (aAPCs) induced brisk expansion of $CD4^+$ populations but not $CD8^+$ T cells (Deeths et al. 1999; Laux et al. 2000), demonstrating that the CD28 costimulation may not be sufficient for expansion of $CD8^+$ CTL. Maus et al. (2002) demonstrated that the incorporation of CD137L into an aAPC greatly augmented the capacity for Ag-specific expansion of $CD8^+$ T cells *ex vivo*. Zhang et al. (2007) directly compared the efficacy of CD28 vs. CD137 signaling in the expansion of $CD8^+$ CTL, and showed that anti-CD3/CD137L aAPCs preferentially expand memory $CD8^+$ T cells, resulting in an increased frequency of cells responding to viral recall antigens in the expanded cultures from healthy donors, whereas anti-CD3/anti-CD28 aAPCs preferentially expand naïve $CD8^+$ cells and therefore do not enrich for viral-specific CTL. The CTL expanded using CD137 costimulation mediate enhanced cytolytic capacity compared with using CD28 costimulation. For more effectively expanding tumor-specific CTL, the recombinant replication-defective adenovirus and HSV amplicons encoding CD137L were constructed and used to convert autologous monocytes or tumor cells into efficient APC (Serghides et al. 2005; Yi et al. 2007). These systems provide theoretical means to selectively expand tumor-specific effector populations without the need for pre-sorting for tumor-reactive T cells.

As an alternative to deliver the CD137 signal, Stephan and colleagues (Stephan et al. 2007) recently employed a genetic approach to constitutively co-express CD80 and CD137L in primary human cytomegalovirus (CMV)-specific T cells and prostate-specific membrane antigen (PSMA)-targeted T cells, substituting for the lack of these ligands on APCs. The T cells expressing CD80 and CD137L vigorously respond to tumor cells lacking costimulatory ligands and provoked potent rejection of large, systemic tumors in immunodeficient mice. These findings obtained in a very challenging tumor model, underscore the remarkable biological activity and potency of constitutive, high-level expression of costimulatory ligands on T cells.

4 The Coinhibitory B7-H1/PD-1 Signaling Pathway

4.1 Expression of B7-H1, B7-DC and PD-1

B7-H1 (CD274) (Dong et al. 1999) and B7-DC (CD273) (Tseng et al. 2001) were initially identified as a potential costimulatory molecule that could stimulate T cell responses in the presence of TCR signaling. While the overall expression of B7-H1 and B7-DC transcripts is similarly found in various lymphoid and nonlymphoid tissues (Dong et al. 1999; Freeman et al. 2000; Latchman et al. 2001; Tamura et al. 2001), the expression profiles of cell surface proteins are quite distinct. The expression of B7-H1 protein, although virtually absent in normal tissues except macrophage and dendritic cell-like cells, could be induced in a variety of tissues and cell types, such as DCs, macrophages, B cells, T cells, NK cells, and bone marrow-derived mast cells, epithelial cells, muscle cells, trophoblast, endothelial cells and various tumor cells (Dong et al. 1999; Tamura et al. 2001). On the contrary, cell surface B7-DC was mainly detected on several types of myeloid cells including DCs and macrophages (Tseng et al. 2001). Cell surface expression of both B7-H1 and B7-DC could be up-regulated upon activation or IFN-γ treatment of human monocytes and DCs (Tseng et al. 2001; Dong et al. 2002).

PD-1 is a distant homologue of CTLA-4 molecule, which was originally identified as a gene that was highly expressed by cell lines undergoing programmed cell death (Ishida et al. 1992). PD-1 is not detectable on naive T cells but its expression goes up in T cells, B cells, and myeloid cells after activation (Freeman et al. 2000; Agata et al. 1996). PD-1 expression is also upregulated on purified human T cells by cytokines using the common gamma chain including IL-2, IL-7, IL-15, and IL-21 in the absence of TCR ligation (Kinter et al. 2008). PD-1 is retained in an intracellular compartment of freshly isolated regulatory T cells, but is translocated to the cell surface after TCR stimulation (Raimondi et al. 2006). The expression of PD-1 is particularly high on the surface of functionally exhausted $CD8^+$ effector T cells during persistent viral infections in both mice and humans (Barber et al. 2006; Day et al. 2006).

4.2 Complex Interactions Among B7-H1, B7-DC, B7-1, PD-1, and Possible Additional Binding Partners

Both B7-H1 and B7-DC were found to bind PD-1 and, therefore, were renamed as PD ligand 1 (PD-L1) and PD ligand 2 (PD-L2), respectively, to emphasize PD-1 as a receptor (Freeman et al. 2000; Latchman et al. 2001). This nomenclature, however, undermines the complex costimulatory interactions within this pathway because subsequent studies demonstrated that B7-H1 could suppress T cell responses by interacting with another independent receptor B7-1 (Butte et al. 2007, 2008). Furthermore, B7-H1 was shown to be a receptor and could utilize PD-1 as a ligand to deliver an anti-apoptotic signal (Azuma et al. 2008).

The predominant role of PD-1 is inhibitory for immune responses, and this notion is supported by the phenotypes of lymphoproliferative/autoimmune diseases in PD-1-deficient mice (Okazaki and Honjo 2006). There is ample evidence that the major ligand for the suppressive function of PD-1 *in vivo* appears to be B7-H1 because results obtained from PD-1 or B7-H1 deficient mice as well as blocking antibodies against PD-1 or B7-H1 are often similar (Nishimura et al. 1999, 2001). However, B7-H1 deficient mice do not develop autoimmune diseases, albeit mild to moderate levels of $CD8^+$ T cell accumulation are common in peripheral organs (Dong et al. 2004). In T cell culture systems, studies reveal either positive or negative function of B7-H1 and B7-DC in T cell growth and cytokine production, highlighting a lack of reliable *in vitro* models for the prediction of their functions *in vivo*. Possible interpretations for these somewhat confusing data are either additional receptor(s) for B7-H1 and B7-DC or possible receptor functions of these so-called "ligand" molecules. B7-H1 was recently shown to mediate suppressive functions through B7-1 on T cells (Butte et al. 2007). Our studies using structural biology and site-directed mutagenesis approaches have led to the characterization of B7-H1 and B7-DC mutants with abolished PD-1 binding capacity (Wang et al. 2003b). Interestingly, several such mutants are still able to costimulate proliferation and cytokine production of T cells from normal or even PD-1$^{-/-}$ mice at a comparable level to wild type B7-H1 and B7-DC. The costimulation of B7-DC in conjunction with B7-1 for cytokine production is also shown to be PD-1 independent (Shin et al. 2003). Therefore, B7-H1 and B7-DC may costimulate T cell growth through a receptor other than PD-1 and B7-1. In addition to being a ligand, B7-H1 could also act as a receptor and utilize PD-1 as the ligand. By transfection of intracellular domain-deficient B7-H1 or PD-1 into tumor cells or T cells, respectively, cancer cells expressing truncated B7-H1 lost their resistance to lysis by tumor antigen-specific CD8^{+} T cells. In contrast, truncated PD-1 on T cells was still able to act as a ligand for full length B7-H1 on cancer cells to deliver an anti-apoptotic signal (Azuma et al. 2008). Therefore, it is premature to conclude that the interaction between B7-H1 and PD-1 is exclusively suppressive.

4.3 B7-H1/PD-1 Interaction in the Suppression of Immune Responses

The broad distribution of B7-H1 in non-lymphoid organs and the autoimmune phenotype of PD-1$^{-/-}$ mice suggest a role of PD-1 signaling in the regulation of peripheral self-tolerance of T cells. PD-1$^{-/-}$ mice on the C57BL/6 background develop a lupus-like arthritis (Nishimura et al. 1999), while BALB/c mice develop a cardiomyopathy secondary to the production of an autoantibody directed against cardiac troponin (Nishimura et al. 2001; Okazaki et al. 2003). The autoimmunity that occurred in PD-1$^{-/-}$ mice is different from that which developed in CTLA-4$^{-/-}$ mice. The CTLA-4 deficient mice died within 3∼4 weeks of birth from massive lymphocytic infiltration and tissue destruction in critical organs (Waterhouse et al. 1995; Tivol et al. 1995), while PD-1$^{-/-}$ mice developed strain-specific autoimmunity in old age (Nishimura et al. 1999, 2001). These differences may reflect the different regulatory roles of these two negative cosignaling pathways in self-reactive T cells. CTLA-4 signaling controls the activation of self-reactive T cells, while PD-1 signaling plays critical roles in regulating the effector functions of activated self-reactive T cells in peripheral tissues. In addition, PD-1 and B7-H1 have also been shown to be involved in fetomaternal tolerance (Guleria et al. 2005), the regulation of alloimmune responses (Sandner et al. 2005), graft-versus-host disease (Blazar et al. 2003), and autoimmune disease in multiple mouse models (Wang et al. 2005; Salama et al. 2003; Ansari et al. 2003; Matsumoto et al. 2004). These results suggest a predominant role of B7-H1 and PD-1 interactions in the establishment and/or maintenance of peripheral tolerance.

B7-H1/PD-1 interaction appears to play a critical role in regulation of exhausted virus-specific $CD8^+$ effector T cells during persistent viral infections. PD-1 is upregulated upon activation, and a functionally significant high level of expression is maintained by exhausted $CD8^+$ T cells in mice chronically infected with lymphocytic choriomeningitis virus (LCMV) (Barber et al. 2006). *In vivo* administration of antibodies that block the interaction of B7-H1 and PD-1 restores the ability of the exhausted $CD8^+$ T cells to proliferate, secrete cytokines, kill infected targets, and decrease viral load in the animals. Similarly, PD-1 is expressed at high levels on non-functional T cells during human immunodeficiency virus (HIV) infections, and anti-PD-1 or anti-B7-H1 antibodies are able to restore their proliferation and effector functions, at least *in vitro* (Day et al. 2006; Trautmann et al. 2006). Comparable findings have been observed during chronic infections with hepatitis B and C viruses (Boni et al. 2007; Urbani et al. 2006; Penna et al. 2007), Helicobacter pylori (Das et al. 2006), and Mycobacterium tuberculosis (Jurado et al. 2008). PD-1 expression was dramatically upregulated on effector $CD8^+$ T cells in acute and chronic LCMV infection, and was then rapidly downregulated after the virus is cleared in acutely infected mice. In contrast, PD-1 expression continued to increase on virus-specific $CD8^+$ T cells in chronically infected mice, and the high level of expression was sustained (Barber et al. 2006).

5 Manipulation of B7-H1/PD-1 Pathway in Tumor Immunotherapy

5.1 B7-H1/PD-1 Pathway in the Evasion of Tumor Immunity

Our early observation that multiple human tumor lines and freshly isolated cancer cells over-express B7-H1 (Dong et al. 2002) has prompted the investigation of the potential role of B7-H1/PD-1 pathway in the regulation of tumor immunity. Many human cancers have been reported to aberrantly express B7-H1 (Dong et al. 2002; Hamanishi et al. 2007). Upregulation of B7-H1 is strongly associated with local inflammatory and immune responses because IFN-γ is found to be the most potent inducer of B7-H1 (Keir et al. 2008). Retrospective studies showed a significant correlation of intra-tumor B7-H1 expression with poor prognosis in ovarian cancer (Hamanishi et al. 2007), renal cancer (Thompson et al. 2004, 2006), pancreatic cancer (Nomi et al. 2007), breast cancer (Ghebeh et al. 2006), and bladder urothelial carcinoma (Inman et al. 2007; Nakanishi et al. 2007). In addition, 41% of TILs expressed B7-H1 in breast cancer, which was associated with a large tumor size and Her2/neu–positive status (Ghebeh et al. 2006). In renal cell cancer, a high expression level of B7-H1 on both tumor cells and TILs correlated with aggressive tumor behavior and was associated with a 4.5-fold higher risk of cancer-related death than patients with low B7-H1 (Thompson et al. 2004). Interestingly, the expression level of B7-H1 on tumor cells was found to correlate inversely with numbers of ovarian intraepithelial $CD8^+$ T cells, the presence of which was associated with improved patient outcomes (Hamanishi et al. 2007). In contrast to B7-H1, expression of B7-DC in tumors was much less frequent, which is due to the fact that B7-DC is generally limited to myeloid cells.

To test whether over-expression of B7-H1 on tumor cells impaired anti-tumor immunity, murine immunogenic P815 cells were transfected to express B7-H1. B7-H1 expressing tumor cells were relatively resistant to *in vitro* cytolysis of tumor-specific CTL compared with control P815 cells (Iwai et al. 2002; Hirano et al. 2005) and resistant to immunotherapy of anti-CD137 mAb. But blockade with anti-B7-H1 restores the response to anti-CD137 treatment (Hirano et al. 2005). In a different model, the effect of over expression of B7-H1 on the murine squamous cell cancer cell line SCCVII resulted in diminished immune-mediated control that was restored upon B7-H1 blockade (Strome et al. 2003). Tumor outgrowth of the naturally B7-H1-expressing J558L myeloma cell line was controlled in syngeneic PD-$1^{-/-}$ mice and in wild type mice treated with anti-B7-H1 mAb (Iwai et al. 2002).

In addition to a direct effect by B7-H1 expressed on tumor cells, tumor-associated APCs can also utilize the B7-H1/PD-1 pathway to control antitumor T cell responses. Myeloid DCs (MDCs) generated from peripheral blood of ovarian cancer patients express high levels of B7-H1, which could be upregulated by tumor environmental factors IL-10 and vascular endothelial growth factor (VEGF) *in vitro*. T cells stimulated in the presence of autologous tumor MDCs and anti-B7-H1 mAb augmented T-cell effector function and led to improved control of the growth of human ovarian carcinomas inoculated in non-obese diabetic (NOD)/ severe combined immunodeficiency (SCID) mice (Curiel et al. 2003). Plasmacytoid DCs in the TDLN of B16 melanoma express IDO, which strongly activates the suppressive activity of regulatory T cells. The suppressive activity of IDO-treated regulatory T cells required cell contact with IDO-expressing DCs and was abrogated by B7-H1 blockade (Sharma et al. 2007).

Although the outcome of B7-H1 expression on cancer microenvironment, especially on cancer cells, remains to be determined in a prospective study, ample evidence supports that aberrant over-expression of B7-H1 on tumor cells impairs antitumor immunity – resulting in the immune evasion in cancer microenvironment. The mechanisms by which tumor-associated B7-H1 might protect tumors from T-cell-mediated immune destruction have been explored by the induction of tumor-specific T cell death (Dong et al. 2002) or by making the tumor cells resistant to T-cell-mediated destruction (Hirano et al. 2005). Like the "exhausted" viral antigen-specific T cells in chronic viral infection, the majority of TILs express high level of PD-1 compared with the T cells in normal tissues and peripheral blood lymphocytes. The overwhelming majority of CD8 T cells specific for the tumor differentiation antigen MART-1/ Melan-A (hereafter, MART-1) expressed high levels of PD-1 in tumors compared with MART-specific T cells in peripheral blood in the same patients. PD-1 expression correlated with an exhausted phenotype and impaired effector function (Ahmadzadeh et al. 2009). Two independent groups (Zhang et al. 2009; Mumprecht et al. 2009) also showed that tumor-specific CTLs express high levels of PD-1 and have impaired function in a mouse model of chronic myelogenous leukemia (CML) and acute myelogenous leukemia (AML). They confirmed not only that PD-1 expression is a marker of T-cell exhaustion, but also that B7-H1 expressed by tumor cells contributes to T-lymphocyte dysfunction. These findings suggest that the tumor microenvironment can lead to up-regulation of PD-1 on tumor-reactive T cells and contribute to impaired antitumor immune responses.

5.2 *Blocking B7-H1/PD-1 Pathway in Cancer Therapy*

With extensive data showing that the B7-H1/PD-1 pathway plays a critical role in evasion of tumor immunity, ironically, blockade of B7-H1 or PD-1 by mAb as single agent is often not very effective in treating established tumors induced by transplantable murine tumor lines. In several tumor models using highly immunogenic murine tumors, marginal to moderate therapeutic effects were observed (Nomi et al. 2007; Iwai et al. 2002, 2005; Strome et al. 2003; Webster et al. 2007). These findings, however, are not totally unexpected because blockade of B7-H1 or PD-1 is not expected to directly stimulate immune responses, but protect ongoing T cell responses to tumor antigens. In the majority of transplantable tumor models, rapid growth of transplanted tumors in syngeneic mice may not allow development of a significant T cell response against the tumor, and the majority of tumor antigen-specific T cells remain ignorant (Chen 1998). To support this notion, immunization of tumor-bearing mice with cancer vaccines (Webster et al. 2007) or other means to stimulate T cell response (Nomi et al. 2007; Hirano et al. 2005; Strome et al. 2003) together with blockade of anti-B7-H1 or anti-PD-1 mAb often gives dramatic synergistic effects. These observations highlight the importance of mechanism–based design of cancer therapeutics to maximize efficacy.

Two phase I clinical trials using anti-PD-1 antibodies have been completed for the treatment of patients with advanced malignancies. CT-011 is a humanized antibody against PD-1, and the ability of CT-011 to enhance the function of human tumor-specific T cells has been tested *in vitro* (Wong et al. 2007). Blockade of PD-1 with this mAb during *in vitro* stimulation with melanoma peptide increased the numbers and effector activity of tumor-specific human T cells. Both Th1 and Th2 cytokine production were increased. PD-1 blockade did not change the percentage of apoptotic antigen-specific human T cells, suggesting that the increase in number was due to increased proliferation, not decreased death. A phase I clinical trial in 17 patients with advanced hematologic malignancies showed that this antibody was well tolerated and has had clinical benefit in 33% of patients with one complete remission. Development of autoimmunity was not reported in this trial (Berger et al. 2008). In a phase I study of MDX-1106, a fully human mAb against PD-1, in patients with advanced solid cancer, 39 patients with colorectal cancer, melanoma, prostate cancer, non-small cell lung carcinoma and renal cell carcinoma were treated with MDX-1106 from 0.3 to 10 mg/kg. Administration of MDX-1106 was safe in general and even high doses of antibody were well tolerated. Toxicities include grade 2–3 anemia, lymphopenia, colitis, and arthritis. Clinical responses include one durable complete response (CR), two partial response (PR) and two mixed responses in 39 patients (Brahmer et al. 2008).

Experimental and clinical results indicates that manipulation of B7-H1/PD-1 pathway provides a new class of agents and represents a promising new strategy for tumor therapy that might be able to synergize with other therapeutic approaches to increase efficacy of the cancer treatments.

References

Agata Y, Kawasaki A, Nishimura H, Ishida Y, Tsubata T, Yagita H, Honjo T (1996) Expression of the PD-1 antigen on the surface of stimulated mouse T and B lymphocytes. Int Immunol 8: 765–772

Ahmadzadeh M, Johnson LA, Heemskerk B, Wunderlich JR, Dudley ME, White DE, Rosenberg SA (2009) Tumor antigen-specific CD8 T cells infiltrating the tumor express high levels of PD-1 and are functionally impaired. Blood 114:1537–1544

Alderson MR, Smith CA, Tough TW, Davis-Smith T, Armitage RJ, Falk B, Roux E, Baker E, Sutherland GR, Din WS (1994) Molecular and biological characterization of human 4-1BB and its ligand. Eur J Immunol 24:2219–2227

Ansari MJ, Salama AD, Chitnis T, Smith RN, Yagita H, Akiba H, Yamazaki T, Azuma M, Iwai H, Khoury SJ, Auchincloss H Jr, Sayegh MH (2003) The programmed death-1 (PD-1) pathway regulates autoimmune diabetes in nonobese diabetic (NOD) mice. J Exp Med 198:63–69

Azuma T, Yao S, Zhu G, Flies AS, Flies SJ, Chen L (2008) B7-H1 is a ubiquitous antiapoptotic receptor on cancer cells. Blood 111:3635–3643

Barber DL, Wherry EJ, Masopust D, Zhu B, Allison JP, Sharpe AH, Freeman GJ, Ahmed R (2006) Restoring function in exhausted CD8 T cells during chronic viral infection. Nature 439: 682–687

Berger R, Rotem-Yehudar R, Slama G, Landes S, Kneller A, Leiba M, Koren-Michowitz M, Shimoni A, Nagler A (2008) Phase I safety and pharmacokinetic study of CT-011, a humanized antibody interacting with PD-1, in patients with advanced hematologic malignancies. Clin Cancer Res 14:3044–3051

Bertram EM, Lau P, Watts TH (2002) Temporal segregation of 4-1BB versus CD28-mediated costimulation: 4-1BB ligand influences T cell numbers late in the primary response and regulates the size of the T cell memory response following influenza infection. J Immunol 168:3777–3785

Blazar BR, Carreno BM, Panoskaltsis-Mortari A, Carter L, Iwai Y, Yagita H, Nishimura H, Taylor PA (2003) Blockade of programmed death-1 engagement accelerates graft-versus-host disease lethality by an IFN-gamma-dependent mechanism. J Immunol 171:1272–1277

Bollard CM, Aguilar L, Straathof KC, Gahn B, Huls MH, Rousseau A, Sixbey J, Gresik MV, Carrum G, Hudson M, Dilloo D, Gee A, Brenner MK, Rooney CM, Heslop HE (2004) Cytotoxic T lymphocyte therapy for Epstein-Barr virus^{+} Hodgkin's disease. J Exp Med 200:1623–1633

Boni C, Fisicaro P, Valdatta C, Amadei B, Di Vincenzo P, Giuberti T, Laccabue D, Zerbini A, Cavalli A, Missale G, Bertoletti A, Ferrari C (2007) Characterization of hepatitis B virus (HBV)-specific T-cell dysfunction in chronic HBV infection. J Virol 81:4215–4225

Brahmer JR, Topalian S, Wollner I, Powderly JD, Picus J, Drake C, Covino J, Korman A, Pardoll D, Lowy I (2008) Safty and activity of MDX-1106 (ONO-4538), an anti-PD-1 monoclonal antibody, in patients with slected refractory or relapsed malignancies. J Clin Oncol 26(May 20 suppl 15S):3006

Broll K, Richter G, Pauly S, Hofstaedter F, Schwarz H (2001) CD137 expression in tumor vessel walls. High correlation with malignant tumors. Am J Clin Pathol 115:543–549

Butte MJ, Keir ME, Phamduy TB, Sharpe AH, Freeman GJ (2007) Programmed death-1 ligand 1 interacts specifically with the B7-1 costimulatory molecule to inhibit T cell responses. Immunity 27:111–122

Butte MJ, Pena-Cruz V, Kim MJ, Freeman GJ, Sharpe AH (2008) Interaction of human PD-L1 and B7-1. Mol Immunol 45:3567–3572

Carreno BM, Collins M (2002) The B7 family of ligands and its receptors: new pathways for costimulation and inhibition of immune responses. Annu Rev Immunol 20:29–53

Chen L (1998) Immunological ignorance of silent antigens as an explanation of tumor evasion. Immunol Today 19:27–30

Chen L (2004) Co-inhibitory molecules of the B7-CD28 family in the control of T-cell immunity. Nat Rev 4:336–347

Chen L, McGowan P, Ashe S, Johnston J, Li Y, Hellstrom I, Hellstrom KE (1994) Tumor immunogenicity determines the effect of B7 costimulation on T cell-mediated tumor immunity. J Exp Med 179:523–532

Curiel TJ, Wei S, Dong H, Alvarez X, Cheng P, Mottram P, Krzysiek R, Knutson KL, Daniel B, Zimmermann MC, David O, Burow M, Gordon A, Dhurandhar N, Myers L, Berggren R, Hemminki A, Alvarez RD, Emilie D, Curiel DT, Chen L, Zou W (2003) Blockade of B7-H1 improves myeloid dendritic cell-mediated antitumor immunity. Nat Med 9:562–567

Das S, Suarez G, Beswick EJ, Sierra JC, Graham DY, Reyes VE (2006) Expression of B7-H1 on gastric epithelial cells: its potential role in regulating T cells during Helicobacter pylori infection. J Immunol 176:3000–3009

Day CL, Kaufmann DE, Kiepiela P, Brown JA, Moodley ES, Reddy S, Mackey EW, Miller JD, Leslie AJ, DePierres C, Mncube Z, Duraiswamy J, Zhu B, Eichbaum Q, Altfeld M, Wherry EJ, Coovadia HM, Goulder PJ, Klenerman P, Ahmed R, Freeman GJ, Walker BD (2006) PD-1 expression on HIV-specific T cells is associated with T-cell exhaustion and disease progression. Nature 443:350–354

DeBenedette MA, Shahinian A, Mak TW, Watts TH (1997) Costimulation of CD28- T lymphocytes by 4-1BB ligand. J Immunol 158:551–559

Deeths MJ, Kedl RM, Mescher MF (1999) $CD8^+$ T cells become nonresponsive (anergic) following activation in the presence of costimulation. J Immunol 163:102–110

Dong H, Zhu G, Tamada K, Chen L (1999) B7-H1, a third member of the B7 family, co-stimulates T-cell proliferation and interleukin-10 secretion. Nat Med 5:1365–1369

Dong H, Strome SE, Salomao DR, Tamura H, Hirano F, Flies DB, Roche PC, Lu J, Zhu G, Tamada K, Lennon VA, Celis E, Chen L (2002) Tumor-associated B7-H1 promotes T-cell apoptosis: a potential mechanism of immune evasion. Nat Med 8:793–800

Dong H, Zhu G, Tamada K, Flies DB, van Deursen JM, Chen L (2004) B7-H1 determines accumulation and deletion of intrahepatic $CD8(^+)$ T lymphocytes. Immunity 20:327–336

Dudley ME, Wunderlich JR, Robbins PF, Yang JC, Hwu P, Schwartzentruber DJ, Topalian SL, Sherry R, Restifo NP, Hubicki AM, Robinson MR, Raffeld M, Duray P, Seipp CA, Rogers-Freezer L, Morton KE, Mavroukakis SA, White DE, Rosenberg SA (2002) Cancer regression and autoimmunity in patients after clonal repopulation with antitumor lymphocytes. Science 298:850–854

Freeman GJ, Long AJ, Iwai Y, Bourque K, Chernova T, Nishimura H, Fitz LJ, Malenkovich N, Okazaki T, Byrne MC, Horton HF, Fouser L, Carter L, Ling V, Bowman MR, Carreno BM, Collins M, Wood CR, Honjo T (2000) Engagement of the PD-1 immunoinhibitory receptor by a novel B7 family member leads to negative regulation of lymphocyte activation. J Exp Med 192:1027–1034

Futagawa T, Akiba H, Kodama T, Takeda K, Hosoda Y, Yagita H, Okumura K (2002) Expression and function of 4-1BB and 4-1BB ligand on murine dendritic cells. Int Immunol 14:275–286

Ghebeh H, Mohammed S, Al-Omair A, Qattan A, Lehe C, Al-Qudaihi G, Elkum N, Alshabanah M, Bin Amer S, Tulbah A, Ajarim D, Al-Tweigeri T, Dermime S (2006) The B7-H1 (PD-L1) T lymphocyte-inhibitory molecule is expressed in breast cancer patients with infiltrating ductal carcinoma: correlation with important high-risk prognostic factors. Neoplasia 8:190–198

Guinn BA, DeBenedette MA, Watts TH, Berinstein NL (1999) 4-1BBL cooperates with B7-1 and B7-2 in converting a B cell lymphoma cell line into a long-lasting antitumor vaccine. J Immunol 162:5003–5010

Guleria I, Khosroshahi A, Ansari MJ, Habicht A, Azuma M, Yagita H, Noelle RJ, Coyle A, Mellor AL, Khoury SJ, Sayegh MH (2005) A critical role for the programmed death ligand 1 in fetomaternal tolerance. J Exp Med 202:231–237

Hamanishi J, Mandai M, Iwasaki M, Okazaki T, Tanaka Y, Yamaguchi K, Higuchi T, Yagi H, Takakura K, Minato N, Honjo T, Fujii S (2007) Programmed cell death 1 ligand 1 and tumor-infiltrating $CD8^+$ T lymphocytes are prognostic factors of human ovarian cancer. Proc Natl Acad Sci U S A 104:3360–3365

Harding FA, McArthur JG, Gross JA, Raulet DH, Allison JP (1992) CD28-mediated signalling co-stimulates murine T cells and prevents induction of anergy in T-cell clones. Nature 356: 607–609

Hirano F, Kaneko K, Tamura H, Dong H, Wang S, Ichikawa M, Rietz C, Flies DB, Lau JS, Zhu G, Tamada K, Chen L (2005) Blockade of B7-H1 and PD-1 by monoclonal antibodies potentiates cancer therapeutic immunity. Cancer Res 65:1089–1096

Hurtado JC, Kim YJ, Kwon BS (1997) Signals through 4-1BB are costimulatory to previously activated splenic T cells and inhibit activation-induced cell death. J Immunol 158:2600–2609

Inman BA, Sebo TJ, Frigola X, Dong H, Bergstralh EJ, Frank I, Fradet Y, Lacombe L, Kwon ED (2007) PD-L1 (B7-H1) expression by urothelial carcinoma of the bladder and BCG-induced granulomata: associations with localized stage progression. Cancer 109:1499–1505

Ishida Y, Agata Y, Shibahara K, Honjo T (1992) Induced expression of PD-1, a novel member of the immunoglobulin gene superfamily, upon programmed cell death. EMBO J 11:3887–3895

Ito F, Li Q, Shreiner AB, Okuyama R, Jure-Kunkel MN, Teitz-Tennenbaum S, Chang AE (2004) Anti-CD137 monoclonal antibody administration augments the antitumor efficacy of dendritic cell-based vaccines. Cancer Res 64:8411–8419

Iwai Y, Ishida M, Tanaka Y, Okazaki T, Honjo T, Minato N (2002) Involvement of PD-L1 on tumor cells in the escape from host immune system and tumor immunotherapy by PD-L1 blockade. Proc Natl Acad Sci U S A 99:12293–12297

Iwai Y, Terawaki S, Honjo T (2005) PD-1 blockade inhibits hematogenous spread of poorly immunogenic tumor cells by enhanced recruitment of effector T cells. Int Immunol 17: 133–144

Jiang D, Chen Y, Schwarz H (2008) CD137 induces proliferation of murine hematopoietic progenitor cells and differentiation to macrophages. J Immunol 181:3923–3932

Jurado JO, Alvarez IB, Pasquinelli V, Martinez GJ, Quiroga MF, Abbate E, Musella RM, Chuluyan HE, Garcia VE (2008) Programmed death (PD)-1:PD-ligand 1/PD-ligand 2 pathway inhibits T cell effector functions during human tuberculosis. J Immunol 181:116–125

Kawai K, Saijo K, Oikawa T, Morishita Y, Noguchi M, Ohno T, Akaza H (2003) Clinical course and immune response of a renal cell carcinoma patient to adoptive transfer of autologous cytotoxic T lymphocytes. Clin Exp Immunol 134:264–269

Keir ME, Butte MJ, Freeman GJ, Sharpe AH (2008) PD-1 and its ligands in tolerance and immunity. Annu Rev Immunol 26:677–704

Kim JA, Averbook BJ, Chambers K, Rothchild K, Kjaergaard J, Papay R, Shu S (2001) Divergent effects of 4-1BB antibodies on antitumor immunity and on tumor-reactive T-cell generation. Cancer Res 61:2031–2037

Kinter AL, Godbout EJ, McNally JP, Sereti I, Roby GA, O'Shea MA, Fauci AS (2008) The common gamma-chain cytokines IL-2, IL-7, IL-15, and IL-21 induce the expression of programmed death-1 and its ligands. J Immunol 181:6738–6746

Latchman Y, Wood CR, Chernova T, Chaudhary D, Borde M, Chernova I, Iwai Y, Long AJ, Brown JA, Nunes R, Greenfield EA, Bourque K, Boussiotis VA, Carter LL, Carreno BM, Malenkovich N, Nishimura H, Okazaki T, Honjo T, Sharpe AH, Freeman GJ (2001) PD-L2 is a second ligand for PD-1 and inhibits T cell activation. Nat Immunol 2:261–268

Laux I, Khoshnan A, Tindell C, Bae D, Zhu X, June CH, Effros RB, Nel A (2000) Response differences between human CD4($^{+}$) and CD8($^{+}$) T-cells during CD28 costimulation: implications for immune cell-based therapies and studies related to the expansion of double-positive T-cells during aging. Clin Immunol 96:187–197

Lee PP, Yee C, Savage PA, Fong L, Brockstedt D, Weber JS, Johnson D, Swetter S, Thompson J, Greenberg PD, Roederer M, Davis MM (1999) Characterization of circulating T cells specific for tumor-associated antigens in melanoma patients. Nat Med 5:677–685

Lee SW, Park Y, So T, Kwon BS, Cheroutre H, Mittler RS, Croft M (2008) Identification of regulatory functions for 4-1BB and 4-1BBL in myelopoiesis and the development of dendritic cells. Nat Immunol 9:917–926

Lenschow DJ, Walunas TL, Bluestone JA (1996) CD28/B7 system of T cell costimulation. Annu Rev Immunol 14:233–258

Li Q, Carr A, Ito F, Teitz-Tennenbaum S, Chang AE (2003) Polarization effects of 4-1BB during CD28 costimulation in generating tumor-reactive T cells for cancer immunotherapy. Cancer Res 63:2546–2552

Li B, Lin J, Vanroey M, Jure-Kunkel M, Jooss K (2007) Established B16 tumors are rejected following treatment with GM-CSF-secreting tumor cell immunotherapy in combination with anti-4-1BB mAb. Clin Immunol 125:76–87

Lin GH, Sedgmen BJ, Moraes TJ, Snell LM, Topham DJ, Watts TH (2009) Endogenous 4-1BB ligand plays a critical role in protection from influenza-induced disease. J Immunol 182: 934–947

Lynch DH (2008) The promise of 4-1BB (CD137)-mediated immunomodulation and the immunotherapy of cancer. Immunol Rev 222:277–286

Mack DG, Lanham AK, Palmer BE, Maier LA, Watts TH, Fontenot AP (2008) 4-1BB enhances proliferation of beryllium-specific T cells in the lung of subjects with chronic beryllium disease. J Immunol 181:4381–4388

Manjunath N, Shankar P, Wan J, Weninger W, Crowley MA, Hieshima K, Springer TA, Fan X, Shen H, Lieberman J, von Andrian UH (2001) Effector differentiation is not prerequisite for generation of memory cytotoxic T lymphocytes. J Clin Invest 108:871–878

Martinet O, Ermekova V, Qiao JQ, Sauter B, Mandeli J, Chen L, Chen SH (2000) Immunomodulatory gene therapy with interleukin 12 and 4-1BB ligand: long- term remission of liver metastases in a mouse model. J Natl Cancer Inst 92:931–936

Matsumoto K, Inoue H, Nakano T, Tsuda M, Yoshiura Y, Fukuyama S, Tsushima F, Hoshino T, Aizawa H, Akiba H, Pardoll D, Hara N, Yagita H, Azuma M, Nakanishi Y (2004) B7-DC regulates asthmatic response by an IFN-gamma-dependent mechanism. J Immunol 172: 2530–2541

Maus MV, Thomas AK, Leonard DG, Allman D, Addya K, Schlienger K, Riley JL, June CH (2002) Ex vivo expansion of polyclonal and antigen-specific cytotoxic T lymphocytes by artificial APCs expressing ligands for the T-cell receptor, CD28 and 4-1BB. Nat Biotechnol 20:143–148

May KF Jr, Chen L, Zheng P, Liu Y (2002) Anti-4-1BB monoclonal antibody enhances rejection of large tumor burden by promoting survival but not clonal expansion of tumor-specific CD8^{+} T cells. Cancer Res 62:3459–3465

McMillin DW, Hewes B, Gangadharan B, Archer DR, Mittler RS, Spencer HT (2006) Complete regression of large solid tumors using engineered drug-resistant hematopoietic cells and anti-CD137 immunotherapy. Hum Gene Ther 17:798–806

Melero I, Shuford WW, Newby SA, Aruffo A, Ledbetter JA, Hellstrom KE, Mittler RS, Chen L (1997) Monoclonal antibodies against the 4-1BB T-cell activation molecule eradicate established tumors. Nat Med 3:682–685

Melero I, Johnston JV, Shufford WW, Mittler RS, Chen L (1998a) NK1.1 cells express 4-1BB (CDw137) costimulatory molecule and are required for tumor immunity elicited by anti-4-1BB monoclonal antibodies. Cell Immunol 190:167–172

Melero I, Bach N, Hellstrom KE, Aruffo A, Mittler RS, Chen L (1998b) Amplification of tumor immunity by gene transfer of the co-stimulatory 4-1BB ligand: synergy with the CD28 co-stimulatory pathway. Eur J Immunol 28:1116–1121

Miller RE, Jones J, Le T, Whitmore J, Boiani N, Gliniak B, Lynch DH (2002) 4-1BB-specific monoclonal antibody promotes the generation of tumor-specific immune responses by direct activation of CD8 T cells in a CD40-dependent manner. J Immunol 169:1792–1800

Morgan RA, Dudley ME, Wunderlich JR, Hughes MS, Yang JC, Sherry RM, Royal RE, Topalian SL, Kammula US, Restifo NP, Zheng Z, Nahvi A, de Vries CR, Rogers-Freezer LJ, Mavroukakis SA, Rosenberg SA (2006) Cancer regression in patients after transfer of genetically engineered lymphocytes. Science 314:126–129

Mumprecht S, Schurch C, Schwaller J, Solenthaler M, Ochsenbein AF (2009) Programmed death 1 signaling on chronic myeloid leukemia-specific T cells results in T-cell exhaustion and disease progression. Blood 114:1528–1536

Nakanishi J, Wada Y, Matsumoto K, Azuma M, Kikuchi K, Ueda S (2007) Overexpression of B7-H1 (PD-L1) significantly associates with tumor grade and postoperative prognosis in human urothelial cancers. Cancer Immunol Immunother 56:1173–1182

Nishimura H, Nose M, Hiai H, Minato N, Honjo T (1999) Development of lupus-like autoimmune diseases by disruption of the PD-1 gene encoding an ITIM motif-carrying immunoreceptor. Immunity 11:141–151

Nishimura H, Okazaki T, Tanaka Y, Nakatani K, Hara M, Matsumori A, Sasayama S, Mizoguchi A, Hiai H, Minato N, Honjo T (2001) Autoimmune dilated cardiomyopathy in PD-1 receptor-deficient mice. Science 291:319–322

Nomi T, Sho M, Akahori T, Hamada K, Kubo A, Kanehiro H, Nakamura S, Enomoto K, Yagita H, Azuma M, Nakajima Y (2007) Clinical significance and therapeutic potential of the programmed death-1 ligand/programmed death-1 pathway in human pancreatic cancer. Clin Cancer Res 13:2151–2157

Okazaki T, Honjo T (2006) The PD-1-PD-L pathway in immunological tolerance. Trends Immunol 27:195–201

Okazaki T, Tanaka Y, Nishio R, Mitsuiye T, Mizoguchi A, Wang J, Ishida M, Hiai H, Matsumori A, Minato N, Honjo T (2003) Autoantibodies against cardiac troponin I are responsible for dilated cardiomyopathy in PD-1-deficient mice. Nat Med 9:1477–1483

Pardoll D (2003) Does the immune system see tumors as foreign or self? Annu Rev Immunol 21:807–839

Penna A, Pilli M, Zerbini A, Orlandini A, Mezzadri S, Sacchelli L, Missale G, Ferrari C (2007) Dysfunction and functional restoration of HCV-specific CD8 responses in chronic hepatitis C virus infection. Hepatology 45:588–601

Pollok KE, Kim YJ, Zhou Z, Hurtado J, Kim KK, Pickard RT, Kwon BS (1993) Inducible T cell antigen 4-1BB. Analysis of expression and function. J Immunol 150:771–781

Pollok KE, Kim YJ, Hurtado J, Zhou Z, Kim KK, Kwon BS (1994) 4-1BB T-cell antigen binds to mature B cells and macrophages, and costimulates anti-mu-primed splenic B cells. Eur J Immunol 24:367–374

Pulle G, Vidric M, Watts TH (2006) IL-15-dependent induction of 4-1BB promotes antigen-independent CD8 memory T cell survival. J Immunol 176:2739–2748

Radoja S, Saio M, Frey AB (2001) $CD8^+$ tumor-infiltrating lymphocytes are primed for Fas-mediated activation-induced cell death but are not apoptotic in situ. J Immunol 166:6074–6083

Raimondi G, Shufesky WJ, Tokita D, Morelli AE, Thomson AW (2006) Regulated compartmentalization of programmed cell death-1 discriminates $CD4^+CD25^+$ resting regulatory T cells from activated T cells. J Immunol 176:2808–2816

Sabbagh L, Snell LM, Watts TH (2007) TNF family ligands define niches for T cell memory. Trends Immunol 28:333–339

Sabbagh L, Pulle G, Liu Y, Tsitsikov EN, Watts TH (2008) ERK-dependent Bim modulation downstream of the 4-1BB-TRAF1 signaling axis is a critical mediator of CD8 T cell survival *in vivo*. J Immunol 180:8093–8101

Salama AD, Chitnis T, Imitola J, Ansari MJ, Akiba H, Tushima F, Azuma M, Yagita H, Sayegh MH, Khoury SJ (2003) Critical role of the programmed death-1 (PD-1) pathway in regulation of experimental autoimmune encephalomyelitis. J Exp Med 198:71–78

Sandner SE, Clarkson MR, Salama AD, Sanchez-Fueyo A, Domenig C, Habicht A, Najafian N, Yagita H, Azuma M, Turka LA, Sayegh MH (2005) Role of the programmed death-1 pathway in regulation of alloimmune responses *in vivo*. J Immunol 174:3408–3415

Schwartz RH (2003) T cell anergy. Annu Rev Immunol 21:305–334

Schwarz H, Valbracht J, Tuckwell J, von Kempis J, Lotz M (1995) ILA, the human 4-1BB homologue, is inducible in lymphoid and other cell lineages. Blood 85:1043–1052

Seo SK, Park HY, Choi JH, Kim WY, Kim YH, Jung HW, Kwon B, Lee HW, Kwon BS (2003) Blocking 4-1BB/4-1BB ligand interactions prevents herpetic stromal keratitis. J Immunol 171:576–583

Seo SK, Choi JH, Kim YH, Kang WJ, Park HY, Suh JH, Choi BK, Vinay DS, Kwon BS (2004) 4-1BB-mediated immunotherapy of rheumatoid arthritis. Nat Med 10:1088–1094

Serghides L, Bukczynski J, Wen T, Wang C, Routy JP, Boulassel MR, Sekaly RP, Ostrowski M, Bernard NF, Watts TH (2005) Evaluation of OX40 ligand as a costimulator of human antiviral memory CD8 T cell responses: comparison with B7.1 and 4-1BBL. J Immunol 175:6368–6377

Sharma MD, Baban B, Chandler P, Hou DY, Singh N, Yagita H, Azuma M, Blazar BR, Mellor AL, Munn DH (2007) Plasmacytoid dendritic cells from mouse tumor-draining lymph nodes directly activate mature Tregs via indoleamine 2, 3-dioxygenase. J Clin Invest 117:2570–2582

Sharpe AH, Freeman GJ (2002) The B7-CD28 superfamily. Nat Rev 2:116–126

Shi W, Siemann DW (2006) Augmented antitumor effects of radiation therapy by 4-1BB antibody (BMS-469492) treatment. Anticancer Res 26:3445–3453

Shin T, Kennedy G, Gorski K, Tsuchiya H, Koseki H, Azuma M, Yagita H, Chen L, Powell J, Pardoll D, Housseau F (2003) Cooperative B7-1/2 (CD80/CD86) and B7-DC costimulation of $CD4^+$ T cells independent of the PD-1 receptor. J Exp Med 198:31–38

Shuford WW, Klussman K, Tritchler DD, Loo DT, Chalupny J, Siadak AW, Brown TJ, Emswiler J, Raecho H, Larsen CP, Pearson TC, Ledbetter JA, Aruffo A, Mittler RS (1997) 4-1BB costimulatory signals preferentially induce $CD8^+$ T cell proliferation and lead to the amplification *in vivo* of cytotoxic T cell responses. J Exp Med 186:47–55

Stephan MT, Ponomarev V, Brentjens RJ, Chang AH, Dobrenkov KV, Heller G, Sadelain M (2007) T cell-encoded CD80 and 4-1BBL induce auto- and transcostimulation, resulting in potent tumor rejection. Nat Med 13:1440–1449

Straathof KC, Bollard CM, Popat U, Huls MH, Lopez T, Morriss MC, Gresik MV, Gee AP, Russell HV, Brenner MK, Rooney CM, Heslop HE (2005) Treatment of nasopharyngeal carcinoma with Epstein-Barr virus–specific T lymphocytes. Blood 105:1898–1904

Strome SE, Martin B, Flies D, Tamada K, Chapoval AI, Sargent DJ, Shu S, Chen L (2000) Enhanced therapeutic potential of adoptive immunotherapy by *in vitro* CD28/4-1BB costimulation of tumor-reactive T cells against a poorly immunogenic, major histocompatibility complex class I-negative A9P melanoma. J Immunother 23:430–437

Strome SE, Dong H, Tamura H, Voss SG, Flies DB, Tamada K, Salomao D, Cheville J, Hirano F, Lin W, Kasperbauer JL, Ballman KV, Chen L (2003) B7-H1 blockade augments adoptive T-cell immunotherapy for squamous cell carcinoma. Cancer Res 63:6501–6505

Sun Y, Lin X, Chen HM, Wu Q, Subudhi SK, Chen L, Fu YX (2002a) Administration of agonistic anti-4-1BB monoclonal antibody leads to the amelioration of experimental autoimmune encephalomyelitis. J Immunol 168:1457–1465

Sun Y, Chen HM, Subudhi SK, Chen J, Koka R, Chen L, Fu YX (2002b) Costimulatory molecule-targeted antibody therapy of a spontaneous autoimmune disease. Nat Med 8:1405–1413

Takahashi C, Mittler RS, Vella AT (1999) Cutting edge: 4-1BB is a bona fide CD8 T cell survival signal. J Immunol 162:5037–5040

Tamura H, Dong H, Zhu G, Sica GL, Flies DB, Tamada K, Chen L (2001) B7-H1 costimulation preferentially enhances CD28-independent T-helper cell function. Blood 97:1809–1816

Tan JT, Ha J, Cho HR, Tucker-Burden C, Hendrix RC, Mittler RS, Pearson TC, Larsen CP (2000) Analysis of expression and function of the costimulatory molecule 4-1BB in alloimmune responses. Transplantation 70:175–183

Thompson RH, Gillett MD, Cheville JC, Lohse CM, Dong H, Webster WS, Krejci KG, Lobo JR, Sengupta S, Chen L, Zincke H, Blute ML, Strome SE, Leibovich BC, Kwon ED (2004) Costimulatory B7-H1 in renal cell carcinoma patients: Indicator of tumor aggressiveness and potential therapeutic target. Proc Natl Acad Sci USA 101:17174–17179

Thompson RH, Kuntz SM, Leibovich BC, Dong H, Lohse CM, Webster WS, Sengupta S, Frank I, Parker AS, Zincke H, Blute ML, Sebo TJ, Cheville JC, Kwon ED (2006) Tumor B7-H1 is associated with poor prognosis in renal cell carcinoma patients with long-term follow-up. Cancer Res 66:3381–3385

Tivol EA, Borriello F, Schweitzer AN, Lynch WP, Bluestone JA, Sharpe AH (1995) Loss of CTLA-4 leads to massive lymphoproliferation and fatal multiorgan tissue destruction, revealing a critical negative regulatory role of CTLA-4. Immunity 3:541–547

Trautmann L, Janbazian L, Chomont N, Said EA, Gimmig S, Bessette B, Boulassel MR, Delwart E, Sepulveda H, Balderas RS, Routy JP, Haddad EK, Sekaly RP (2006) Upregulation of PD-1 expression on HIV-specific $CD8^+$ T cells leads to reversible immune dysfunction. Nat Med 12:1198–1202

Tseng SY, Otsuji M, Gorski K, Huang X, Slansky JE, Pai SI, Shalabi A, Shin T, Pardoll DM, Tsuchiya H (2001) B7-DC, a new dendritic cell molecule with potent costimulatory properties for T cells. J Exp Med 193:839–846

Tsuboi K, Saijo K, Ishikawa E, Tsurushima H, Takano S, Morishita Y, Ohno T (2003) Effects of local injection of ex vivo expanded autologous tumor-specific T lymphocytes in cases with recurrent malignant gliomas. Clin Cancer Res 9:3294–3302

Uno T, Takeda K, Kojima Y, Yoshizawa H, Akiba H, Mittler RS, Gejyo F, Okumura K, Yagita H, Smyth MJ (2006) Eradication of established tumors in mice by a combination antibody-based therapy. Nat Med 12:693–698

Urbani S, Amadei B, Tola D, Massari M, Schivazappa S, Missale G, Ferrari C (2006) PD-1 expression in acute hepatitis C virus (HCV) infection is associated with HCV-specific CD8 exhaustion. J Virol 80:11398–11403

Vinay DS, Cha K, Kwon BS (2006) Dual immunoregulatory pathways of 4-1BB signaling. J Mol Med 84:726–736

Wang S, Chen L (2004) Co-signaling molecules of the B7-CD28 family in positive and negative regulation of T lymphocyte responses. Microbes Infect 6:759–766

Wang J, Guo Z, Dong Y, Kim O, Hart J, Adams A, Larsen CP, Mittler RS, Newell KA (2003a) Role of 4-1BB in allograft rejection mediated by $CD8^+$ T cells. Am J Transplant 3:543–551

Wang S, Bajorath J, Flies DB, Dong H, Honjo T, Chen L (2003b) Molecular modeling and functional mapping of B7-H1 and B7-DC uncouple costimulatory function from PD-1 interaction. J Exp Med 197:1083–1091

Wang J, Yoshida T, Nakaki F, Hiai H, Okazaki T, Honjo T (2005) Establishment of NOD-Pdcd1-/- mice as an efficient animal model of type I diabetes. Proc Natl Acad Sci U S A 102: 11823–11828

Waterhouse P, Penninger JM, Timms E, Wakeham A, Shahinian A, Lee KP, Thompson CB, Griesser H, Mak TW (1995) Lymphoproliferative disorders with early lethality in mice deficient in Ctla-4. Science 270:985–988

Webster WS, Thompson RH, Harris KJ, Frigola X, Kuntz S, Inman BA, Dong H (2007) Targeting molecular and cellular inhibitory mechanisms for improvement of antitumor memory responses reactivated by tumor cell vaccine. J Immunol 179:2860–2869

Wen T, Bukczynski J, Watts TH (2002) 4-1BB ligand-mediated costimulation of human T cells induces CD4 and CD8 T cell expansion, cytokine production, and the development of cytolytic effector function. J Immunol 168:4897–4906

Wilcox RA, Chapoval AI, Gorski KS, Otsuji M, Shin T, Flies DB, Tamada K, Mittler RS, Tsuchiya H, Pardoll DM, Chen L (2002) Cutting edge: Expression of functional CD137 receptor by dendritic cells. J Immunol 168:4262–4267

Wong RM, Scotland RR, Lau RL, Wang C, Korman AJ, Kast WM, Weber JS (2007) Programmed death-1 blockade enhances expansion and functional capacity of human melanoma antigen-specific CTLs. Int Immunol 19:1223–1234

Xu DP, Sauter BV, Huang TG, Meseck M, Woo SL, Chen SH (2005) The systemic administration of Ig-4-1BB ligand in combination with IL-12 gene transfer eradicates hepatic colon carcinoma. Gene Ther 12:1526–1533

Ye Z, Hellstrom I, Hayden-Ledbetter M, Dahlin A, Ledbetter JA, Hellstrom KE (2002) Gene therapy for cancer using single-chain Fv fragments specific for 4-1BB. Nat Med 8:343–348

Yee C, Thompson JA, Byrd D, Riddell SR, Roche P, Celis E, Greenberg PD (2002) Adoptive T cell therapy using antigen-specific $CD8^+$ T cell clones for the treatment of patients with metastatic melanoma: *in vivo* persistence, migration, and antitumor effect of transferred T cells. Proc Natl Acad Sci USA 99:16168–16173

Yi KH, Nechushtan H, Bowers WJ, Walker GR, Zhang Y, Pham DG, Podack ER, Federoff HJ, Tolba KA, Rosenblatt JD (2007) Adoptively transferred tumor-specific T cells stimulated ex vivo using herpes simplex virus amplicons encoding 4-1BBL persist in the host and show antitumor activity *in vivo*. Cancer Res 67:10027–10037

Zhang H, Snyder KM, Suhoski MM, Maus MV, Kapoor V, June CH, Mackall CL (2007) 4-1BB is superior to CD28 costimulation for generating $CD8^+$ cytotoxic lymphocytes for adoptive immunotherapy. J Immunol 179:4910–4918

Zhang L, Gajewski TF, Kline J (2009) PD-1/PD-L1 interactions inhibit antitumor immune responses in a murine acute myeloid leukemia model. Blood 114:1545–1552

Zhu Y, Zhu G, Luo L, Flies AS, Chen L (2007) CD137 stimulation delivers an antigen-independent growth signal for T lymphocytes with memory phenotype. Blood 109:4882–4889

LAG-3 in Cancer Immunotherapy

Monica V. Goldberg and Charles G. Drake

Contents

1 Structural Aspects of LAG-3 ... 270
1.1 Basic Structure ... 270
1.2 LAG-3 Expression ... 270
1.3 Binding of Class II MHC ... 271
1.4 Localization of LAG-3 in T Cells ... 272
2 LAG-3 Function ... 272
2.1 Role in CD4 T Cell Function and Expansion ... 272
2.2 Role of LAG-3 on Regulatory T Cells ... 273
2.3 Role of LAG-3 on CD8 T Cells ... 273
2.4 LAG-3 Mechanism of Action ... 274
3 LAG-3 in Cancer Immunotherapy ... 275
3.1 Preclinical Studies ... 275
3.2 Clinical Studies ... 275
4 Conclusions ... 276
References ... 277

Abstract LAG-3 (CD223) is a cell surface molecule expressed on activated T cells (Huard et al. Immunogenetics 39:213–217, 1994), NK cells (Triebel et al. J Exp Med 171:1393–1405, 1990), B cells (Kisielow et al. Eur J Immunol 35:2081–2088, 2005), and plasmacytoid dendritic cells (Workman et al. J Immunol 182:1885–1891, 2009) that plays an important but incompletely understood role in the function of these lymphocyte subsets. In addition, the interaction between LAG-3 and its major ligand, Class II MHC, is thought to play a role in modulating dendritic

M.V. Goldberg
Johns Hopkins Kimmel Cancer Center, 1650 Orleans Street – CRB 423, Baltimore, MD 21231, USA

C.G. Drake (✉)
Johns Hopkins Kimmel Cancer Center, 1650 Orleans Street – CRB 410, Baltimore, MD 21231, USA
e-mail: cdrake@jhmi.edu

G. Dranoff (ed.), *Cancer Immunology and Immunotherapy*,
Current Topics in Microbiology and Immunology 344, DOI 10.1007/82_2010_114

cell function (Andreae et al. J Immunol 168:3874–3880, 2002). Recent preclinical studies have documented a role for LAG-3 in CD8 T cell exhaustion (Blackburn et al. Nat Immunol 10:29–37, 2009), and blockade of the LAG-3/Class II interaction using a LAG-3 Ig fusion protein is being evaluated in a number of clinical trials in cancer patients. In this review, we will first discuss the basic structural and functional biology of LAG-3, followed by a review of preclinical and clinical data pertinent to a role for LAG-3 in cancer immunotherapy.

Keywords Anergy · CD4 lymphocyte · CD8 lymphocyte · Checkpoint · Tolerance · Treg · Tumor immunology · LAG-3

1 Structural Aspects of LAG-3

LAG-3 was initially discovered in an experiment designed to selectively isolate molecules expressed in an IL-2-dependent NK cell line (Triebel et al. 1990). A unique, 489-amino acid membrane protein was found, and further analyses showed that the coding region for this protein was located on the distal portion of the short arm of human chromosome 12, adjacent to the coding region for CD4. Analysis of the amino acid sequence of LAG-3 revealed an Ig superfamily member, with four IgG loops, similar to that of CD4, and subsequent studies have been, to a large part, guided by this homology.

1.1 Basic Structure

The structure of LAG-3 is shown in Fig. 1. As above, both LAG-3 and CD4 molecules include four IgG domains. Although this structural homology is high, at the amino acid level LAG-3 is less than 20% homologous to CD4, indicating that the two genes likely diverged early in evolution (Dijkstra et al. 2006). The membrane-distal D1 domain of LAG-3 contains a unique "extra loop," to which antibodies have been raised (Baixeras et al. 1992), and which is not present on any CD4 molecules thus sequenced. As will be discussed below, LAG-3 has been demonstrated to bind to Class II MHC primarily through a small set of amino acids localized to the D1 domain (Huard et al. 1997) – this is in sharp contrast to CD4 which interacts with Class II MHC through a fairly large surface involving multiple residues (Fleury et al. 1991; Moebius et al. 1993). In addition, the intracellular portion of LAG-3 is relatively short, containing a unique motif (KIEELE) that is required for LAG-3 modulation of T cell function (Workman and Vignali 2003).

1.2 LAG-3 Expression

LAG-3 is in many ways a T cell activation marker, expressed on both CD4 and CD8 T cells 3–4 days post activation (Huard et al. 1994). It is also expressed on natural

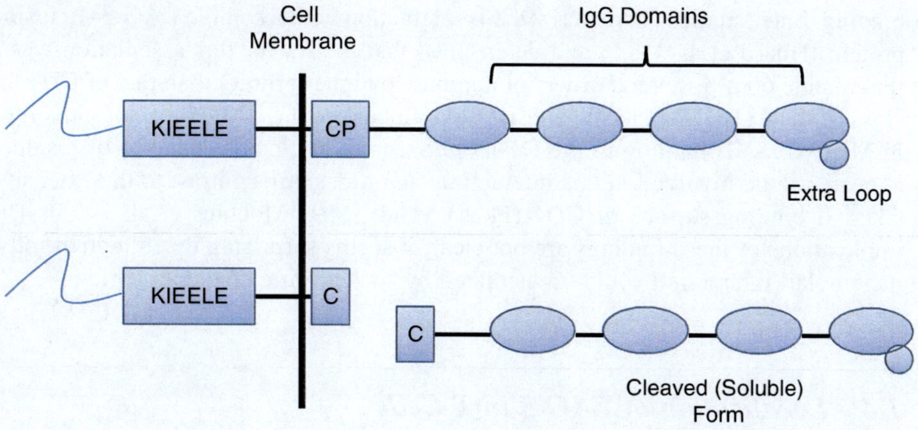

Fig. 1 LAG-3 structure: LAG-3 is a transmembrane protein with structural homology to CD4, in which it includes four extracellular IgG domains. The membrane-distal IgG domain contains a short amino acid sequence, the so-called extra loop that is not found in other IgG superfamily proteins. The intracellular domain contains a unique amino acid sequence (KIEELE) that is required for LAG-3 to exert a negative effect on T cell function. LAG-3 can be cleaved at the connecting peptide (CP) by metalloproteases to generate a soluble form, which is detectable in serum

killer (NK) cells, although its function on that cell type is of uncertain significance (Huard et al. 1998). One study suggests expression on activated B cells, although those data have not been widely replicated (Kisielow et al. 2005). Finally, LAG-3 mRNA can also be found in the thymic medulla, the splenic red pulp, and the base of the cerebellum (Workman et al. 2002). When T cells are activated, LAG-3 expression is first detectable approximately 24 h post activation, peaking around day 2 and then gradually declining by day 8. Early studies on LAG-3 suggested that its expression might serve to distinguish T_H1 from T_H2 CD4 T cells (Annunziato et al. 1996); i.e., IL-12 potently stimulated LAG-3 expression, and blockade of IFN-γ decreased LAG-3 expression (Annunziato et al. 1997). More recently, these findings have been called into question, with one study showing that LAG-3 expression might not reliably distinguish T_H1 from T_H2 cells, at least in humans (Rogala et al. 2002).

1.3 Binding of Class II MHC

Based on the structural (but not amino acid) homology between LAG-3 and CD4, early studies were performed to determine whether LAG-3 might interact with Class II MHC. COS-7 cells were transfected with human LAG-3 and shown to rosette human B cell tumors (Baixeras et al. 1992). This interaction could be blocked via antibodies to either LAG-3 or HLA-DR, indicating the specificity of binding. Later studies characterized this interaction with a soluble LAG-3–Ig fusion protein (Huard et al. 1995) and determined that the K_d for this association was a remarkable 60 nM, several orders of magnitude higher affinity than that of CD4 for class II MHC (10^{-4} M). Mutagenesis studies localized the LAG-3 residues involved in MHC Class II binding to the D1 loop. Surprisingly, only a handful of residues appeared to be involved in this interaction, again in sharp contrast to the extensive Class II binding surface of CD4 (Fleury et al. 1991; Moebius et al. 1993). The implications of these findings are not clear; it seems surprising that a high affinity, nanomolar, interaction could be mediated by such a limited contact region.

1.4 Localization of LAG-3 in T Cells

Because LAG-3 bears structural homology to CD4, it seemed logical to hypothesize that LAG-3 might co-segregate with CD4 in T cell activation. Instead, initial studies showed that LAG-3 does not co-segregate with CD4 but rather localizes with CD8 and CD3/TCR complexes (Hannier and Triebel 1999). These results have been recently readdressed using a new murine anti-LAG-3 antibody, and once again it was found that LAG-3 was not co-localized with CD4 either at the cell surface or intracellularly (Woo et al. 2010). Interestingly, a significant fraction of the LAG-3 molecules in a CD4 T cell was stored in intracellular compartments in close association with the microtubule organizing center, potentially facilitating rapid transit to the T cell surface during activation.

2 LAG-3 Function

2.1 Role in CD4 T Cell Function and Expansion

Early studies using a monoclonal antibody to LAG-3 showed that human CD4 T cell clones exhibited more persistent proliferation when LAG-3 was blocked in vitro (Huard et al. 1995). This proliferation was accompanied by enhanced cytokine production with a mixed pattern (IL-2, IL-4, IFN-γ). These pro-inflammatory effects were limited to antigen-dependent stimuli and were not noted in CD8 T cells. These data were the first to suggest a negative regulatory effect of LAG-3 on T cell function, a role confirmed by later studies using human cells (Macon-Lemaitre and Triebel 2005). However, the development of LAG-3 knockout (Miyazaki et al. 1996) animals allowed a more precise inquiry into the role of LAG-3 on T cells in murine models. These experiments showed a role for LAG-3 in regulating the in vitro and in vivo expansion of both CD4 and CD8 T cells, thus confirming its role as a negative regulator (Workman et al. 2002). Further studies with a LAG-3 molecule lacking the KIEELE domain demonstrated a critical role for this motif in the negative regulatory function of LAG-3; i.e., LAG-3 molecules lacking this domain could not negatively modulate T cell function in vitro or in vivo (Workman and Vignali 2003).

A negative regulatory role for the LAG-3/Class II MHC interaction, however, is not without controversy. Using a series of mixed lymphocyte reactions, one group showed that soluble LAG-3 clearly down-modulated human CD4 T cell function in vitro, suggesting that the interaction between LAG-3 and Class II MHC in these culture conditions was a stimulatory one (Subramanyam et al. 1998). Interestingly, this down-modulation of the MLR response was not noted in human CD8 T cells, suggesting that the interaction between Class II and LAG-3 on CD8 T cells might be functionally distinct from that on CD4 cells. These results are seemingly contradictory to a subsequent series of experiments (see below), in which soluble LAG-3–Ig was shown to function in vitro and in vivo as an activator of dendritic cells.

2.2 *Role of LAG-3 on Regulatory T Cells*

Using microarray analyses, our group found that LAG-3 was relatively upregulated on CD4 T cells that encounter self-antigen in vivo and adopt a regulatory phenotype (Huang et al. 2004). In this model of self-tolerance, we found that a LAG-3-blocking antibody appeared to mitigate regulatory T cell (Treg) function in vivo, and transfection of antigen-specific CD4 T cells with full-length, but not truncated, LAG-3 could confer in vitro regulatory properties. This finding is supported by studies in patients with Hodgkins lymphoma, showing elevated Treg levels when patients' disease was active. In vitro studies showed that depletion of LAG-3+ CD4 T cells enhanced tumor-specific CD8 T cell reactivity, consistent with a role for LAG-3 in suppressing antitumor immunity (Gandhi et al. 2006). This finding is supported by more recent studies showing an enhanced suppressive capacity of LAG-3+ CD4+ CD25+ cells versus LAG-3− cells from the tumor sites of cancer patients (Camisaschi et al. 2010). A recent study also reports a role for LAG-3 in a FoxP3+ subset of CD8 T cells with regulatory function (Joosten et al. 2007), a novel finding that is especially interesting as regulatory CD8 T cells enjoy a resurgent interest (Kapp and Bucy 2008).

2.3 *Role of LAG-3 on CD8 T Cells*

Although early studies questioned a role for LAG-3 in CD8 T cells, such findings were curious given the five- to eightfold increased expression of LAG-3 in activated CD8 versus CD4 cells, as well as the relative co-localization of LAG-3 and CD8 in activated T cells. Studies using LAG-3 knockout animals confirmed a role for LAG-3 in regulating CD8 T cell homeostatic proliferation, as well as in the in vivo response to a superantigen (Workman et al. 2004). We confirmed this role by adoptively transferring antigen-specific CD8 T cells to mice bearing their cognate antigen as either a self or a tumor antigen (Grosso et al. 2007). In this setting, LAG-3 knockout CD8 T cells showed enhanced proliferation and cytokine production. Interestingly, administration of a LAG-3-blocking antibody around the time of adoptive T cell transfer showed a similar enhancement of immune function, suggesting a potential direct role for the blocking antibody on CD8 T cells. This was verified by administering the blocking antibody to mice receiving an adoptive transfer of LAG-3 knockout T cells, although here no additional effects were noted. Recent studies using antibodies that block CTLA-4 found evidence for a similar direct role on effector T cells, confirming that immune checkpoint blockade may, in some circumstances, function via a cell-intrinsic mechanism (Peggs et al. 2009). In terms of the intersection of LAG-3 with other immune checkpoints, it is important to note a recent seminal study involving exhausted CD8 T cells in a model of chronic viral infection. Here, it was found that nonfunctional CD8 T cells could express multiple checkpoint molecules, and that some cells co-expressed both LAG-3 and the well-described immune checkpoint molecule PD-1 (Blackburn et al. 2009). In this model, blockade of both PD-1 and LAG-3 resulted in an improved antiviral immune response as compared to either molecule alone. We observed a similar phenotype in our model of self-antigen tolerance (Grosso et al. 2009), demonstrating a population of nonfunctional CD8 T cells that express both LAG-3 and PD-1. These studies have recently been extended to human ovarian carcinoma samples, where a significant fraction of tumor antigen-specific CD8 T cells co-express LAG-3 and PD-1 (Matsuzaki et al. 2010). Taken together, these important studies suggest that immunotherapy of chronic infections and cancer may require the blockade of multiple immune checkpoints.

2.4 LAG-3 Mechanism of Action

The precise mechanisms by which LAG-3 negatively modulates T cell function are not completely understood. As above, it is clear that the unique intracellular KIELLE domain is required for these effects. However, early studies on LAG-3 were able to demonstrate a soluble form of the molecule in the sera of certain patients, suggesting that cleavage of LAG-3 might play some physiological role (Triebel et al. 2006). In an elegant series of studies, the Vignali group expanded on these findings, showing that LAG-3 is cleaved near the cell surface by two members of the TNF alpha converting enzyme (TACE) family of metalloproteases known as ADAM 10 and ADAM 17 (Li et al. 2007). Expression of a non-cleavable form of LAG-3 mediated an irreversible defect in T cell function, showing that LAG-3 cleavage was a major mechanism by which its negative regulatory function was mitigated. Interestingly, these studies revealed no role for the cleaved form of LAG-3, in sharp contrast to the studies below involving a LAG-3–Ig fusion protein.

3 LAG-3 in Cancer Immunotherapy

3.1 *Preclinical Studies*

Shortly after the generation of a LAG-3–Ig fusion protein for use in biochemical and functional studies, this reagent was studied in vivo in a murine tumor model. In contrast to the findings in a human mixed lymphocyte reaction, as well as to those involving the cleaved portion of the molecule, soluble LAG-3–Ig mediated tumor control and regression in mice bearing RENCA (kidney), MCA 205 (sarcoma), or TS/A (mammary) tumors (Prigent et al. 1999). These findings could be replicated by transduction of tumor cells with LAG-3, suggesting that LAG-3 might mediate an antitumor effect by binding to Class II MHC on antigen-presenting cells and potentially mediating their maturation or function. Indeed, in vitro studies using human monocyte-derived dendritic cells confirmed this hypothesis, showing that LAG-3–Ig upregulated the expression of co-stimulatory molecules and increased IL-12 expression in dendritic cells (Andreae et al. 2002). These phenotypic changes resulted in an enhanced ability of LAG-3–Ig-matured dendritic cells to mediate T_H1 response, as documented by an increased production of IFN-γ by responding T cells. These results also suggested that LAG-3–Ig could potentially function as an adjuvant, potentiating a vaccine response. This was indeed the case, as LAG-3–Ig was shown to markedly enhance the CD8 T cell response to a soluble antigen vaccine (Ovalbumin), as well as the humoral response to a particulate antigen (hepatitis B surface antigen) in mice (El and Triebel 2000). This adjuvant effect was extended to a cancer vaccine setting; here LAG-3–Ig was able to prevent mammary carcinogenesis when administered along with a weak DNA vaccine in HER-2/neu transgenic mice (Cappello et al. 2003). It should be appreciated that these results, though exiting, seem to be somewhat contradictory to the fairly well-documented negative role of LAG-3 on T cell proliferation and function. Indeed, it seems counterintuitive that the interaction between LAG-3 and Class II could on one hand mediate T cell downregulation, yet on the other hand send a pro-inflammatory maturation signal to the class II expressing dendritic cells. In this context, one recent study appears to contradict a pro-immune effect of LAG-3/Class II engagement on dendritic cells, suggesting that LAG-3 on regulatory CD4 T cells in fact inhibits dendritic cell function (Liang et al. 2008).

3.2 *Clinical Studies*

Shortly after the discovery of LAG-3, it was noted that some renal cell cancer (RCC) patients have a dramatic expansion of LAG-3+ CD4+ tumor infiltrating lymphocytes (Angevin et al. 1997). In follow-up work, it was found that LAG-3 expression in RCC TIL varied from 11% to 48%, whereas significant levels of CTLA-4 or the checkpoint molecule 4-1BB could not be detected (Demeure et al. 2001).

However, LAG-3 blockade did not seem to augment CD8 T cell lysis in these studies, suggesting that LAG-3 blockade might perhaps be more important in the early, i.e., priming phase of T cell activation, or perhaps reflecting the technical limitations inherent in using expanded human TIL as a reagent.

Based on the interesting murine studies using LAG-3–Ig, this reagent is being commercially developed (IMP321, Immutep, Paris) and tested in several clinical trials. In the first Phase I trial, IMP321 was administered in increasing doses with a standard influenza vaccine (Brignone et al. 2007a). No dose-limiting toxicity was observed, and adverse effects were minimal. No augmentation of the humoral vaccine response was noted, but a TH1 CD4 T cell response could be detected in several participants. A second, similar trial combined IMP321 with a commercial hepatitis B vaccine (Brignone et al. 2007b). Interestingly, at higher dose levels, CD4 and CD8 T cell responses could be detected after a single IMP321 treatment. These results were subsequently extended to patients with renal cell carcinoma in a single-agent, dose-escalation trial (Brignone et al. 2009). The agent was once again well tolerated, and treatment appeared to correlate with the development of an effector phenotype in CD8 but not CD4 T cells in the periphery. As is typical of Phase I trials in cancer immunotherapy, no objective responses were noted, but several patients showed stable disease. A more innovative trial combined IMP321 with taxane-based chemotherapy in women with breast cancer (Brignone et al. 2010). This single-armed trial demonstrated an objective response rate of 50%, as compared with a historical response rate of approximately 25%. Although single-armed studies in cancer immunotherapy must be interpreted with caution, a number of additional phase II trials are either underway or in the planning phase (www.clinicaltrials.gov; www.immutep.com).

4 Conclusions

On a basic level, LAG-3 is a remarkably interesting cell surface molecule. Phylogenetic studies show that it arose early, most likely sharing a common ancestor with CD4. LAG-3 plays an important role in modulating T cell expansion and function, and blockade of LAG-3 with monoclonal antibodies can augment T cell function in multiple models. The mechanisms by which LAG-3 exerts its physiological function are relatively poorly understood, but cleavage of LAG-3 by metalloproteases is one way in which LAG-3 function can be attenuated. The intracellular signaling pathways underlying LAG-3 function have been relatively poorly investigated and may yield future insight into its role in T cell phenotype and polarization. Although several key preclinical studies suggest a role for LAG-3 blocking antibodies in cancer immunotherapy, the majority of research in this area revolves around LAG-3–Ig, which modulates dendritic cell function in vitro and in vivo. The ultimate test of LAG-3–Ig as a clinical reagent depends on the completion of several clinical trials, some of which are currently underway, and for which final results are eagerly awaited.

References

Andreae S, Piras F et al (2002) Maturation and activation of dendritic cells induced by lymphocyte activation gene-3 (CD223). J Immunol 168:3874–3880

Angevin E, Kremer F et al (1997) Analysis of T-cell immune response in renal cell carcinoma: polarization to type 1-like differentiation pattern, clonal T-cell expansion and tumor-specific cytotoxicity. Int J Cancer 72:431–440

Annunziato F, Manetti R et al (1996) Expression and release of LAG-3-encoded protein by human CD4+ T cells are associated with IFN-gamma production. FASEB J 10:769–776

Annunziato F, Manetti R et al (1997) Opposite role for interleukin-4 and interferon-gamma on CD30 and lymphocyte activation gene-3 (LAG-3) expression by activated naive T cells. Eur J Immunol 27:2239–2244

Baixeras E, Huard B et al (1992) Characterization of the lymphocyte activation gene 3-encoded protein. A new ligand for human leukocyte antigen class II antigens. J Exp Med 176:327–337

Blackburn SD, Shin H et al (2009) Coregulation of CD8+ T cell exhaustion by multiple inhibitory receptors during chronic viral infection. Nat Immunol 10:29–37

Brignone C, Grygar C et al (2007a) IMP321 (sLAG-3) safety and T cell response potentiation using an influenza vaccine as a model antigen: a single-blind phase I study. Vaccine 25:4641–4650

Brignone C, Grygar C et al (2007b) IMP321 (sLAG-3), an immunopotentiator for T cell responses against a HBsAg antigen in healthy adults: a single blind randomised controlled phase I study. J Immune Based Ther Vaccines 5:5

Brignone C, Escudier B et al (2009) A phase I pharmacokinetic and biological correlative study of IMP321, a novel MHC class II agonist, in patients with advanced renal cell carcinoma. Clin Cancer Res 15:6225–6231

Brignone C, Gutierrez M et al (2010) First-line chemoimmunotherapy in metastatic breast carcinoma: combination of paclitaxel and IMP321 (LAG-3Ig) enhances immune responses and antitumor activity. J Transl Med 8:71

Camisaschi C, Casati C et al (2010) LAG-3 expression defines a subset of CD4(+)CD25(high) Foxp3(+) regulatory T cells that are expanded at tumor sites. J Immunol 184:6545–6551

Cappello P, Triebel F et al (2003) LAG-3 enables DNA vaccination to persistently prevent mammary carcinogenesis in HER-2/neu transgenic BALB/c mice, 1. Cancer Res 63:2518–2525

Demeure CE, Wolfers J et al (2001) T Lymphocytes infiltrating various tumour types express the MHC class II ligand lymphocyte activation gene-3 (LAG-3): role of LAG-3/MHC class II interactions in cell-cell contacts 1. Eur J Cancer 37:1709–1718

Dijkstra JM, Somamoto T et al (2006) Identification and characterization of a second CD4-like gene in teleost fish. Mol Immunol 43:410–419

El MS, Triebel F (2000) A soluble lymphocyte activation gene-3 molecule used as a vaccine adjuvant elicits greater humoral and cellular immune responses to both particulate and soluble antigens. J Immunol 164:5583–5589

Fleury S, Lamarre D et al (1991) Mutational analysis of the interaction between CD4 and class II MHC: class II antigens contact CD4 on a surface opposite the gp120-binding site. Cell 66:1037–1049

Gandhi MK, Lambley E et al (2006) Expression of LAG-3 by tumor-infiltrating lymphocytes is coincident with the suppression of latent membrane antigen-specific CD8+ T-cell function in Hodgkin lymphoma patients. Blood 108:2280–2289

Grosso JF, Kelleher CC et al (2007) LAG-3 regulates CD8+ T cell accumulation and effector function in murine self- and tumor-tolerance systems. J Clin Invest 117:3383–3392

Grosso JF, Goldberg MV et al (2009) Functionally distinct LAG-3 and PD-1 subsets on activated and chronically stimulated CD8 T cells. J Immunol 182:6659–6669

Hannier S, Triebel F (1999) The MHC class II ligand lymphocyte activation gene-3 is co-distributed with CD8 and CD3-TCR molecules after their engagement by mAb or peptide-MHC class I complexes. Int Immunol 11:1745–1752

Huang CT, Workman CJ et al (2004) Role of LAG-3 in regulatory T cells. Immunity 21:503–513
Huard B, Gaulard P et al (1994) Cellular expression and tissue distribution of the human LAG-3-encoded protein, an MHC class II ligand. Immunogenetics 39:213–217
Huard B, Prigent P et al (1995) CD4/major histocompatibility complex class II interaction analyzed with CD4- and lymphocyte activation gene-3 (LAG-3)-Ig fusion proteins. Eur J Immunol 25:2718–2721
Huard B, Mastrangeli R et al (1997) Characterization of the major histocompatibility complex class II binding site on LAG-3 protein. Proc Natl Acad Sci USA 94:5744–5749
Huard B, Tournier M et al (1998) LAG-3 does not define a specific mode of natural killing in human. Immunol Lett 61:109–112
Joosten SA, van Meijgaarden KE et al (2007) Identification of a human CD8+ regulatory T cell subset that mediates suppression through the chemokine CC chemokine ligand 4. Proc Natl Acad Sci USA 104:8029–8034
Kapp JA, Bucy RP (2008) CD8+ suppressor T cells resurrected. Hum Immunol 69:715–720
Kisielow M, Kisielow J et al (2005) Expression of lymphocyte activation gene 3 (LAG-3) on B cells is induced by T cells 2. Eur J Immunol 35:2081–2088
Li N, Wang Y et al (2007) Metalloproteases regulate T-cell proliferation and effector function via LAG-3. EMBO J 26:494–504
Liang B, Workman C et al (2008) Regulatory T cells inhibit dendritic cells by lymphocyte activation gene-3 engagement of MHC class II. J Immunol 180:5916–5926
Macon-Lemaitre L, Triebel F (2005) The negative regulatory function of the lymphocyte-activation gene-3 co-receptor (CD223) on human T cells. Immunology 115:170–178
Matsuzaki J, Gnjatic S et al (2010) Tumor-infiltrating NY-ESO-1-specific CD8+ T cells are negatively regulated by LAG-3 and PD-1 in human ovarian cancer. Proc Natl Acad Sci USA 107:7875–7880
Miyazaki T, Dierich A et al (1996) LAG-3 is not responsible for selecting T helper cells in CD4-deficient mice. Int Immunol 8:725–729
Moebius U, Pallai P et al (1993) Delineation of an extended surface contact area on human CD4 involved in class II major histocompatibility complex binding. Proc Natl Acad Sci USA 90:8259–8263
Peggs KS, Quezada SA et al (2009) Blockade of CTLA-4 on both effector and regulatory T cell compartments contributes to the antitumor activity of anti-CTLA-4 antibodies. J Exp Med 206:1717–1725
Prigent P, El MS et al (1999) Lymphocyte activation gene-3 induces tumor regression and antitumor immune responses. Eur J Immunol 29:3867–3876
Rogala B, Gluck J et al (2002) Do the molecules CD26 and lymphocytes activation gene-3 differentiate between type 1 and 2 T cell response? J Investig Allergol Clin Immunol 12:198–203
Subramanyam M, Wands G et al (1998) Soluble human lymphocyte activation gene-3 modulates allospecific T cell responses. Int Immunol 10:679–689
Triebel F, Jitsukawa S et al (1990) LAG-3, a novel lymphocyte activation gene closely related to CD4. J Exp Med 171:1393–1405
Triebel F, Hacene K et al (2006) A soluble lymphocyte activation gene-3 (sLAG-3) protein as a prognostic factor in human breast cancer expressing estrogen or progesterone receptors. Cancer Lett 235:147–153
Woo SR, Li N et al (2010) Differential subcellular localization of the regulatory T-cell protein LAG-3 and the coreceptor CD4. Eur J Immunol 40:1768–1777
Workman CJ, Vignali DA (2003) The CD4-related molecule, LAG-3 (CD223), regulates the expansion of activated T cells, 1. Eur J Immunol 33:970–979
Workman CJ, Dugger KJ et al (2002) Cutting edge: molecular analysis of the negative regulatory function of lymphocyte activation gene-3, 2. J Immunol 169:5392–5395
Workman CJ, Cauley LS et al (2004) Lymphocyte activation gene-3 (CD223) regulates the size of the expanding T cell population following antigen activation in vivo. J Immunol 172:5450–5455
Workman CJ, Wang Y et al (2009) LAG-3 regulates plasmacytoid dendritic cell homeostasis. J Immunol 182:1885–1891

Immunologically Active Biomaterials for Cancer Therapy

Omar A. Ali and David J. Mooney

Contents

1 The Challenge of Cancer Immunotherapy 280
2 Sources and Inspiration for Biomaterials 282
 2.1 Raw Materials 282
 2.2 Controlled Delivery and Cell Targeting 283
 2.3 Synthetic ECMs 284
3 Antigen Delivery and DC Targeting 285
4 Adjuvant Materials 288
5 Three-Dimensional Niches That Regulate Immune Responses In Situ 291
6 Conclusions and Future Prospects 292
References 293

Abstract Our understanding of immunological regulation has progressed tremendously alongside the development of materials science, and at their intersection emerges the possibility to employ immunologically active biomaterials for cancer immunotherapy. Strong and sustained anticancer, immune responses are required to clear large tumor burdens in patients, but current approaches for immunotherapy are formulated as products for delivery in bolus, which may be indiscriminate and/ or shortlived. Multifunctional biomaterial particles are now being developed to target and sustain antigen and adjuvant delivery to dendritic cells *in vivo*, and these have the potential to direct and prolong antigen-specific T cell responses. Three-dimensional immune cell niches are also being developed to regulate the recruitment, activation and deployment of immune cells in situ to promote potent

O.A. Ali (✉) and D.J. Mooney
Harvard School of Engineering and Applied Sciences, Harvard University, 58 Oxford St., 415, Cambridge, MA 02138, USA

Wyss Institute for Biologically Inspired Engineering, Cambridge, MA, USA
e-mail: alio@seas.harvard.edu

O.A. Ali
InCytu Inc, 701 George Washington Hwy, Lincoln, RI 02865, USA

G. Dranoff (ed.), *Cancer Immunology and Immunotherapy*,
Current Topics in Microbiology and Immunology 344, DOI 10.1007/82_2010_69

antitumor responses. Recent studies demonstrate that materials with immune targeting and stimulatory capabilities can enhance the magnitude and duration of immune responses to cancer antigens, and preclinical results utilizing material-based immunotherapy in tumor models show a strong therapeutic benefit, justifying translation to and future testing in the clinic.

1 The Challenge of Cancer Immunotherapy

Effective cancer immunotherapy induces the killing of tumor cells by cytotoxic T lymphocytes (CTLs), resulting in tumor regression and a survival benefit for patients. Malignant tumors are often characterized by an intense proliferative capacity, and local to systemic invasiveness (Mbeunkui and Johann 2009; Curiel and Curiel 2002), and these lethal characteristics have rendered surgical resection, radiation treatment, and chemotherapy ineffective for many cancer patients. Tumors are also replete with antigens, resulting in immune recognition and significant immune-cell infiltrates, but tumor cells create microenvironments (e.g., production of immunosuppressive cytokines) that suppress anticancer activity (Mbeunkui and Johann 2009; Curiel and Curiel 2002). The potential for the innate immune system to react specifically and systemically against local and metastatic lesions (Curiel and Curiel 2002), and to obtain memory that may prevent tumor recurrence (Klebanoff et al. 2006) has inspired the development of immunotherapies that seek to reprogram anticancer responses (Curiel and Curiel 2002; Klebanoff et al. 2006). A key challenge is to formulate treatment modalities that provide specific and persistent immunostimulation to sustain immune attack against tumor cells (predominantly by CTLs) until patients' tumors are completely cleared (Curiel and Curiel 2002; Klebanoff et al. 2006; Banchereau and Steinman 2007; Schuler et al. 2003).

Current immunotherapeutic approaches are of two main types: cancer vaccines and adoptive T cell transfer (Curiel and Curiel 2002; Klebanoff et al. 2006; Banchereau and Steinman 2007; Schuler et al. 2003). Cancer vaccines introduce tumor-associated antigens at the vaccine site and seek to cause tumor regression by relying on a cascade of events that are orchestrated by dendritic cells (DCs) (Banchereau and Steinman 2007; Schuler et al. 2003). Innate antigen recognition and processing is the responsibility of DCs, which, upon activation, have a potent ability to present tumor-antigens processed onto major histocompatibility complexes (MHC), and to translate pathogenic danger signals (e.g., lipopolysaccharides and bacterial DNA) into the expression of specific stimulatory molecules and cytokines (Banchereau and Steinman 1998, 2007; Mellman and Steinman 2001; Holger et al. 2007). Activated DCs then migrate to lymphoid tissues to interact with naïve T cells by presenting MHC-antigen peptides and immunostimulatory cytokines, which signal and propagate antigen-specific T cell differentiation and expansion (Banchereau and Steinman 1998, 2007; Mellman and Steinman 2001; Holger et al. 2007; Sozzani et al. 1998). The type and potency of the T cell response elicited by activated DCs, and, by extrapolation, cancer vaccines, depends on several factors: the type of antigen (endogenous versus exogenous), the microenvironment of the DC-antigen encounter, the extent of DC activation and the number of DCs that stimulate CTL differentiation and expansion (Curiel and Curiel 2002; Klebanoff et al. 2006; Banchereau and Steinman 1998, 2007; Schuler et al. 2003; Mellman and Steinman 2001; Holger et al. 2007; Sozzani et al. 1998). In contrast to vaccines, adoptive T cell transfer bypasses antigen delivery and mediators of T cell activation, by transfusing autologous or allogenic T cells that have been modified in ex vivo cultures and selected to target specific cancer antigens (Klebanoff et al. 2006; Celluzzi et al. 1996; Jenne et al. 2000; Plautz et al. 1998; Hinrichs et al. 2009).

Although cancer vaccines and adoptive T cell transfers have induced CTL responses to specific tumor-associated antigens, and tumor regression in a subset of cancer patients (Curiel and Curiel 2002; Klebanoff et al. 2006; Banchereau and Steinman 2007; Schuler et al. 2003; Celluzzi et al. 1996; Jenne et al. 2000; Plautz et al. 1998; Hinrichs et al. 2009; Yu et al. 2004), these treatments have failed to confer reproducible survival benefit (Klebanoff et al. 2006; Rosenberg et al. 2004). Clinical tests of cancer vaccines have utilized a variety of methods to deliver antigen, including delivery of bulk antigen in the form of tumor lysates (Jenne et al. 2000; Nestle et al. 1998) and irradiated tumor cells (Jinushi et al. 2008; Nemunaitis et al. 2006) or patient-derived DCs pulsated with tumor antigen in ex vivo cultures (Celluzzi et al. 1996). Adjuvants and toll-like receptor (TLR) agonists are often mixed into vaccines to provide danger signals (factors associated with infectious microenvironments) in order to enhance DC maturation and amplify effector responses (Banchereau and Steinman 2007; Holger et al. 2007). However, the limitations of current approaches include short term antigen presentation and immunostimulation due to short, *in vivo* half-lives (within tissues and immune cells), and in the case of DC or T cell transplantation therapies, there is a rapid loss in cell viability and no control over cell function upon transplantation (Curiel and Curiel 2002; Klebanoff et al. 2006; Banchereau and Steinman 2007; Schuler et al. 2003). The indiscriminate targeting and rapid loss of bioavailability and bioactivity in relation to current therapies likely reduces their efficiency, which limits DC and CTL activation resulting in transient to ineffective tumor attack. Intuitively, persistent induction of antitumor CTL activity is required to mediate tumor regression, and to clear large tumor burdens (Curiel and Curiel 2002; Klebanoff et al. 2006; Banchereau and Steinman 2007; Schuler et al. 2003; Rosenberg et al. 2004).

This review will discuss the development and application of immunologically active biomaterials that specifically target DCs and T cells, and regulate their responses to antigens and tumors. We specifically focus on two biomaterial approaches that enable specific and sustained regulation of immune activity, and controlled immunostimulation: drug delivery and three-dimensional cell niches. Biopolymers of many different types have been formulated into particulate systems that control the bioavailability, the pharmacokinetics and the localization of proteins and nucleic acids, and we will discuss work to develop material vectors for antigen and adjuvants with DC targeting ability. Moreover, as an alternative to approaches that utilize ex vivo cell manipulation (e.g., DC-based vaccines and Adoptive T cell transfer), biomaterials have been fashioned into biofunctional, three-dimensional matrices that create distinct, immunostimulatory microenvironments and regulate DC and T cell trafficking and activation in situ. We also highlight the use of these delivery systems and niches to prime DC and T cell responses to tumors in animal models, and the prospects for their clinical impact in cancer immunotherapy.

2 Sources and Inspiration for Biomaterials

Biomaterials are derived from various combinations of natural or synthetic components, and, by definition, are intended to interact with biological systems. Biomaterials have historically been designed to augment cellular behavior that promotes tissue regeneration [e.g., skin grafts (Powell and Boyce 2006; Marston et al. 2003)] or to replace tissue function [e.g., stents and prosthetics (Huebsch and Mooney 2009; Dibra et al. 2010)]; traditionally, these materials were fabricated to minimize host inflammatory and immune responses, due to their potentially destructive affects (Dibra et al. 2010). However, our understanding of immunological regulation has progressed tremendously alongside the development of materials science, and at their intersection emerges the possibility to employ immunologically active biomaterials for cancer immunotherapy. In this section we discuss the sources and raw materials for the fabrication of biomaterial systems and the inspiration underlying their design as drug delivery agents and synthetic extracellular matrices to control cell processes.

2.1 Raw Materials

Nature provides numerous sources of structural proteins and polysaccharides, derived from plants and animals, that may be modified into immuno-active biomaterials. Natural materials, including collagen protein derived from the connective tissue of animals, chitosan polysaccharides extracted from the exoskeleton of crustaceans and alginate polysaccharides isolated from seaweed, have been fashioned into gels and utilized as drug delivery devices or as depots for cell transplantation (Huebsch and Mooney 2009; Ali and Mooney 2006; Eiselt et al. 2000; Miyata et al. 1992; Li and Xu 2002). These materials have been utilized in the clinic for cosmetic and wound care applications with established biocompatibility (Ali and Mooney 2006; Eiselt et al. 2000; Rogero et al. 2003; Majeti and Kuma 2000; Li et al. 2005). Further, the concentrations, molecular weight and crosslinking density of collagen, chitosan and alginate macromolecules can be modified to develop gels with defined degradation rates, stiffness, and functional groups, which can influence the release kinetics or binding of immunostimulatory biomolecules for drug delivery, or the viability and activation state of cells interacting with the material matrix (Ali and Mooney 2006; Eiselt et al. 2000; Miyata et al. 1992; Li and Xu 2002; Rogero et al. 2003; Majeti and Kuma 2000; Li et al. 2005; Lee et al. 2000a; Chevallay and Herbage 2000; Borzacchiello et al. 2001; Bodnar et al. 2005).

Biodegradable devices may also be fabricated from a variety of synthetic polymers, and are frequently used as drug delivery vehicles. Polyglycolide (PGA), polylactide (PLA), and their copolymers polylactide-*co*-glycolide (PLG) which degrade, by hydrolysis, into the natural metabolites, lactic and glycolic acid (Healy et al. 1999; Griffith 2002), have been widely used in the clinic setting as biodegradable sutures, and are commonly fabricated into particulate systems for the controlled delivery of biomolecules (Huebsch and Mooney 2009; Ali and Mooney 2006; Healy et al. 1999; Griffith 2002). Polyanhydrides are another class of biodegradable materials that have been utilized as drug delivery vehicles, such as wafers for the clinical delivery of chemotherapeutic agents at the site of glioblastoma resection (Gliadel) (Brem et al. 1995) and as investigative vaccine carriers (Kipper et al. 2006). In addition, liposome particles (phospholipid bilayers) and block copolymers with hydrophobic and hydrophilic domains are assembled into vesicles or micelle carriers that encapsulate proteins and nucleic acids to protect them from *in vivo* degradation and for their controlled release (Huebsch and Mooney 2009; Ali and Mooney 2006; Hubbell et al. 2009; Torchilin 2005).

2.2 Controlled Delivery and Cell Targeting

Engineering solutions are needed for delivering therapeutic biomolecules to specific sites of treatment with controlled kinetics, which has inspired the development of biomaterials as delivery vehicles (Lee et al. 2000b; Gombotz and Pettit 1995; Langer 1998; Boontheekul and Mooney 2003). Molecular therapeutics form the basis for the prevention and treatment of many human diseases; however, their use is limited by short *in vivo* half-lives which limits their bioavailability to target cells and tissues (Langer 1998; Boontheekul and Mooney 2003). Therefore, in some cases, multiple, systemic administrations of therapeutic molecules are utilized to prolong therapeutic stimulation but this increases nonspecific cell/tissue exposure and may cause severe adverse reactions, which limits the time-course and benefit of treatment.

Biomaterials are now tailored with defined physical properties such as degradation mechanisms and rates Manmohan et al. (2005), and specialized surface characteristics, that protect encapsulated bioactive molecules against degradation *in vivo*, control their release kinetics and allow for specific cellular targeting *in vivo* (Hubbell et al. 2009; Lee et al. 2000b; Gombotz and Pettit 1995; Langer 1998; Boontheekul and Mooney 2003). To efficiently target therapeutic agents (e.g., immunostimulatory cytokines), researchers are developing sophisticated micro- and nano-particulate systems that carry particular surface molecules (e.g., antibodies) to recognize and bind to specific cells. The size and surface properties of these particulate systems are also modified to control particle localization within specified tissues and body compartments (e.g., lymphoid tissues) (Hubbell et al. 2009; Torchilin 2005; Lee et al. 2000b; Gombotz and Pettit 1995; Langer 1998; Boontheekul and Mooney 2003). Material carriers are not only designed to encapsulate and protect proteins and nucleic acids from degradation *in vivo*, but they may also be designed with specific degradation properties allowing the delivery of its bioactive load at specific tissue locations or, for intercellular delivery, at defined intervals within the cell-internalization pathway (Hubbell et al. 2009).

2.3 Synthetic ECMs

The natural extracellular matrix (ECM), in structure and function, has inspired the development and application of three-dimensional biomaterial systems that produce distinct microenvironments that transmit chemical and mechanical cues to cells in situ (Huebsch and Mooney 2009; Ali and Mooney 2006; Chevallay and Herbage 2000; Borzacchiello et al. 2001; Griffith 2002; Silva and Mooney 2004). The interstitial space of tissues contains fibrous ECM proteins (for example, collagens and laminins), and gels of polysaccharides (e.g., glycosaminoglycan and heparin sulfate) (Silva and Mooney 2004; Kallur 2003; Discher et al. 2009). The ECM presents a variety of cell adhesion ligands, provides support and anchorage for cells, regulates cellular communication/migration, and sequesters a wide range of cellular growth factors – to act as a local depot (Discher et al. 2009; Discher et al. 2005). The ECM components and the corresponding degradative enzymes are produced by resident cells in response to local stimuli (e.g., inflammation), which may cause ECM remodeling and a redistribution of cell signals until homeostasis is reachieved between cells and matrix (Silva and Mooney 2004; Kallur 2003; Discher et al. 2009; Discher et al. 2005). Thus, the ECM interacts dynamically with cells to regulate their processes, and this ability may be translated to biomaterial systems.

Three-dimensional biomaterial constructs are now engineered to provide the necessary structural support as synthetic ECMs for cell transplantation and delivery, as long-term depots for the controlled presentation of bioactive molecules, and as niches with controlled microenvironments that regulate cell function (Huebsch and Mooney 2009; Ali and Mooney 2006; Chevallay and Herbage 2000; Borzacchiello et al. 2001; Griffith 2002; Silva and Mooney 2004). The porosity and degradation rate of these materials may be optimized to provide a residence for cells, and to regulate host cell infiltration or cell deployment for therapy. Adhesion ligands may be patterned onto biomaterial surfaces to orient the spatial distribution of cells and cell–cell communication (e.g., immune synapes) (Boontheekul and Mooney 2003; Silva and Mooney 2004; Doh and Irvine 1990). Synthetic matrices are also modified to regulate the spatial and temporal

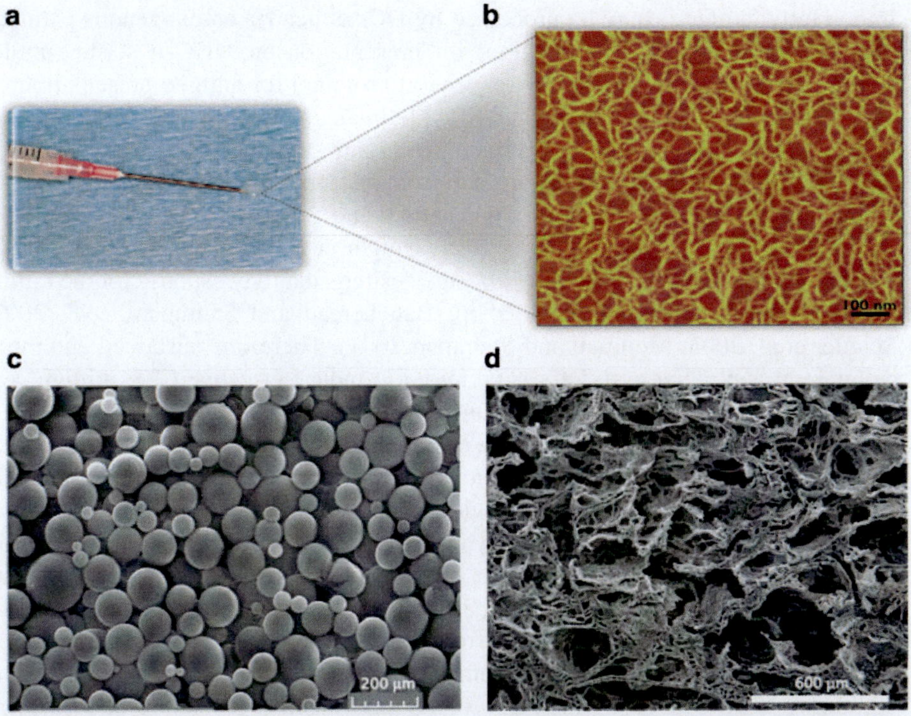

Fig. 1 *Examples of biomaterial systems*. (**a**) An image of an injectable alginate hydrogel system for controlled drug delivery and cell transplantation. Courtesy of Dr. Eduardo Silva, Wyss Institute for Bioinspired Materials, Harvard University. (**b**) Atomic force microscopy (AFM) height image of thin RGD modified alginate hydrogel layer, revealing branched polysaccharide chains and a random nanoporous architecture (~40 nm) typical of polysaccharide gels. Courtesy of Dr. Susan Hsiong. (**c**) SEM micrograph of PLG microspheres (~5–100 µm) that can be utilized to encapsulate and sustain delivery of proteins and nucleic acids. Courtesy of Edward Doherty, InCytu, Inc. (**d**) SEM micrograph of a cross section of a macroporous (10–250 µm size pores) PLG matrix that may be modified to present growth and programming factors to act as a local three-dimensional cell niche *in vivo* (as cells reside within the porous material)

presentation of multiple soluble cues to create distinct microenvironments that can mimic developmental/pathological pathways and regulate cell processes in situ (Fig. 1).

3 Antigen Delivery and DC Targeting

Immature DCs are sentinel-like cells capable of processing and presenting antigens, and priming antigen-specifc, adaptive immune responses (when they encounter antigen with danger signaling), and they traffic through all the tissues of the body, with relatively dense populations located in lymphoid tissues (Banchereau and Steinman 1998, 2007; Schuler et al. 2003; Mellman and Steinman 2001).

Importantly, antigens may be processed by DCs either via an exogenous pathway (e.g., soluble antigens in circulation) for presentation on MHC-II surface molecules, or an endogenous pathway (e.g., viral proteins) for antigen presentation on MHC-I (Banchereau and Steinman 2007; Mellman and Steinman 2001). Targeting intracellular antigen release and antigen processing (as conducted by cells infected with viruses) with material vectors can promote antigen presentation on MHC-I, which stimulates CTL responses (Banchereau and Steinman 1998, 2007; Schuler et al. 2003; Mellman and Steinman 2001; Holger et al. 2007; Sozzani et al. 1998; Celluzzi et al. 1996; Jenne et al. 2000) – the desired adaptive response for the killing of tumor cells (Klebanoff et al. 2006; Banchereau and Steinman 1998, 2007; Schuler et al. 2003; Mellman and Steinman 2001). Therefore, sustained and intracellular antigen delivery to DCs is preferred to induce effective CTL priming and expansion, and long-term cancer immunotherapy.

Biomaterial particulate systems are designed to mediate antigen delivery to DCs with a variety of mechanisms that promote the sustained induction of cytotoxic, CD8+ T cell responses. There is evidence that particles between the sizes of 1–10 μm are preferentially phagocytosed by antigen presenting cells (APCs), including DCs and not by other cells, allowing for passive DC targeting (Tabata and Ikada 1990). Biomaterial-based particulates are also capable of extending the *in vivo* half-life of antigen delivery from days to weeks by providing protection against protein degradation (within both extra- and intra-cellular environments) and sustaining their delivery, which allows for prolonged DC loading and antigen-presentation by the DCs (Hubbell et al. 2009; Tabata and Ikada 1990; Waeckerle-Men et al. 2005).

The delivery of antigen encapsulated in biodegradable polymer particles is driven by diffusion of the antigen and material degradation, allowing for adjustable and sustained release kinetics that mimic the priming and boosting injections of conventional immunization regimens. The natural materials, collagen and alginate, have been processed into antigen-loaded microparticles that reduced the amount of antigen necessary to stimulate humoral immunity, and sustained this response for extended periods (Lofthouse et al. 2001; Suckow et al. 1999). Hydrophilic PLG microspheres of various molecular weights were demonstrated to control the release of antigen over 30–60 days, dependent on the period of time when the polymeric material was completely degraded by hydrolysis (Thomasin et al. 1996). Moreover, the *in vitro* uptake of these PLG microparticles (0.5–5 μm) by primary DCs did not produce a negative effect on cell viability (Nemunaitis et al. 2006; Waeckerle-Men et al. 2005; Thomasin et al. 1996). Consequently, upon cell internalization, these microspheres can serve as antigen reservoirs in DCs, and it was demonstrated that they promote MHC-antigen presentation by DCs for extended periods of time (up to 9 days), compared to the much shorter delivery of free, soluble antigen (2–3 days) (Audran et al. 2003). Importantly, in comparison to soluble proteins, MHC-I and MHC-II antigen presentation of PLGA-MS-encapsulated antigen peptides by murine DCs was significantly prolonged, and proteins were presented 50-fold more efficiently on class I molecules important for priming CTL responses (Waeckerle-Men et al. 2005; Thomasin et al. 1996;

Audran et al. 2003). The vaccination of mice with primary DCs loaded with PLGA-MS-encapsulating influenza antigen or the cancer-associated antigen MUC-1 raised strong and persisting cytotoxic T cell responses for up to 10–16 days *in vivo* (Waeckerle-Men et al. 2005; Audran et al. 2003). The prolonged antigen presentation and CTL stimulation in these models is likely due to the slow hydrolysis (i.e., degradation) of PLG microparticles within DCs, which provides a continuous supply of antigens for processing and presentation onto MHC-class I molecules. The effects of pulsing DCs with antigen-loaded biomaterials were translated to human derived DCs, as they are able to internalized PLG particles in high numbers, which promoted persistent antigen presentation and DC activation on similar time-scales as murine DCs (Waeckerle-Men et al. 2006).

The degradation mechanisms of particulate systems have been optimized to control the timing of the release of nucleic acids and antigens within DCs. Materials sensitive to pH levels, similar to the levels found within cellular compartments, are now being developed to time antigen release coinciding with material degradation. Poly (ortho) ester (POE) biomaterial particles are stable at physiologically neutral pH but degrade rapidly at pH 5, or the levels associated with the phagosome compartment of DCs, and this property was exploited to deliver DNA vaccines (Wang et al. 2004). Plasmid DNA encoding the peptide antigen, SIYRYYGL called SIY, was loaded into pH POE microparticles ($\sim$5 μm) that protected the DNA from degradative enzymes and effectively transfected APCs, *in vivo*, promoting the production and presentation of the SIY antigen, and specific T cell activation that was greater than the delivery of free DNA or the use of particles insensitive to acidic conditions (Wang et al. 2004). Importantly, these POE microparticles were tested as a prophylactic, DNA vaccine, and significantly suppressed the growth of SIY-expressing thymoma cells. This response was demonstrated to be dependent on the generation of SIY-specific immunity (Wang et al. 2004). Similarly, other pH and oxidation sensitive materials have been developed to stably deliver proteins and nucleic acids to DCs, by facilitating endosomal and lysosomal disruption that prevents intracellular degradation, and causes the release of these bioactive molecules into the cytosol for antigen processing or antigen-encoding transfection (Napoli et al. 2004; Paramonov et al. 2008; Cohen et al. 2009; Meyer and Wagner 2006).

The surfaces of biomaterial drug carriers can be modified with ligands to target antigen delivery to host DCs in situ. DEC-205 is an endocytosis receptor expressed by DCs, and ph-sensitive microparticles conjugated to anti-DEC-205 antibodies were shown to be internalized by DCs with an approximately threefold difference in efficiency as compared to control particles (Kwon et al. 2005). Moreover, by utilizing ovalbumin (OVA) as a model antigen, studies demonstrated that anti-DEC-205 conjugated microparticles enhance antigen uptake and MHC-I processing by DCs *in vivo*, and significantly increased the levels of anti-OVA CTL responses in mice (Kwon et al. 2005). Similarly, anti-CD11c and anti-DEC-205 antibodies were attached to liposomal particles that targeted DCs both *in vitro* and *in vivo* with enhanced efficiency (Van Broekhoven et al. 2004). Therefore, antibody conjugation to particulate vehicles offers a potential approach to efficiently target antigen delivery to host DCs.

Another method of antigen targeting involves passively targeting lymphoid tissues rich in DCs by simply optimizing particle sizing, which facilitates lymphatic transport. To achieve effective transport into lymph vessels, particles must be fabricated on the nano-scale, as liposome and other synthetic particles larger than 200 nm generally remain at the injection site, whereas smaller particles (~20–30 nm), due to the dynamics of interstitial flow, can be drained well into lymphoid tissues (Nishioka and Yoshino 2001; Oussoren and Storm 2001; Oussoren et al. 1997; Reddy et al. 2007). Intradermal injection of pluronic-stabilized polypropylene sulfide (PPS) nanoparticles, 25 nm in size, which degrade under the oxidative conditions within lysosomes, were able to target 50% of the DCs in the draining lymph node (100 nm particles targeted only 10%). When these particles were conjugated to a model antigen, they were able to promote specific humoral and CTL immunity, offering a promising strategy for cancer vaccination (Reddy et al. 2007).

4 Adjuvant Materials

Adjuvants initiate and enhance immune responses to antigens, and it has become clear that cancer vaccines will require delivery vehicles that can deliver multiple signals that will elicit and amplify "danger-like" responses to cancer antigens (Banchereau and Steinman 2007; Hubbell et al. 2009). It is understood that DCs continuously sample self-antigens within all tissues, and will not mount anti-antigen responses without secondary signals that indicate a threat to the body. The study of the immune response to various infections and cell damage has revealed "danger signaling" that activates DCs, and these signals are now being utilized as candidate adjuvants. Pathogenic associated molecular patterns (PAMPs), including lipopolysaccharide (LPS), and cytosine–guanosine (CpG) dinucleotide sequences are potent "danger signals". Dying or damaged cells also release signals (damage associated molecular patterns; DAMPs), such as heat shock proteins, that activate DCs and can propagate immune responses (Janeway and Medzhitov 2002; Sansonetti 2006; Meylan et al. 2006; Akira et al. 2006).

The family of DC receptors that recognize "danger signals" are TLRs (ten members in humans), and they explain the DC capacity to respond to many danger signals. Each TLR binds to distinct PAMPs, e.g., TLR4 detects the LPS molecule specific for gram negative bacteria, TLR3 recognizes double-stranded RNA derived from viral infection, and the natural ligands for TLR9 are CpG-rich DNA motifs found frequently in bacterial and viral DNA (Holger et al. 2007; Akira et al. 2006). The triggering of different TLRs mediates DC activation and DC production of distinct immunostimulatory cytokines that propagate specific T cell responses. For example, DCs activated via the byproducts of intracellular pathogens, dsRNA and CpG-rich nucleotide sequences that ligate TLR3 and TLR9, respectively, produce interferons (IFN-α and IFN-γ) and IL-12 that are important in promoting Th1 responses and CTL differentiation/expansion, and cell-mediated attack on infected cells and tumor cells (Holger et al. 2007; Janeway and Medzhitov 2002; Sansonetti 2006; Meylan et al. 2006; Akira et al. 2006). Since one of the main goals of cancer immunotherapy is to produce specific, cytotoxic T cells that kill tumor cells, we will focus on DC adjuvant technology and DC responses that direct these Th1 responses and cytotoxic T cell responses, to kill tumor cells in particular. Additionally, the development of synthetic analogs of TLR agonists, including various CpG oligonucleotides (ODN), and poly(I:C) (substitute for dsRNA), provide opportunities for the development of material systems that co-deliver "danger signals" with antigen to amplify specific immune responses to tumors (Holger et al. 2007).

Biomaterials are now being synthesized with adjuvant activity (including materials that engage TLRs) to complement their ability to control antigen delivery for vaccination. Biomaterials may also inherently be strong adjuvants that enhance immune responses. Polyester microparticles taken up by DCs have demonstrated the ability to promote an activated morphology, upregulate antigen presentation and the expression of costimulatory molecules and immunostimulatory cytokines, and enhance T cell activation when co-delivered with antigen (not encapsulated into the microparticles) (Bennewitz and Babensee 2005; Yoshida and Babensee 2004; Todd et al. 1998; Little et al. 2004). In addition, hydrophobic surface coatings on relatively inert, antigen-loaded nanoparticles promote complement activation and adjuvant effects that enhanced DC activation and the priming of adaptive immune responses (Hubbell et al. 2009; Reddy et al. 2007). The polycationic polymer polyethylenimine (PEI), which forms positively charged colloidal particles when utilized to condense nucleic acids, has been utilized extensively as a transfection vector due to its ability to enhance cell uptake, and has been also shown to trigger selective TLR5 activation *in vitro* and elicit the production of hallmark TLR5-inducible cytokines in WT mice, but not in Tlr5-/- littermates (Cubillos-Ruiz et al. 2009). In an interesting study, PEI complexed with siRNA (silencing immunosuppressive mechanisms) to form nanoparticles that engaged both TLR5 and TLR7 silenced local immunosuppressive mechanisms, activated regulatory DCs into potent stimulators of CTLs, and led to significant antitumor immunity in mouse models of ovarian cancer (Cubillos-Ruiz et al. 2009). This result motivates testing current biomaterials for their ability to engage TLRs, and design of biomaterial carriers that not only efficiently deliver antigen but also act as TLR agonists to enhance immune responses.

Controlled release particles may also be utilized to co-deliver immunostimulatory cytokines and TLR agonists that modulate DC and T cell responses to cancer antigens. Additionally, particulate systems containing immobilized danger signals, including LPS derivatives(Elamanchili et al. 2007), poly (I:C) (Wischke et al. 2009) and CpG-ODN (Kaiser-Schulz et al. 2007) or that provide the sustained release of cytokine adjuvants, such as GM-CSF (Nair et al. 2006), IFNs (Gu et al. 2005), and IL-12(Nair et al. 2006), have been utilized to enhance DC activation and T cell antitumor activity in mouse models. For example, intravesical delivery of chitosan incorporating IL-12 induced T cell infiltration into orthotopic bladder tumors in mice, resulting in significant cure rates (88%) after four therapeutic treatments (Zaharoff et al. 2009). Additionally, vaccine formulations utilizing

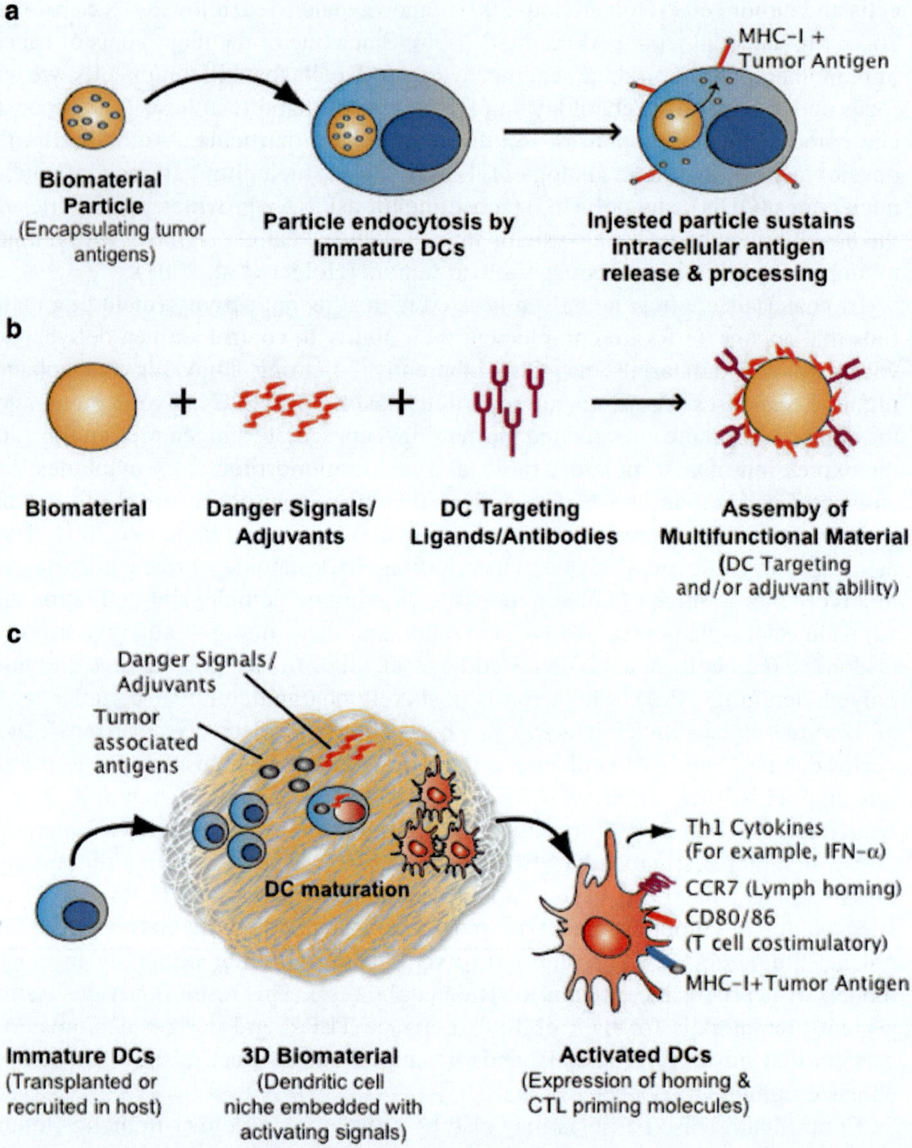

Fig. 2 *Design of immunologically active biomaterials for cancer immunotherapy*. (**a**) Tumor antigens are encapsulated into biomaterial particles that are sized or modified for preferential phagocytosis or endocytosis by APCs, including DCs. The particles protect antigen from degradative enzymes and can sustain their release into the cytosol (antigen reservoir) for intracellular processing and presentation onto MHC-I molecules that can prime CTL responses. (**b**) Biomaterial delivery vehicles are often made into multifunctional materials by conjugation with adjuvants and DC targeting ligands to control the kinetics and localization of adjuvant presentation, in order to enhance and direct DC or T cell migration and activation *in vivo*. These materials may be utilized to co-deliver antigen. (**c**) Three-dimensional biomaterials are fabricated into porous matrices that produce defined microenvironments. Illustrated is a model schematic of an activating DC niche

PLG microparticles that co-deliver the melanoma associated antigen, Trp-2, and a TLR-4 agonist (7-acyl lipid A) activated Th1-polarizing interferon production, Trp-2 specific CTL responses, and suppressed the growth of B16 melanoma tumors in mice (Hamdy et al. 2008). In a clinical application, patients with advanced staged follicular lymphoma were vaccinated after chemotherapy-induced remission with liposomal vaccines delivering both a lymphoma antigen and IL-12, which promoted antigen-specific T cell responses that persisted for 18 months following the completion of vaccination; and at 50 months, six of ten patients remained in complete, continuous remission (Neelapu et al. 2004) (Fig. 2).

5 Three-Dimensional Niches That Regulate Immune Responses In Situ

As a promising alternative to cell-based approaches (e.g., DC-based vaccines and adoptive T cell transfer) for cancer immunotherapy, biomaterials may be fashioned into three-dimensional matrices that regulate immune cell trafficking and activation in situ (Huebsch and Mooney 2009). Immune mechanisms have evolved to recognize and defend against pathogenic infection, and now infection-mimicking microenvironments may be developed using synthetic ECMs and immune cell niches aimed at promoting effective immune responses to cancer antigens. Three-dimensional biomaterial constructs may be designed to support DC and T cell transplantation or recruitment for extended periods while providing a distinct activating niche, via the controlled presentation of antigens and adjuvants while DCs reside within the matrix.

Vaccine nodes were developed by utilizing injectable alginate hydrogels that crosslinked *in vivo* into a supporting matrix containing activated DCs. These transplanted DCs produced cytokines that recruited both host DCs and T cells to the injection site, and the vaccine site subsequently transformed into a potent T cell effector site that could be useful for local tumor immunotherapy (Hori et al. 2008). Moreover, these three-dimensional, DC niches were able to maintain cell viability, and DC and T cell in situ recruitment for over a week (Hori et al. 2008). Similar alginate hydrogel systems were also used to control the release of immunocytokines (IL-15 superagonist) and danger signaling to recruit and activate cytotoxic T cells, and peritumoral injections of these systems significantly enhanced the survival of melanoma-bearing mice (Hori et al. 2009).

Fig.2 (continued) embedded with programming factors (tumor antigens and adjuvants) to activate resident DCs (recruited or transplanted) in situ into an antitumor state with upregulated antigen expression and costimulatory molecules (for T cell priming). These activated DCs may be deployed and home to lymphoid tissue to stimulate antigen-specific CTL responses. These systems may continuously produce activated DCs in situ for sustain periods, prolonging the induction of antitumor responses. Alternative approaches include three-dimensional biomaterials developed to deliver tumor specific T cells or to act as CTL effector sites for local tumor therapy

A recent series of studies describe the development of implantable, and macroporous polymer matrices (PLG; ~85% of the volume is pores) that mimic infectious microenvironments to regulate DC and T cell trafficking and activation in situ (Ali et al. 2009a). Following subcutaneous implantation, GM-CSF was released from these PLG matrices into the surrounding tissue, to recruit significant numbers of host DCs (~3 $\times$ 10^6 cells) (Ali et al. 2009b). CpG-rich oligonucleotides were also immobilized on the matrices as danger signals, and antigen (tumor lysates within the PLG) was released to matrix resident DCs to program DC development and maturation (Ali et al. 2009b). This coordination of DC migration and activation (as DCs reside within the matrix) induced potent, prolonged, and specific cytotoxic, T cell mediated immunity (both local and systemically) that completely eradicated large B16 melanoma tumors in mice (>25 mm^2 at the time of vaccination; 55% long-term therapeutic cure rate) (Ali et al. 2009a, b).

Interestingly, these systems can also be utilized to determine the cellular and molecular signatures of effective therapeutic immune responses to solid tumors; as a critical number and pattern of DC subset generation at the vaccine site, including plasmacytoid DCs (pDCs) and CD8+ DCs (not commonly included in ex vivo DC vaccines), strongly correlated with vaccine efficacy (Ali et al. 2009b). Moreover, the aforementioned immune niches begin as vaccine nodes and translate into the formation of distinct T cell effector sites, which can be monitored to elucidate the cellular and molecular interactions that govern antitumor activities in the therapeutic setting (Hori et al. 2008; Ali et al. 2009b; Hori et al. 2009). These insights into vaccine and effector immunobiology enabled by this biomaterial approach may provide important design criteria (e.g., CD8+ DCs and pDCs as cellular targets) for future cancer immunotherapy.

6 Conclusions and Future Prospects

Immunologically active biomaterials have the potential to offer *in vivo* control over anticancer immune responses: control over the duration and location of antigen and adjuvant delivery, control over local microenvironments, control over the type and quantity of DC activation in situ, and control over the maintenance of specific, adaptive immunity. To date, preclinical studies in cancer vaccine development have successfully modified the sizing and surface functionality of biomaterial particles to target and regulate antigen and adjuvant delivery to DCs, which enhanced the production and persistence of CTL responses *in vivo*. In some studies, antigen-loaded particulate systems were modified to act as adjuvants themselves or to co-deliver adjuvants that increased the numbers of activated host DCs, and amplified the production of adaptive responses to tumors. Three-dimensional materials were designed into vaccine niches (immuno-active synthetic matrices that transplanted or recruited DCs and activated them within immunostimulatory microenvironments) that transitioned into effector sites augmenting T cell responses and caused significant regression of solid tumors in mice. Other interesting avenues that are emerging for biomaterials include their development as synthetic TLR agonists and danger signals to coincide with antigen targeting abilities, and the development of cell niches that continuously deploy transplanted cells that may be utilized to deliver activated DCs and anticancer T cells (Huebsch and Mooney 2009; Silva et al. 2008). An exciting prospect is the emerging application of materials systems/assays to elucidate important cellular and molecular mechanisms in immunobiology that direct the fate of immune responses.

Developments in materials science and immunology research will significantly enable the transformation of biomaterial technologies from the laboratory to clinical use for cancer immunotherapy. Although material-based vaccine formulations have shown compelling preclinical results, translation to clinical testing is virtually nonexistent at present, as material design has historically focused on other medical applications for a variety of technical and economic reasons. However, as the limitations of current cancer immunotherapies (molecular and cell-based therapies delivered in bolus) are becoming clear, including inadequate bioavailability and control, immunologically active and multifunctional biomaterials vectors are becoming more attractive. It is worth noting, in addition, that the material backbones of many of the systems discussed in this review have extensive and safe histories of clinical testing and use in other medical applications, which will likely facilitate their use in immunotherapies. The future clinical implementation of biomaterials for immunotherapy will likely be as novel combination products, which include both materials and biomolecules and/or cells. The biodistribution and dose of molecules and cells delivered by novel immuno-active materials, such as the systems discussed in this review, still need to be evaluated for safety and optimized in animal models, and, ultimately, in cancer patients. In sum, as the limitations of current cancer immunotherapies are becoming clear, including inadequate bioavailability and control, the design capabilities of immunologically active and multifunctional biomaterials are becoming more promising and exciting.

References

Akira S, Uematsu S, Takeuchi O (2006) Pathogen recognition and innate immunity. Cell 124: 783–801

Ali OA, Mooney DJ (2006) "Converging cell therapy with biomaterials". Cell transplantation from laboratory to clinic. Elsevier Inc., Burlington, MA, pp 591–609

Ali OA, Huebsch N, Cao L (2009a) Infection-mimicking materials to program dendritic cells in situ. Nat Mater 2:151–158

Ali OA, Emerich D, Dranoff G, Mooney DJ (2009b) In situ regulation of DC subsets and T cells mediates tumor regression in mice. Sci Transl Med 1:8–19

Audran R, Peter K, Dannull J et al (2003) Encapsulation of peptides in biodegradable microspheres prolongs their MHC class-I presentation by dendritic cells and macrophages *in vitro*. Vaccine 21(11–12):1250–1255

Banchereau J, Steinman RM (1998) Dendritic cells and the control of immunity. Nature 6673:245–252

Banchereau J, Steinman RM (2007) Taking dendritic cells into medicine. Nature 49:419–426

Bennewitz N, Babensee JE (2005) The effect of the physical form of poly(lactic-co-glycolic acid) carriers on the humoral immune response to co-delivered antigen. Biomaterials 26:2991–2999

Bodnar M, Hartmann JF, Borbely J (2005) Preparation and characterization of chitosan-based nanoparticles. Biomacromolecules 6(5):2521–2527

Boontheekul T, Mooney DJ (2003) Protein-based signaling systems in tissue engineering. Curr Opin Biotechnol 14:559–565

Borzacchiello A, Ambrosio L, Netti PA (2001) Chitosan-based hydrogels: synthesis and characterization. J Mater Sci Mater Med 12(10–12):861–864

Brem H, Piantadosi S, Burger PC et al (1995) Placebo-controlled trial of safety and efficacy of intraoperative controlled delivery by biodegradable polymers of chemotherapy for recurrent gliomas. The polymer-brain tumor treatment group. Lancet 345:1008–1012

Celluzzi CM, Mayordomo JI, Storkus WJ et al (1996) Peptide- pulsed dendritic cells induce antigen-specific, CTL-mediated protective tumor immunity. J Exp Med 183:283–287

Chevallay B, Herbage D (2000) Collagen-based biomaterials as 3D scaffold for cell cultures: applications for tissue engineering and gene therapy. Med Biol Eng Comput 38(2):211–218

Cohen JA, Neaudette TT, Tseng WW et al (2009) T-cell activation by antigen-loaded pH-sensitive hydrogel particles *in vivo*: the effect of particle size. Bioconjug Chem 20:111–119

Cubillos-Ruiz JR, Engle X, Scarlett UK et al (2009) Polyethylenimine-based siRNA nanocomplexes reprogram tumor-associated dendritic cells via TLR5 to elicit therapeutic antitumor immunity. J Clin Invest 119(8):2231–2244

Curiel TJ, Curiel DT (2002) Tumor immunotherapy: inching toward the finish line. J Clin Invest 109:311–312

Dibra A, Tiroch K, Schulz S et al (2010) Drug-eluting stents in acute myocardial infarction: updated meta-analysis of randomized trials. Clin Res Cardiol [Epub ahead of print]

Discher DE, Janmey P, Wang Y (2005) Tissue cells feel and respond to the stiffness of their substrate. Science 310(5751):1139–1143

Discher DE, Mooney DJ, Zandstra PW (2009) Growth factors, matrices, and forces combine and control stem cells. Science 324(5935):1673–1677

Doh J, Irvine DJ (1990) Immunological synapse arrays: patterned protein surfaces that modulate immunological synapse structure formation in T cells. Proc Natl Acad Sci USA 15:5700–5705

Eiselt P, Yeh J, Latvala RK et al (2000) Porous carriers for biomedical applications based on alginate hydrogels. Biomaterials 21:1921–1927

Elamanchili P, Lutsiak CME, Hamdy S et al (2007) Pathogen-mimicking nanoparticles for vaccine delivery to dendritic cells. J Immunother 30(4):378–395

Gombotz WR, Pettit DK (1995) Biodegradable polymers for protein and peptide drug delivery. Bioconjug Chem 6:332–351

Griffith LG (2002) Emerging design principles in biomaterials and scaffolds for tissue engineering. Ann NY Acad Sci 961:83–95

Gu F, Younes HM, El-Kadi AO et al (2005) Sustained interferon-gamma delivery from a photocrosslinked biodegradable elastomer. J Control Release 102(3):607–617

Hamdy S, Molavi O, Ma Z et al (2008) Co-delivery of cancer-associated antigen and Toll-like receptor 4 ligand in PLGA nanoparticles induces potent $CD8^+$ T cell-mediated anti-tumor immunity. Vaccine 26:5046–5057

Healy KE, Rezania A, Stile RA (1999) Designing biomaterials to direct biological responses. Ann NY Acad Sci 875:24–35

Hinrichs CS, Borman ZA, Cassard L et al (2009) Adoptively transferred effector cells derived from naive rather than central memory CD8+ T cells mediate superior antitumor immunity. Proc Natl Acad Sci USA 106(41):17469–17474

Holger K, Frank B, Hessel E, Coffman RL (2007) Therapeutic targeting of innate immunity with Toll-like receptor agonists and antagonists. Nat Med 13:552–559

Hori Y, Winans AM, Huang CC et al (2008) Dendritic cell-carrying alginate gels for immunization and immunotherapy. Biomaterials 27:3671–3682

Hori Y, Stern PJ, Hynes RO, Irvine DJ (2009) Engulfing tumors with synthetic extracellular matrices for cancer immunotherapy. Biomaterials 30(35):6757–6767

Hubbell JA, Thomas SN, Swartz MA (2009) Materials engineering for immunomodulation. Nature 462(7272):449–460

Huebsch N, Mooney DJ (2009) Inspiration and application in the evolution of biomaterials. Nature 462:426–432

Janeway CA Jr, Medzhitov R (2002) Innate immune recognition. Annu Rev Immunol 20:197–216

Jenne L, Arrighi JF, Jonuleit H et al (2000) Dendritic cells containing apoptotic melanoma cells prime human CD8+ T cells for efficient tumor cell lysis. Cancer Res 60:4446–4452

Jinushi M, Hodi SF, Dranoff G (2008) Enhancing the clinical activity of granulocyte-macrophage colony-stimulating factor-secreting tumor cell vaccines. Immunol Rev 222:287–298

Kaiser-Schulz G, Heit A, Quintanilla-Martinez L et al (2007) Polylactide-coglycolide microspheres co-encapsulating recombinant tandem prion protein with CpG-oligonucleotide break self-tolerance to prion protein in wild-type mice and induce CD4 and CD8 T cell responses. J Immunol 179(5):2797–2807

Kallur R (2003) Angiogenesis: basement membranes: structure, assembly and role in tumour angiogenesis. Nat Rev Cancer 3:422–433

Kipper MJ, Wilson JH, Wannemuehler MJ, Narasimhan B (2006) Single dose vaccine based on biodegradable polyanhydride microspheres can modulate immune response mechanism. J Biomed Mat Res 76A:798–810

Klebanoff CA, Gattinoni L, Restifo NP (2006) CD8+ T-cell memory in tumor immunology and immunotherapy. Immunol Rev 211:214–224

Kwon YJ, James E, Shastri N, Frechet JMJ (2005) In vivo targeting of dendritic cells for activation of cellular immunity using vaccine carriers based on pH-responsive microparticles. Proc Natl Acad Sci USA 102(51):18264–18268

Langer R (1998) Drug delivery and targeting. Nature 392:5–10

Lee KY, Rowley J, Moy E et al (2000a) Controlling mechanical and swelling properties of alginate hydrogels independently by cross-linker type and cross-linking density. Macromolecules 33:4291–4294

Lee KY, Peters MC, Anderson KW, Mooney DJ (2000b) Controlled growth factor release from synthetic extracellular matrices. Nature 408:998–1000

Li J, Xu Z (2002) Physical characterization of a chitosan-based hydrogel delivery system. J Pharm Sci 91(7):1669–1677

Li GY, Fukunaga S, Takenouch K, Nakamura F (2005) Comparative study of the physiological properties of collagen, gelatin and collagen hydrolysate as cosmetic materials. Int J Cosmet Sci 27:101–106

Little SR, Lynn DM, Ge Q et al (2004) Poly-b amino ester-containing microparticles enhance the activity of nonviral genetic vaccines. Proc Natl Acad Sci USA 101:9534–9539

Lofthouse S, Nagahara S, Sedgmen B et al (2001) The application of biodegradable collagen minipellets as vaccine delivery vehicles in mice and sheep. Vaccine 19:4318–4327

Majeti NV, Kuma R (2000) A review of chitin and chitosan applications. React Funct Polym 46(1):1–27

Manmohan S, Jina K, Mildred U et al (2005) Charged polylactide co-glycolide microparticles as antigen delivery systems. Expert Opin Biol Ther 4(4):483–491

Marston WA, Hanft J, Norwood P et al (2003) The efficacy and safety of dermagraft in improving the healing of chronic diabetic foot ulcers: results of a prospective randomized trial. Diabetes Care 26:1701

Mbeunkui F, Johann DJ Jr (2009) Cancer and the tumor microenvironment: a review of an essential relationship. Cancer Chemother Pharmacol 63(4):571–582

Mellman I, Steinman RM (2001) Dendritic cells: specialized and regulated antigen processing machines. Cell 106(3):255–258

Meyer M, Wagner E (2006) pH-responsive shielding of non-viral gene vectors. Expert Opin Drug Deliv 3:563–571

Meylan E, Tschopp J, Karin M (2006) Intracellular pattern recognition receptors in the host response. Nature 442:39–44
Miyata T, Taira T, Noishiki Y (1992) Collagen engineering for biomaterial use. Clin Mater 9(3–4):139–148
Nair RE, Jong YS, Jones SA et al (2006) IL-12 + GM-CSF microsphere therapy induces eradication of advanced spontaneous tumors in her-2/neu transgenic mice but fails to achieve long-term cure due to the inability to maintain effector T-cell activity. J Immunother 29(1):10–20
Napoli A, Valentini M, Tirelli N et al (2004) Oxidation-responsive polymeric vesicles. Nat Mater 3:183–189
Neelapu SS, Baskar S, Gause BL et al (2004) Human autologous tumor-specific T-cell responses induced by liposomal delivery of a lymphoma antigen. Clin Cancer Res 24:8309–8317
Nemunaitis J, Jahan T, Ross H et al (2006) Phase 1/2 trial of autologous tumor mixed with an allogeneic GVAX vaccine in advanced-stage non-small-cell lung cancer. Cancer Gene Ther 13(6):555–562
Nestle FO, Alijagic S, Gillet M et al (1998) Vaccination of melanoma patients with peptide- or tumor lysate-pulsed dendritic cells. Nat Med 4(3):328–332
Nishioka Y, Yoshino H (2001) Lymphatic targeting with nanoparticulate system. Adv Drug Deliv Rev 47:55–64
Oussoren C, Storm G (2001) Liposomes to target the lymphatics by subcutaneous administration. Adv Drug Deliv Rev 50:143–156
Oussoren C, Zuidema J, Crommelin DJA, Storm G (1997) Lymphatic uptake and biodistribution of liposomes after subcutaneous injection. 2. Influence of liposomal size, lipid composition and lipid dose. Biochim Biophys Acta 1328:261–272
Paramonov SE, Bachelder EM, Beaudette TT (2008) Fully acid-degradable biocompatible polyacetal microparticles fordrug delivery. Bioconjug Chem 19:911–919
Plautz GE, Barnett GH, Miller DW et al (1998) Systemic T cell adoptive immunotherapy of malignant gliomas. J Neurosurg 89:42–51
Powell HM, Boyce ST (2006) EDC cross-linking improves skin substitute strength and stability. Biomaterials 27(34):5821–5827
Reddy ST, Van Der Vlies AJ, Simeon E et al (2007) Exploiting lymphatic transport and complement activation in nanoparticle vaccines. Nat Biotechnol 2:1159–1164
Rogero SO, Malmonge SM, Lugao AB et al (2003) Biocompatibility Study of Polymeric Biomaterials. Artif Organs 27(5):424–427
Rosenberg SA, Yang JC, Restifo NP (2004) Cancer immunotherapy: moving beyond current vaccines. Nat Med 10:909–915
Sansonetti PJ (2006) The innate signaling of dangers and the dangers of innate signaling. Nat Immunol 7:1237–1242
Schuler G, Schuler-Thurner B, Steinman RM (2003) The use of dendritic cells in cancer immunotherapy. Curr Opin Immunol 15:138–147
Silva EA, Mooney DJ (2004) Synthetic extracellular matrices for tissue engineering and regeneration. Curr Top Dev Biol 64:181–205
Silva EA, Kim ES, Kong HJ, Mooney DJ (2008) Material-based deployment enhances efficacy of endothelial progenitor cells. Proc Natl Acad Sci USA 38:14347–14352
Sozzani S, Allavena P, D'Amica G et al (1998) Differential regulation of chemokine receptors during dendritic cell maturation: a model for their trafficking properties. J Immunol 161:1083–1086
Suckow MA, Siger L, Bowersock TL et al (1999) Alginate microparticles for vaccine delivery. Polysaccharide Appl 737(1):1–14
Tabata I, Ikada Y (1990) Phagocytosis of polymer microspheres by macrophages. Adv Polym Sci 94:107–141
Thomasin C, Giampietro Corradin G, Men Y et al (1996) Tetanus toxoid and synthetic malaria antigen containing poly(lactide)/poly(lactide-co-glycolide) microspheres: importance of polymer degradation and antigen release for immune response. J Control Release 41:131–145

Todd CW, Pozzi LA, Guarnaccia JR et al (1998) Development of adjuvant-active nonionic block copolymers. Adv Drug Deliv Rev 32:199–223

Torchilin VP (2005) Recent advances with liposomes as pharmaceutical carriers. Nat Rev Drug Discov 4:145–160

Van Broekhoven CL, Parish CR, Demangel C et al (2004) Targeting dendritic cells with antigen-containing liposomes: a highly effective procedure for induction of antitumor immunity and for tumor immunotherapy. Cancer Res 64:4357–4365

Waeckerle-Men Y, Gander B, Groettrup M (2005) Delivery of tumor antigens to dendritic cells using biodegradable microspheres. Methods Mol Med 109:35–46

Waeckerle-Men Y, Uetz-von Allmen E, Gander B et al (2006) Encapsulation of proteins and peptides into biodegradable poly(d, l-lactide-co-glycolide) microspheres prolongs and enhances antigen presentation by human dendritic cells. Vaccine 24:1847–1857

Wang C, Ge Q, Ting D, Nguyen D et al (2004) Molecularly engineered poly(ortho ester) microspheres for enhanced delivery of DNA vaccines. Nat Mater 3:190–196

Wischke C, Zimmermann J, Wessinger B et al (2009) Poly(I:C) coated PLGA microparticles induce dendritic cell maturation. Int J Pharm 365:61–68

Yoshida M, Babensee JE (2004) (2004) Poly(lactic-co-glycolic acid) enhances maturation of human monocyte-derived dendritic cells. J Biomed Mater Res 71A:45–51

Yu JS, Liu G, Ying H et al (2004) Vaccination with tumor lysate-pulsed dendritic cells elicits antigen specific cytotoxic T cells in patients with malignant glioma. Cancer Res 64:4973–4979

Zaharoff DA, Hoffman BS, Hooper HB et al (2009) Intravesical immunotherapy of superficial bladder cancer with chitosan/interleukin-12. Cancer Res 69:6192–6199

Erratum: Identification of Human Idiotype-Specific T Cells in Lymphoma and Myeloma

Jinsheng Weng, Sattva S. Neelapu, Alison F. Woo, and Larry W. Kwak

Erratum to: Current Topics in Microbiology and Immunology
DOI: 10.1007/82_2010_70

The original version of this article unfortunately contained two mistakes. Figures 1 and 2 were incorrect. The correct versions are given below:

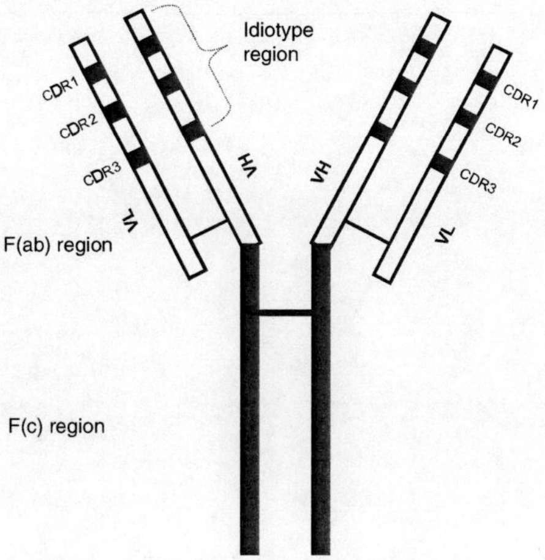

Fig. 1 The term idiotype refers to the unique amino acid sequences within the highly variable regions of the heavy and light chains of the surface immunoglobulin expressed on B cell malignancies. Idiotype includes both three complementarity-determining regions (CDR) and three framework region (FR) of immunoglobulin

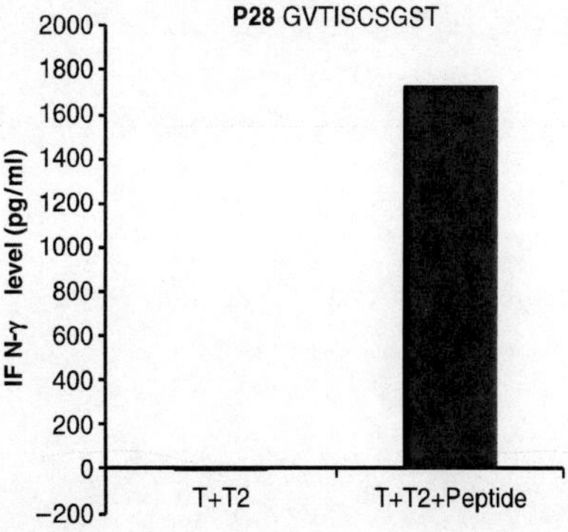

Fig. 2 IFN-γ ELISA. 1×10^5 idiotype light chain peptide-specific T cells secreted a large amount of IFN-γ when cocultured with 1×10^5 T2 cells loaded with 10 μM corresponding peptide (P28) compared with T2 loaded with 10 μM HIV peptide

The online version of the original chapter can be found under
DOI: 10.1007/82_2010_70

J. Weng (✉), S.S. Neelapu, A.F. Woo, and L.W. Kwak
Department of Lymphoma and Myeloma, The University of Texas M. D. Anderson Cancer Center, Houston, TX 77030, USA
e-mail: jweng@mdanderson.org

G. Dranoff (ed.), *Cancer Immunology and Immunotherapy*,
Current Topics in Microbiology and Immunology 344, DOI 10.1007/82_2010_120

Index

A

Activation induced cell death (AICD), 220
ADAM–17, 14
Adhesion molecule expression, 137–138
Adjuvant materials, 288–291
Adoptive transfer, 47, 253–254
AG490, 49
Anaplastic large cell lymphoma (ALCL), 50
Angiogenesis, 131–132
Antibody responses and IL–12, 175–177
Anti-CD137 antibodies
  autoimmune, 251
  memory T cells, 249, 250
  tumor therapy, 249–252
Anti-CTLA–4 blockade, 219
Antigen delivery and DC targeting, 285–288
Antigen-presenting cells (APC), 133
Antigen-specific immune responses, 180–181
Antigen-specific T cells, 155
Antitumor immune modulators
  adhesion molecule expression, 137–138
  angiogenesis, 131–132
  tumor endothelium, 138–141
  vascular endothelium, 137
  VEGF effects, leukocytes, 133–137
Autologous transplantation, 162

B

4–1BB, 153
BCR-ABL kinase inhibitors, 50
B7-H1 expression, 257, 258
B7-H1/PD–1 pathway, blocking, 259–260
B7-H1/PD–1 signaling pathway, 254–257
Blocking antibodies, CTLA–4
  active/passive immunization, 217–218
  chemotherapy/radiotherapy/tumor ablation, 218
  immunostimulatory strategies, 218–219
  monotherapy, 217
Bronchus-associated lymphoid tissues (BALT), 9

C

Cachexia, 26, 28
Cancer immunotherapy
  adjuvant materials, 288–291
  antigen delivery and DC targeting, 285–288
  cell targeting, 283–284
  raw materials, 282–283
  synthetic ECMs, 284–285
Cancer therapy,
CD28, 153
CD3/CD28 costimulated activated T cell, 158
CD3/CD45RO infiltration, 6
CD137 expression, 248
CD137L expression, 248, 249
CD137 signaling, effector/memory T cells, 249–250
CD4 T cell function and expansion, 272–273
CD8 T cells, 15
CD8+ T cells, 25
  exhausted, 255, 257
Cell-based therapy, activated immune cells, 110
Cell engineering, 159
Cell extrinsic suppression, 215–217
Cell intrinsic suppression, 215
Cell manufacturing, 154–155

G. Dranoff (ed.), *Cancer Immunology and Immunotherapy*,
Current Topics in Microbiology and Immunology 344, DOI 10.1007/82_2010

Cell targeting, 283–284
Central memory (TCM), 152
Class II MHC binding, 271–272
Clinical trials, anti-PD–1 antibodies, 259
Coinhibitory signaling, 247
Colon cancer, immune infiltrates, 5
Complex interaction, 255–256
Costimulation, 253–254
Costimulatory signaling, 246, 247, 249, 250, 252
CTLA–4, 64, 68, 70–72, 75, 76, 81
Cyclooxygenase 2 (COX–2), 16
Cytokines, 27
Cytokine secretion, 17
Cytotoxic, 25
Cytotoxic CD8+ T cells, 29
Cytotoxic T cells, 32
Cytotoxic T-lymphocyte antigen–4 modulation
  antibody responses, 232–233
  antigen-specific T cell activity, 229–230
  cellular phenotype analysis, 230
  clinical application, 222–229
  combinations, 226
  Foxp3, 231
  HLA-DR, 231–232
  ICOS, 231
  IDO, 232
  immune related adverse effects, 227
  immunogram, 233
  ipilimumab, 227–228
  postsurgical adjuvant therapy, 225
  preclinical data, 213–219
  tremelimumab, 226–227

D

Dacarbazine (DTIC), 212
Dendritic cell defects, 133–135
Dendritic cell subsets
  antigen-specific immune responses, 180–181
  human dendritic cell subsets, 175–178
  ideal antigens, 182–183
  immune intervention, cancer, 185
  optimal DCs, 181–182
  therapies, 183–184
  tumor environment, 178–179
  type 1 and 2 response, 175
  vaccination trials, 180
Diffuse large B-cell lymphoma (DLCBL), 17
Disease free survival (DFS), 4

E

Effector memory (T_{EM}), 152
Effector T cells
  functional corruptions, 248
  survival, 248, 250
Endothelin. *See* Antitumor immune modulators
Endothelin and tumor angiogenesis, 139–140
Endothelin system, 138–139
Epidermal growth factor receptor (EGFR), 42
ET_BR, 140–141
Expansion, 152
Ex vivo culture, 156

F

Foxp3, 231
Foxp3+ regulatory T cells, 34

G

Genotoxicity, 160
GITR modulation
  and active immunization, 221–222
  monotherapy, 221
Graft-*versus*-host disease (GVHD), 156

H

Hematological malignancies, 69–71
HLA-DR, 231–232
Homeostatic proliferation, 161
Human dendritic cell subsets
  antibody responses and IL–12, 175–177
  LCs and $CD8^+$ T cell responses, 177
  plasmacytoid DCs, 177–178

I

ICOS, 231
Ideal antigens, 182–183
Idiotype, 194–206
IDO, 232
IFN-γ. *See* Interferon (IFNγ)
IL–12, 30
IL–17, 31
IL–22, 32
IL–23, 30
IL–15 Rα, 2
Immune contexture, 4
Immune infiltration
  in situ immune contexture, 4–8

intraocular lymphoma, 16–18
lung carcinoma, 8–11
paradoxical control, 13–16
tertiary lymphoid structures (TLS), 2
toll like receptors (TLR), 11–13
Immune intervention, cancer, 185
Immune response
adaptive, 112
innate, 98, 99
Immune scoring, 8
Immune suppression, Stat3
immunologic signaling pathways, 45–46
myeloid-derived suppressor cells (MDSCs), 46–47
regulatory T-cells (Tregs), 47–48
Th1 immune response, 43–44
Immune surveillance, 34
Immunogram, 233
Immunologic signaling pathways, 45–46
Immunosuppressive cytokines, 68
Immunosurveillance, 30
Immunotherapy, 194, 201, 204–206
tumor, 247, 252
viral infection, 247, 255, 257, 258
Induced Treg (iTreg), 63, 64, 78, 83
Inflammatory bowel disease, 31
Inflammatory milieu, 35
Inflammatory niche, 31–32
Interferon (IFNγ), 3, 35
Interleukin–6 (IL–6), 42
Intraocular lymphoma, 16–18
In vivo T cell survival, 14
Ipilimumab, 227–228

J
JAK inhibitors, 49–50
Jak2/Stat3 inhibitor, 49

L
LAG–3 (CD223), 269
cancer immunotherapy, 275–276
CD8 T cells, 273–274
expression, 270–271
regulatory T cells, 273
structural of, 270
LCs and $CD8^+$ T cell responses, 177
Lentiviral vector, 159
Leukocytes, 133–137
Ligand-receptor interactions, 98
Lung carcinoma, 8–11
neo-adjuvant polychemotherapy, 13

M
MDSC. *See* Myeloid derived suppressor cells (MDSC)
MHC, 26
Microenvironnment
chronic inflammation, 103–105
stroma, 105
Molecule-based therapy
immune response augmentory molecules, 114
tumor growth inhibitory molecules, 103
Mouse models
LCMV, 107–109
L12R4, 110–111
SR/CR, 110–113
Myeloid derived suppressor cells (MDSC), 46–47, 77, 78, 80

N
Natural Treg (nTreg), 63, 64, 66, 83
Neoplastic cells, 102–103, 107, 112, 117
Neuroblastoma, 158
NKT, 67, 77–79
NPM/ALK, 50

O
Oncogenic kinase inhibitors, 50–51
Optimal DCs, 181–182

P
Paradoxical control, 13–16
Paraneoplastic cerebellar degeneration (PCD), 183
Pathogen-associated molecular patterns (PAMP), 12
PD–1 expression, 255, 257–259
Peripheral tolerance, 256, 257
Persistence, 152
Pharmacological inhibition of tumor cell growth, 100–101, 117
Placenta growth factor (PlGF), 132
Plasmacytoid DCs, 177–178
Polarization of the adaptive immune system, 27
Polarization of the immune response, 26
Primary intraocular lymphoma (PIOL), 17
PROSTVAC, 174

R
Receptor tyrosine kinases (RTKs), 51
Regulatory T-cells (Tregs), 47–48. *See also* Tregs

RORγt, 32
RTK inhibitors, 51–52

S
siRNA, 52
Solid organ malignancies, 69, 75
STAT3
  activation, 15
  genetic evidence and potential toxicity, 49
  JAK inhibitors, 49–50
  mediated immune suppression, 43–48
  oncogenic kinase inhibitors, 50–51
  RTK inhibitors, 51–52
  siRNA, 52
Synthetic ECMs, 284–285

T
TAM. *See* Tumor associated macrophage (TAM)
T cell immunity, 197–199
T cell infusions, 151
T cell receptor (TCR), 213
Tertiary lymphoid structures (TLS), 2, 4
Th_{17}, 29, 31, 32
Th_{22}, 32
Therapy vaccine, 252
Thymic atrophy, 135
TLR. *See* Toll like receptors (TLR)
TLR7 agonist, 12
TNF-α, 28
TNF-β, 29
Toll like receptors (TLR), 11–13, 66, 81
Transcranial magnetic stimulation
Tregs, 156
  attenuation, 69, 77, 80–82
  cytotoxicity, 69
  lineage, 63–64
  subsets, 64–67
  suppression, 67–68
  surface markers, 64–65
  transcription factors, 67, 82
Tremelimumab, 226–227
Tumor antigen
  expression, 105–107
  MHCI, 98
  presentation, 105–107
  regulation, 113–117
Tumor associated macrophage (TAM), 77, 78
Tumor cell
  development, 101–105
  escape, 102, 114
  recognition, 101, 106, 111, 116
Tumor endothelium, 138–141
Tumor environment, 178–179
Tumor immune surveillance, 25
Tumor immunity, evasion, 257–259
Tumor-induced BALT (Ti-BALT), 9
Tumor infiltrating lymphocytes (TILs), 131, 153
Tumor mediated suppression, 77
Tumor microenvironment, 30, 33

U
Uveitis masquerade syndrome, 17

V
Vaccination against cancer, 109, 113, 116
Vaccine, 194–196, 198–200, 205
Vascular endothelial growth factor (VEGF). *See also* Antitumor immune modulators
  adhesion molecule expression, 137–138
  effects, leukocytes, 133
  gene expression, 6
  placenta growth factor (PlGF), 132
  protein types, 132
Vascular growth factor receptor (VEGFR), 42
VEGF-R2 blockade, 136
VELIPI tumors, 5